Cortisol Excess and Insufficiency

Frontiers of Hormone Research

Vol. 46

Series Editor

Ezio Ghigo Turin

Co-Editor

Federica Guaraldi Turin

Cortisol Excess and Insufficiency

Volume Editors

Emanuela Arvat Turin

Alberto Falorni Perugia

17 figures, 4 in color, and 20 tables, 2016

KARGER Basel · Freiburg · Paris · London · New York · Chennai · New Delhi · Bangkok · Beijing · Shanghai · Tokyo · Kuala Lumpur · Singapore · Sydney

Frontiers of Hormone Research

Founded 1972 by Tj.B. van Wimersma Greidanus, Utrecht
Continued by Ashley B. Grossman, Oxford (1996–2013)

Emanuela Arvat, MD
Division of Oncological Endocrinology
Department of Medical Science
University of Turin, Turin, Italy

Alberto Falorni, MD
Section of Internal Medicine and Endocrine and Metabolic Sciences, Department of Medicine
University of Perugia, Perugia, Italy

Library of Congress Cataloging-in-Publication Data

Names: Arvat, Emanuela, editor. | Falorni, Alberto, editor.
Title: Cortisol excess and insufficiency / volume editors, Emanuela Arvat, Alberto Falorni.
Other titles: Frontiers of hormone research ; v. 46. 0301-3073
Description: Basel ; New York : Karger, [2016] | Series: Frontiers of hormone research, ISSN 0301-3073 ; vol. 46 | Includes bibliographical references and index.
Identifiers: LCCN 2016008853| ISBN 9783318058390 (hard cover : alk. paper) | ISBN 9783318058406 (e-ISBN)
Subjects: | MESH: Adrenal Insufficiency--physiopathology | Adrenocortical Hyperfunction--physiopathology | Hydrocortisone--secretion
Classification: LCC RM292.4.C67 | NLM WK 760 | DDC 615.3/64--dc23 LC record available at http://lccn.loc.gov/2016008853

Bibliographic Indices. This publication is listed in bibliographic services, including Current Contents® and MEDLINE/Pubmed.

www.karger.com
Printed in Germany on acid-free and non-aging paper (ISO 9706) by Kraft Druck, Ettlingen
ISSN 0301–3073
eISSN 1662–3762
ISBN 978–3–318–05839–0
e-ISBN 978–3–318–05840–6

Contents

Preface

Disorders associated with altered cortisol secretion, excessive or insufficient, are associated with important morbidity and mortality.

Cortisol deficiency or Addison's disease was named after the British physician Thomas Addison who, in 1855, first described the typical signs and symptoms of hypoadrenalism, together with autoptic findings, in 11 patients. Almost a century later, the American neurosurgeon Harvey Cushing reported the case of a 23-year-old woman presenting with obesity, hypertrichosis, amenorrhea, overdevelopment of secondary sexual characteristics, abdominal striae rubrae, skin ecchymosis, signs of increased cerebral tension and impaired glucose tolerance, secondary to a corticotroph pituitary adenoma.

Today, hyper- and hypocortisolism are still considered rare disorders; however, because their onset is often insidious with nonspecific signs and symptoms, and the biochemical picture is not so clear, their incidence appears highly underestimated. Hypocortisolism can be life-threatening if not promptly recognized and treated, while detrimental effects of hypercortisolism occur in the long term. Both diagnosis and management are challenging and, even when properly recognized and treated, these disorders still are associated with significant physical and psychological sequelae.

This volume provides a broad overview of the most recent findings – mainly derived from human studies – and present still debated questions for those conditions associated with altered cortisol secretion.

The issue is structured into two main sections. The first 8 chapters focus on hypercortisolism, presenting the new pathophysiology and genetic findings, typical signs, symptoms and comorbidities. They discuss the diagnostic pitfalls and difficulties in the management of chronic hypercortisolism according to the anatomical origin, and look at the long-term impact of the various therapies. Chapters 9–16 are aimed at giving the reader the most recent data on the epidemiology, genetic and molecular mechanisms of autoimmune primary adrenal insufficiency. They focus on the peculiar clinical aspects associated with primary and secondary hypocortisolism, and discuss peculiarities, advantages and limitations of the new cortisone formulations with respect to standard therapy, taking into consideration the balance between good quality of life for the patients and the long-term risk profile, clinical management and costs. Chapters 10 and 15 are also devoted to hypoadrenalism in the context of autoimmune polyendocrine syndromes and congenital adrenal hyperplasia, with a special focus on the new potential in utero diagnostic methods and their impact on patient management.

We hope that this issue of the series *Frontiers of Hormone Research* will be a valuable tool for endocrinologists, as well as for internal medicine doctors and general practitioners, for a reasoned and comprehensive update on the state of the art in the field of disorders associated with hyper- and hypocortisolism, and act as a guide in their management.

The volume and series editors gratefully thank all of the authors who devoted their time and efforts to contribute to this volume, and the staff at Karger who preciously assisted with its timely completion.

Emanuela Arvat, Turin (Volume Editor)
Alberto Falorni, Perugia (Volume Editor)
Ezio Ghigo, Turin (Series Editor)
Federica Guaraldi, Turin (Series Editor)

Arvat E, Falorni A (eds): Cortisol Excess and Insufficiency.
Front Horm Res. Basel, Karger, 2016, vol 46, pp 1–14 (DOI: 10.1159/000443859)

Pseudo-Cushing – A Clinical Challenge?

Francesca Pecori Giraldi · Alberto G. Ambrogio

Department of Clinical Sciences and Community Health, University of Milan, and Neuroendocrinology Research Laboratory, Istituto Auxologico Italiano IRCCS, Milan, Italy

Abstract

The distinction between Cushing's syndrome and pseudo-Cushing is a major clinical challenge. Indeed, any endocrinologist used to dealing with Cushing's syndrome has certainly faced this dilemma more than once and is aware that there are no clear-cut solutions. Several factors contribute to this ongoing quandary, such as unbalanced epidemiology, overlap in clinical features and inherent variability in test responses. Thus, extreme care has to be taken in both excluding and confirming Cushing's syndrome in patients with mild clinical features and borderline laboratory alterations.

Pseudo-Cushing is the moniker applied to patients with features of hypercortisolism due to conditions other than adrenocorticotropic hormone (ACTH)- or cortisol-hypersecreting lesions. These lesions, i.e. pituitary or extrapituitary ACTH-secreting neoplasms, adrenal adenoma or carcinoma, nodular adrenal hyperplasia or adrenal dysplasia, fall under the heading 'Cushing's syndrome', and removal of any such lesion is followed by remission of hypercortisolism. Conversely, in pseudo-Cushing, excess cortisol secretion is secondary to other conditions and removal of a suspicious pituitary or adrenal lesion does not lead to remission. Thus, the distinction between pseudo-Cushing and true Cushing's syndrome carries significant weight in the therapeutic approach.

Historically, pseudo-Cushing is diagnosed in conditions such as obesity, depression and alcoholism, in which excess cortisol secretion is due to activation of the hypothalamic-pituitary-adrenal (HPA) axis, and is thus associated with central overdrive. In recent years, mild signs of excess cortisol have been observed in patients referred for adrenal nodules and this has come to be referred to as 'subclinical Cushing'. This condition [see chapter by Chiodini and Morelli, this vol., pp. 28–38] can be taken to represent pseudo-Cushing due to primary adrenal overactivity, and shares several features and management problems with pituitary-driven pseudo-Cushing.

Causes of Pseudo-Cushing

Obesity

Excess body weight is among the most common features of Cushing's syndrome, with prevalent truncal fat deposition. Glucocorticoids are known to favour preadipocyte differentiation and stimulate lipolysis, acting through the glucocorticoid receptor. This receptor is more abundant in visceral fat than in subcutaneous adipose tissue [1], and it comes as no surprise that alterations of HPA axis parameters are most commonly encountered in patients with truncal obesity [2]. One of the first reported alterations was increased cortisol clearance via hepatic 5-α-reductase in patients with central obesity; indeed, cortisol pharmacokinetic parameters and urinary concentrations are linked to intra-abdominal fat measures [3]. The increased metabolic cortisol removal rate leads to an increased cortisol production rate, which in turn may contribute to heightened HPA reactivity, as observed in response to food and stimulation with either CRH or ACTH [2, 3].

Further contributors to HPA derangements in obesity are non-alcoholic fatty liver disease and obstructive sleep apnoea, both common in severe truncal obesity. The former is associated with increased urinary free cortisol (UFC) and post-dexamethasone cortisol levels, compared to obese subjects without liver disease [4]. Conversely, both altered sleep patterns and hypoxia are associated with higher cortisol levels and enhanced ACTH response to corticotropin-releasing hormone (CRH) compared to non-apnoeic obese. These changes are related to the apnoeic state per se, as long-term continuous positive airway pressure treatment reduces increased evening and night-time cortisol secretion [5] and may revert false-positive responses to the low-dose suppression test [6].

Another recent player to HPA dysregulation in obesity is 11β-hydroxysteroid dehydrogenase (11β-HSD), in particular the liver and adipose tissue type 1 isoenzyme, which acts as a reductase and converts cortisone to cortisol. 11β-HSD type 1 appears overactive in omental compared to subcutaneous fat [2], thus leading to intracellular cortisol excess and the concept of 'Cushing's disease of the omentum'. Given the actions of glucocorticoids on adipose tissue, local cortisol excess may contribute to the development of visceral fat deposition and, indeed, 11β-HSD type 1 inhibitors are being tested in the treatment of obesity-related disorders [7]. However, although 11β-HSD type 1 expression appears positively related to parameters of weight excess [8], this does not lead to clear, BMI-associated changes in serum, salivary or urinary cortisol [9]; indeed, association studies have yielded divergent results suggesting that different obese phenotypes are associated with different patterns of HPA dysregulation [1, 9], with truncal adiposity, metabolic syndrome, fatty liver and sleep apnoea all playing a role.

Overall, the more consistent alterations reported in obese patients are increased urinary cortisol excretion, and up to 5% of patients with obesity present elevated UFC values [3]. False-negative responses to the standard 1-mg overnight test also occur, reportedly in 2–13% obese patients [10, 11], as well as absent circadian rhythmicity [11, 10].

Polycystic Ovary

Polycystic ovary syndrome is a heterogenous androgen excess disorder with varied metabolic abnormalities. The former leads to anovulation, oligo-amenorrhea, hirsutism and acne, while the latter are associated with insulin resistance, diabetes, obesity, hypertension and depressive disorders. Obviously, these features overlap with Cushing's syndrome, and in fact Cushing's syndrome due to either pituitary [12] or adrenal adenoma [13] has initially been mistakenly diagnosed and treated as polycystic ovary syndrome.

HPA dysfunction in polycystic ovary syndrome is consequent to hypersecretion of most if not all adrenocortical precursors associated with increased cortisol metabolism, either by 5α- and -β-reductase or 11β-HSD. This translates into increased excretion of cortisol and cortisol metabolites [14], greater disorderliness in cortisol secretion and loss of correlation with ACTH [15]. Of note, polycystic ovary syndrome is often associated with obesity, thus excess body weight-driven HPA alterations may also come into play.

The diagnosis of polycystic ovary syndrome should theoretically be established upon exclusion of other causes of hyperandrogenism and anovulation [16]. In practice, a minority of referrals are screened for Cushing's syndrome [17], which makes sense given the low degree of clinical suspicion in most patients [18] and overall uncertain specificity of screening tests [10]. In the polycystic ovary population, both normal weight and obese, above normal UFC results were recorded in 25–50% of patients [14, 19], a low-dose dexamethasone suppression test yielded abnormal suppression in 5–15% of patients according to cut-off stringency [19] and circadian rhythmicity was absent in nearly 20% [19].

Depression

Derangements in HPA axis secretion are believed to play a major role in pathogenesis of depression, with central hyperactivity followed by downstream changes in ACTH and cortisol secretion. Indeed, excess HPA activity is now viewed not just an epiphenomenon but rather causal to several depressive symptoms, e.g. memory and cognition. The main findings are increased CRH secretion, reduced sensitivity to steroid-negative feedback and altered circadian rhythmicity [20]. Both clinical and preclinical studies support the key role of excess CRH secretion, as evidenced by increased cerebrospinal fluid levels [21] and greater abundance of CRH neurons in the hypothalamic paraventricular nucleus [22] in depressed individuals. Increased numbers of vasopressin-expressing paraventricular neurons have also been observed in depressed patients, leading to the hypothesis that vasopressin secretion may also be augmented [23]. Excess CRH secretion is linked to the imbalance between mineralocorticoid and glucocorticoid receptors in the hippocampus, limbic system and hypothalamus. In depressed patients, mineralocorticoid receptor activity appears increased, whereas glucocorticoid receptor function is impaired as shown by the divergent sensitivity to dexamethasone (a glucocorticoid receptor agonist) and prednisolone (a glucocorticoid receptor and mineralocorticoid receptor agonist) in depressed patients [24].

Resistance to negative feedback as well as blunted ACTH responses to CRH, possibly a consequence of CRH receptor downregulation [25], are the basis for the dexamethasone-suppressed CRH test. This test is commonly used by psychiatrists to study the HPA axis, and responses may be used to anticipate response to antidepressant treatment and predict suicidal behaviour or relapse [26]. Of note, sensitivity of negative feedback is restored by successful antidepressive therapy [27]. Hyperactivity often reveals itself in an increased cortisol awakening response, a parameter of the HPA axis response to stress. A higher cortisol awakening response has been associated with risk and time to recurrence of major depressive episodes and anxiety disorders [28]. Another common alteration is flattening of the cortisol circadian curve, with absent rhythmicity in some 50% of patients [29]; further, a dysregulated diurnal cortisol pattern is associated with severity of depression.

Of note, not all parameters are equally affected in the different forms of depression, e.g. psychotic depressives more frequently present impaired cortisol rhythmicity [29] and suppression [30]. Further, alterations may vary with the course of depression, and repeatedly recurring depression may even present hypoactive stress responses [31].

One last factor which may affect HPA parameters in depressed patients is medication. Most patients present to the clinic on one or more psychoactive drugs and weaning off any such compound may be hazardous. Thus, testing may have to be performed while on serotonin re-uptake inhibitors, carbamazepine or other agents known to affect results of UFC or dexamethasone suppression [32].

Given the strong link between HPA hyperactivity and depression, it is not surprising that several drugs which act upon the pituitary or adrenal glands have been tried for treatment of depression, e.g. CRH receptor antagonists, metyrapone, ketoconazole and mifepristone. These studies appear promising but have yet to provide data useful for routine clinical practice. Conversely, steroid synthesis inhibitors have proven to be clearly effective in containing psychiatric symptoms due to Cushing's syndrome, both in the acute [33] and long-term phase [34], supporting the link between excess cortisol and psychiatric ailments. Indeed, mood disorders, major depression, frank anxiety, mania and cognitive dysfunctions all may occur in patients with both endogenous and exogenous Cushing's syndrome [34, 35].

Alcoholism

Alcoholism is a complex variant of pseudo-Cushing, as different alterations of the HPA axis occur at various time points in long-term alcohol abuse. Both large alcohol intake, i.e. blood ethanol >30 mg/dl, and acute alcohol withdrawal activate central stress circuits, i.e. CRH and AVP, and are associated with increased ACTH and cortisol levels [36]. To some extent, increased hepatic 11β-HSD type 1 activity and concomitant 11β-HSD type 2 deficiency may also contribute to increased cortisol levels. Cycling through alcohol binges and withdrawals, as is the case in long-standing alcoholism, leads to periods of hypercortisolism which, in turn, translate into increased negative feedback, decreased hypothalamic CRH and pituitary hyporesponsiveness to CRH [37]. As a consequence, upon cessation of alcohol consumption, ACTH secretion may decrease to below the normal range [38]. Indeed, hyporesponsivity of the HPA axis to a variety of hormonal, e.g. Synacthen and CRH [39], and non-hormonal stimuli, i.e. stress tests [40], characterizes abstinent alcoholics. Recovery of normal HPA function may take weeks to months [41, 42].

From a pathophysiological standpoint, excess cortisol appears to play a role in vulnerability to alcoholism [41] and the development of alcohol-related cognitive defects and malnutrition [43]. Further, derangements in cortisol secretion have been used to predict relapse [44].

As regards diagnostic tests, alcoholic patients frequently fail to suppress at the low-dose dexathasone test [42]; indeed, the number of non-suppressors at the 1-mg dexamethasone suppression test may reach 75% of tested alcoholics [45]. Accelerated hepatic dexamethasone clearance is believed to play a role in the high percentage of non-suppressors [46]. Cortisol circadian rhythm is reportedly maintained in actively drinking alcoholics but absent in abstinent alcoholics [42]. Lastly, UFC was up to 2-fold higher in some alcoholics, somewhat less during abstinence and decreased progressively along the alcohol-free time [42].

Clinical Features in Patients with Pseudo-Cushing

In the previous paragraphs, alterations of the HPA axis in individual conditions associated with pseudo-Cushing were discussed. However, in clinical practice, these conditions often occur together and, indeed, Cushing's syndrome may have to be ruled out in patients who are obese and depressed or alcoholics with truncal fat deposition and depression. Cushing's syndrome is rarely suspected in depressed though lean patients, in simple obesity or in normal-weight polycystic ovary patients. It follows, therefore, that patients with pseudo-Cushing will present a combination of HPA axis alterations due to multiple underlying causes.

The timing of disorders is another important indicator, as depressive symptoms developing slowly over time or weight gained over the course of several years are unlikely to be associated with Cushing's syndrome. Conversely, inexplicable weight gain, mood changes, worsening of diabetes or hypertension over a few years or months are suspicious for endogenous Cushing's syndrome [18]. Several studies have shown that the diagnosis of Cushing's syndrome is on average established some 2 years after the appearance of the first symptoms [47, 48] and that patients often consult family practitioners and several specialists, including psychiatrists, internists and gynecologists, prior to an endocrinologist [48], which are the same specialists consulted by depressed, obese and oligomenorrhoic patients. The time to diagnosis is inversely related to the degree of hypercortisolism, as assessed by UFC [49]; therefore, it comes as no surprise that mild hypercortisolism is most difficult to differentiate from pseudo-Cushing in terms of symptom development over time.

Studies comparing prevalence of symptoms suggestive of hypercortisolism among patients with Cushing's syndrome or pseudo-Cushing have shown that some features are more prevalent in one or the other condition. Severe obesity, polycystic ovaries and psychiatric disorders were more frequent among pseudo-Cushing, whereas osteoporosis and ecchymoses occurred with greater prevalence in Cushing's syndrome [32, 50, 51].

In this context, the ongoing debate on the usefulness of screening for occult Cushing's syndrome among patients with obesity, diabetes or hirsutism is worth mentioning. This controversy encompasses both a systematic survey for Cushing's syndrome in all patients referred for these complaints or only patients presenting with specific features, e.g. candidates for bariatric surgery, uncontrolled diabetes and polycystic ovaries. This diagnostic quandary – as yet not entirely resolved [52] – represents the opposite side of the diagnostic spectrum to pseudo-Cushing, i.e. several features of Cushing's syndrome in individuals without pituitary or adrenal lesions. Obviously, in hindsight, some patients screened for occult Cushing's syndrome may indeed present with pseudo-Cushing.

Differential Diagnosis between Cushing's Syndrome and Pseudo-Cushing

The first steps in the diagnostic work-up of Cushing's syndrome rely on the assessment of cortisol secretion, even in ACTH-dependent Cushing's syndrome. Common diagnostic procedures are measurement of cortisol in 24-hour urine collections, in serum or salivary specimens collected at midnight, or in serum samples collected after low-dose dexamethasone suppression [18]. Difficulties relating to the use of these tests in pseudo-Cushing were summarized in a seminal review published in 1998 [53] and, to date, only few advances have been made to aid in the diagnostic process, such as the desmopressin test (where it is in use).

As mentioned above, first-tier tests for Cushing's syndrome, e.g. UFC, midnight cortisol and low-dose suppression tests, all variably provide false-positive results in patients with pseudo-Cushing. Indeed, some alteration of the HPA axis is a prerequisite. Therefore, little reliance can be placed on these tests to accurately distinguish between Cushing's syndrome and pseudo-Cushing. Cut-offs may be varied in order to increase specificity of any screening procedure, but this will inevitably reduce sensitivity, a disquieting trade-off, given the low prevalence and long time to diagnosis for endogenous Cushing's syndrome. This has led to the use of second-tier confirmatory tests: the dexamethasone-suppressed CRH test and the desmopressin test. Use of either is dependent on the expertise of individual centres as, it is worth recalling, neither offers 100% diagnostic accuracy.

Dexamethasone-Suppressed CRH Test

The dexamethasone-suppressed CRH test was first proposed by the NIH in the 1990s as a 100% accurate test for Cushing's syndrome versus pseudo-Cushing [54]. However, as more patients were tested, subsequent large [32, 50, 55, 56] as well as small series [57–60] disproved the initially reported test performance. The rationale for this test is the different sensitivity to pituitary stimulation by CRH under conditions of mild negative feedback, i.e. 2-mg dexamethasone. Patients with endogenous Cushing's syndrome will be insensitive to feedback and mount an adequate pituitary/adrenal response to CRH; conversely, low-dose dexamethasone suppression will prove sufficient to blunt the response in patients with functional hypercortisolism.

In theory, only patients who present serum cortisol less than 1.4 μg/dl (38 nmol/l) after 2-mg dexamethasone for 2 days should be submitted to the test, given that any patient with higher levels does not require CRH stimulation to surpass the response criterion. As the sensitivity of the low-dose dexamethasone test is quite high [18], most patients with Cushing's syndrome will not require this procedure.

Conversely, this test is useful in patients in whom a strong suspicion for Cushing's syndrome persists, notwithstanding inhibition after low-dose dexamethasone as, obviously, inhibition should exclude the diagnosis. Thus, the main point of the test is to confirm the veracity of dexamethasone inhibition, exclude Cushing's syndrome and diagnose pseudo-Cushing.

Analysis of published series totalling some 200 patients with Cushing's syndrome and an equal number of patients with pseudo-Cushing (table 1) revealed that the majority of patients with Cushing's syndrome already surpassed 1.4 μg/dl prior to CRH stimulation and, in hindsight, did not need testing [50, 54]. In the few patients with Cushing's syndrome and misleading inhibition, CRH stimulation reverted the diagnostic response in all but a few cases [50, 55, 56].

On the other hand, among patients in whom the final diagnosis proved to be pseudo-Cushing, some 80% were correctly inhibited by low-dose dexamethasone (table 1), which means that 20% of patients were submitted to the test with serum cortisol levels already higher than the criterion for the CRH response. In these cases, CRH stimulation did not aid in the diagnostic process. Further, results of CRH stimulation proved misleading in a number of patients with pseudo-Cushing. In fact, except for two series in which specificity was equal [32, 54], in all other series specificity of the dexamethasone-suppressed CRH test was lower than for dexamethasone suppression alone

Table 1. Overview of series reporting dexamethasone-suppressed CRH tests in patients with Cushing's syndrome and pseudo-Cushing

	Criteria		Cushing's syndrome					Pseudo-Cushing				
	LDDST, μg/dl	DEX-CRH, μg/dl	pts	LDDST	%	DEX-CRH	%	pts	LDDST	%	DEX-CRH	%
Yanovski [54]	cortisol >1.4	cortisol >1.4	39	35	90	39	100	19	19	100	19	100
Martin [57]	cortisol >1.4	cortisol >1.4	12	12	100	12	100	24	18	75	16	67
Pecori Giraldi [50]	cortisol >1.4	cortisol >1.4	32	30	94	32	100	23	17	74	14	61
Erickson [55]	cortisol >1.8	cortisol >1.4	21	20	95	21	100	30	*25*	83	23	76
		cortisol >2.5				18	90				27	90
Gatta [60]	cortisol >1.4	cortisol >1.4	17	17	100	17	100	14	10	71	7	50
		cortisol >3.9				17	100				12	86
Batista[a] [59]	cortisol >1.4	cortisol >1.4	11	10	91	11	100	21	20	95	15	77
		cortisol >3.2				10	91				20	95
Reimondo [58]	cortisol >1.4	cortisol >1.4	16	13	81	15	94	15	13	87	12	80
Valassi [32]	cortisol >1.4	cortisol >1.4	61	46	75	52	86	46	39	85	39	85
	cortisol >5.0	cortisol >5.0		27	44	36	59		46	100	46	100
Alwani [56]	cortisol >1.8	cortisol >1.8	35	33	94	35	100	19	16	84	15	79
		cortisol >3.1				33	94				19	100
All series	cortisol >1.4	cortisol >1.4	244[b]	163[c]	87	199[c]	95	211[b]	136[c]	84	145[c]	75

LDDST = Low-dose dexamethasone suppression test; DEX-CRH = dexamethasone-suppressed CRH stimulation; pts = number of patients tested. [a] Children. [b] All patients tested. [c] Calculated on the originally reported 1.4 μg/dl criterion [54].

(table 1). Overall, specificity of the test averaged 75.5%, which is inadequate for a second-tier confirmatory test. As a consequence, some authors have proposed alternative cut-offs, i.e. 3.9 μg/dl (110 nmol/l) or 5 μg/dl (138 nmol/l), to increase specificity, but thereby reduced sensitivity [32, 60].

An additional problem with this test is the measurement of low serum cortisol concentrations. Cortisol assays have acceptable precision, but obviously minute differences at the lower end of the assay curve, e.g. 1.3 versus 1.5 μg/dl, may prove random effects or the results of the inherent variability of cortisol secretion [61]. In addition, drugs affecting dexamethasone clearance, e.g. CYP3A4 inhibitors, or cortisol-binding globulin levels, e.g. contraceptive medications, easily induce changes in low, dexamethasone-suppressed cortisol concentrations.

Desmopressin Stimulation

At the same time as the dexamethasone-suppressed CRH test, desmopressin (DDAVP), a long-acting vasopressin analogue, was reported to stimulate ACTH and cortisol secretion in patients with Cushing's disease by Malerbi et al. [62]. DDAVP was shown to have limited value, contrary to initial reports, in the differential diagnosis of ACTH-dependent Cushing's syndrome, but proved highly efficacious for the distinction between Cushing's disease and depressed, obese or frank pseudo-Cushing patients [50, 51, 63–67]. The rationale for the test is the unique sensitivity of patients bearing an ACTH-secreting pituitary adenoma to stimulation by DDAVP, either directly at the

Table 2. Overview of series reporting desmopressin stimulation in patients with Cushing's disease and pseudo-Cushing

	Criteria	Cushing's disease			Pseudo-Cushing		
		pts	response	%	pts	response	%
Malerbi [63]	cortisol increment >36%	14	14	100	11	7	64
Tsagarakis [64]	ACTH increment >50%	25	23	92	20	17	85
Moro [65]	ACTH increment >27 pg/ml	76	66	87	66	60	91
Pecori Giraldi [50]	ACTH increment >27 pg/ml	32	26	81	23	21	90
Tirabassi [51]	ACTH increment >27 pg/ml	52	39	75	28	25	89
	ACTH increment >18 pg/ml and basal cortisol >11 μg/dl		47	90		26	91
Tirabassi [67]	ACTH increment >18 pg/ml and basal cortisol >11 μg/dl	30	29	97	18	18	100
Rollin [66]	ACTH increment >37 pg/ml[a]	68	60	88	56	51	91
	ACTH peak >71 pg/ml		62	91		53	95
All series		297	257	86	222	199	90

pts = Number of patients tested. [a] Used for overall sensitivity/specificity calculations.

pituitary level [68] or indirectly at the suprapituitary level [69]. In patients with Cushing's disease, DDAVP induced a pronounced release of ACTH while, conversely, patients with functional hypercortisolism do not exhibit a significant ACTH or cortisol response. Criteria to differentiate between Cushing's disease and pseudo-Cushing vary (table 2), and given the variability among ACTH assays [70], ACTH increments are likely to represent a more widely applicable response criterion than absolute ACTH values. Currently, there is no uniformly adopted cut-off.

At variance with the dexamethasone-suppressed CRH test, this test can be of use in any patient with equivocal results at first-line testing and measurable ACTH levels; thus, it may prove useful in a much wider patient population and especially in those patients with borderline dexamethasone suppression. Nearly 300 patients with Cushing's disease and over 200 patients with pseudo-Cushing or similar conditions have been reported so far and, on balance, sensitivity is over 85% and specificity approximately 90% (table 2). Given that this test is performed in order to exclude Cushing's disease in patients with high suspicion but equivocal screening tests, high specificity is paramount. Indeed, its use has been advocated by several European experts [71].

On balance, this test may prove useful in the differential diagnosis of Cushing's disease and pseudo-Cushing, but further work needs to be done to identify the optimal criterion.

Plasma ACTH Measurement
Stated causes of pseudo-Cushing are characterized by a variable central overdrive; thus, ACTH levels will be normal notwithstanding increased cortisol concentrations. It follows, therefore, that there will be considerable overlap with patients with Cushing's disease who often present normal ACTH values [47]. Indeed, pseudo-Cushing historically entered the differential diagnosis with Cushing's disease, rather than other causes of endogenous hypercortisolism.

In recent times, however, 'subclinical Cushing' due to adrenal incidentalomas has become a major clinical challenge and this may be taken to represent an adrenal-derived variant of pseudo-Cushing. In this condition, in contrast with centrally driven pseudo-Cushing, ACTH levels will be largely suppressed, although the reliability of plasma ACTH in the low normal range is questionable [70]. The combination of borderline or frankly abnormal cortisol measurements and subnormal ACTH concentrations engenders the same diagnostic dilemmas as in pseudo-Cushing, albeit centred on the adrenal gland. Further, given that enlargement of one or both adrenal glands is apparent, the decision as to the most correct therapeutic approach, i.e. adrenalectomy or surveillance, becomes imperative (for further discussion, see the chapter by Chiodini and Morelli et al. [this vol., pp. 28–38]).

Management of Pseudo-Cushing

Patients in whom Cushing's syndrome is suspected are tested with UFC, a low-dose dexamethasone suppression test and measurement of cortisol at midnight, according to the clinician's preference and assay availability [18, 72]. Equivocal test results may be followed up by dexamethasone-suppressed CRH stimulation and/or a desmopressin test, again according to test suitability and expertise.

From the above it is clear that no single test will reliably exclude Cushing's syndrome from pseudo-Cushing. Further, unless certainty of Cushing's syndrome has been achieved, patients should not embark in further etiological diagnostic work-up. In fact, one of the most worrisome consequences of the difficult differential diagnosis between Cushing's syndrome and pseudo-Cushing is the fact that once a patient is believed to have endogenous Cushing's syndrome, none of the tests used for its etiological diagnosis will cause the clinician to question the diagnosis. In fact, results of plasma ACTH measurements, CRH stimulation or 8-mg dexamethasone suppression will indicate pituitary Cushing's disease, given that patients with pseudo-Cushing present ACTH levels within the normal range and easily fulfil criteria for positive responses to CRH or 8-mg dexamethasone suppression [72]. Even petrosal sinus sampling will not provide a clear distinction [73]. Then again, this is not surprising as these tests are aimed at distinguishing pituitary from extrapituitary ACTH-dependent Cushing's syndrome, and pseudo-Cushing represents a condition of central overdrive.

One further consideration is related to epidemiology. Cushing's syndrome is an extremely rare disease [49], whereas obesity, depression, polycystic ovary syndrome and possibly also alcoholism occur with far greater frequency. Thus, pseudo-Cushing is far more likely than true endogenous hypercortisolism in patients with mild indices of cortisol excess. This should be kept in mind during diagnostic decision-making.

It appears, therefore, that the only reliable strategy is to monitor patients with equivocal tests, treat associated ailments, e.g. depression and obesity, if possible and re-evaluate after some months. Treatment of the underlying cause of HPA derangements usually reverts abnormal tests in patients with pseudo-Cushing, whereas true endogenous Cushing's syndrome may only progress over time. In fact, papers reporting on pseudo-Cushing all state variable length of follow-up, from 1 to 10 years, to exclude further symptom development or worsening of HPA parameters. As clinical and biochemical features are mild, this time span is not wasted; indeed, it may help to avoid needless pituitary surgery in patients with pseudo-Cushing. Conversely, some patients initially believed to have pseudo-Cushing might well prove to have Cushing's syndrome at re-evaluation. For clinicians, follow-up is paramount to both diagnosis and treatment.

Conclusion

The distinction between Cushing's syndrome and pseudo-Cushing is quicksand into which any clinician may fall and indeed some, myself included, admittedly have [74, 75]. Caution and hard-won expertise are required to avoid a misdiagnosis, but we are all aware that Cushing's syndrome is and remains a significant diagnostic challenge.

References

1 Vicennati V, Garelli S, Rinaldi E, Di Dalmazi G, Pagotto U, Pasquali R: Cross-talk between adipose tissue and the HPA axis in obesity and overt hypercortisolemic states. Horm Mol Biol Clin Investig 2014;17:63–77.

2 Björntorp P, Rosmond R: Obesity and cortisol. Nutrition 2000;16:924–936.

3 Pasquali R, Cantorelli S, Casimirri F, Capelli M, Bortoluzzi L, Flamia R, Morselli Labate AM, Barbara L: The hypothalamic-pituitary-adrenal axis in obese women with different patterns of body fat distribution. J Clin Endocrinol Metab 1993;77:341–346.

4 Targher G, Bertolini L, Rodella S, Zoppini G, Zenari L, Falezza G: Associations between liver histology and cortisol secretion in subjects with nonalcoholic fatty liver disease. Clin Endocrinol 2006;64:337–341.

5 Vgontzas AN, Pejovic S, Zoumakis E, Lin HM, Bentley CM, Bixler EO, Sarrigiannidis A, Basta M, Chrousos GP: Hypothalamic-pituitary-adrenal axis activity in obese men with and without sleep apnea: effects of continuous positive airway pressure therapy. J Clin Endocrinol Metab 2007;92:4199–4207.

6 Tamada D, Otsuki M, Kashine S, Hirata A, Onodera T, Kitamura T, Shimomura I: Obstructive sleep apnea syndrome causes a pseudo-Cushing's state in Japanese obese patients with type 2 diabetes mellitus. Endocr J 2013;60:1289–1294.

7 Anagnostis P, Katsiki N, Adamidou F, Athyros VG, Karagiannis A, Kita M, Mikhailidis DP: 11beta-Hydroxysteroid dehydrogenase type 1 inhibitors: novel agents for the treatment of metabolic syndrome and obesity-related disorders? Metabolism 2013;62:21–33.

8 Mariniello B, Ronconi C, Rilli S, Bernante P, Boscaro M, Mantero F, Giacchetti G: Adipose tissue 11β-hydroxysteroid dehydrogenase type 1 expression in obesity and Cushing's syndrome. Eur J Endocrinol 2006;155:435–441.
9 Salehi M, Ferenczi A, Zumoff B: Obesity and cortisol status. Horm Metab Res 2005;37:193–197.
10 Pecori Giraldi F, Ambrogio AG, De Martin M, Fatti LM, Scacchi M, Cavagnini F: Specificity of first-line tests for the diagnosis of Cushing's syndrome: assessment in a large series. J Clin Endocrinol Metab 2007; 92:4123–4129.
11 Baid S, Rubino D, Sinaii N, Ramsey S, Frank A, Nieman LK: Specificity of screening tests for Cushing's syndrome in an overweight and obese population. J Clin Endocrinol Metab 2009;94:3857–3864.
12 Liao CC, Lin SY, Lin HW, Chen KH, Chang LH, Chen ST, Wang J: Menstrual abnormalities in a woman with ACTH-dependent pituitary macroadenoma mimicking polycystic ovary syndrome. Taiwan J Obstet Gynecol 2006;45:176–179.
13 Fegan PG, Sandeman DD, Krone N, Bosman D, Wood PJ, Stewart PM, Hanley N: Cushing's syndrome in women with polycystic ovaries and hyperandrogenism. Nat Clin Pract Endocrinol Metab 2007;3:778–783.
14 Invitti C, Pecori Giraldi F, Dubini A, De Martin M, Cavagnini F: Increased urinary free cortisol and decreased serum corticosteroid-binding globulin in polycystic ovary syndrome. Acta Endocrinol (Copenh) 1991;125:28–32.
15 Invitti C, De Martin M, Delitala G, Veldhuis JD, Cavagnini F: Altered morning and nighttime pulsatile corticotropin and cortisol release in polycystic ovary syndrome. Metabolism 1998;47:143–148.
16 Rotterdam ESHRE/ASRM-Sponsored PCOS Consensus Workshop Group: Revised 2003 consensus on diagnostic criteria and long-term health risks related to polycystic ovary syndrome (PCOS). Hum Reprod 2004;19:41–47.
17 Cussons AJ, Stuckey BG, Walsh JP, Burke V, Norman RJ: Polycystic ovarian syndrome: marked differences between endocrinologists and gynaecologists in diagnosis and management. Clin Endocrinol (Oxf) 2005;62:289–295.
18 Nieman LK, Biller BM, Findling JW, Newell-Price J, Savage MO, Stewart PM, Montori VM: Diagnosis of Cushing's syndrome: an Endocrine Society Clinical Practice Guideline. J Clin Endocrinol Metab 2008; 93:1526–1540.
19 Putignano P, Bertolini M, Losa M, Cavagnini F: Screening for Cushing's syndrome in obese women with and without polycystic ovary syndrome. J Endocrinol Invest 2003;26:539–544.
20 Schatzberg AF: Anna-Monika Award Lecture, DGPPN Kongress, 2013: The role of the hypothalamic-pituitary-adrenal (HPA) axis in the pathogenesis of psychotic major depression. World J Biol Psychiatry 2014;16:1–10.
21 Nemeroff CB, Widerlöv E, Bissette G, Walléus H, Karlsson I, Eklund K, Kilts CD, Loosen PT, Vale W: Elevated concentrations of CSF corticotropin-releasing factor-like immunoreactivity in depressed patients. Science 1984;226:1342–1344.
22 Raadsheer FC, Hoogendijk WJG, Stam FC, Tilders FJH, Swaab DF: Increased numbers of corticotropin-releasing hormone expressing neurons in the hypothalamic paraventricular nucleus of depressed patients. Neuroendocrinology 1994;60:436–444.
23 Scott LV, Dinan TG: Vasopressin as a target for antidepressant development: an assessment of the available evidence. J Affect Disord 2002;72:113–124.
24 Juruena MF, Cleare AJ, Papadopoulos AS, Poon L, Lightman S, Pariante CM: Different responses to dexamethasone and prednisolone in the same depressed patients. Psychopharmacology 2006;189: 225–235.
25 Gold PW, Loriaux DL, Roy A, Kling MA, Calabrese JR, Kellner CH, Nieman LK, Post RM, Pickard D, Gallucci W: Responses to corticotropin-releasing hormone in the hypercortisolism of depression and Cushing's disease. Pathophysiologic and diagnostic implications. N Engl J Med 1986;314:1329–1335.
26 Sher L: Combined dexamethasone suppression-corticotropin-releasing hormone stimulation test in studies of depression, alcoholism, and suicidal behavior. ScientificWorldJournal 2006;6:1398–1404.
27 Pariante CM: The glucocorticoid receptor: part of the solution or part of the problem? J Psychopharmacol 2006;20:79–84.
28 Adam EK, Vrshek-Schallhorn S, Kendall AD, Mineka S, Zinbarg RE, Craske MG: Prospective associations between the cortisol awakening response and first onsets of anxiety disorders over a six-year follow-up. Psychoneuroendocrinology 2014;44: 47–59.
29 Keller J, Flores B, Gomez RG, Sovason HB, Kenna H, Williams GH, Schatzberg AF: Cortisol circadian rhythm alterations in psychotic major depression. Biol Psychiatry 2005;60:275–281.
30 Arana GW, Baldessarini RJ, Ornsteen M: The dexamethasone suppression test for diagnosis and prognosis in psychiatry. Commentary and review. Arch Gen Psychiatry 1985;42:1193–1204.
31 O'Keane V, Frodl T, Dinan TG: A review of atypical depression in relation to the course of depression and changes in HPA axis organization. Psychoneuroendocrinology 2012;37:1589–1599.
32 Valassi E, Swearingen B, Lee H, Nachtigall LB, Donoho DA, Klibanski A, Biller BM: Concomitant medications can confound interpretation of the combined dexamethasone-corticotropin releasing hormone test in Cushing's syndrome. J Clin Endocrinol Metab 2009;94:4851–4859.

33 Bilgin YM, van der Wiel HE, Fischer HRA, De Herder WW: Treatment of severe psychosis due to ectopic Cushing's syndrome. J Endocrinol Invest 2007;30: 776–779.
34 Sonino N, Fava GA: Psychiatric disorders associated with Cushing's syndrome. CNS Drugs 2001;15:361–373.
35 Starkman MN: Neuropsychiatric findings in Cushing syndrome and exogenous glucocorticoid administration. Endocrinol Metab Clin North Am 2013;42: 477–488.
36 Rivier C: Alcohol stimulates ACTH secretion in the rat: mechanisms of action and interactions with other stimuli. Alcohol Clin Exp Res 1996;20:240–254.
37 Costa A, Bono G, Martignoni E, Merlo P, Sances G, Nappi G: An assessment of hypothalamo-pituitary-adrenal axis functioning in non-depressed, early abstinent alcoholics. Psychoneuroendocrinology 1996; 21:263–275.
38 Esel E, Sofuoglu S, Aslan SS, Kula M, Yabanoglu I, Turan MT: Plasma levels of beta-endorphin, adrenocorticotropic hormone and cortisol during early and late alcohol withdrawal. Alcohol Alcohol 2001;36: 572–576.
39 Adinoff B, Krebaum SR, Chandler PA, Ye W, Brown MB, Williams MJ: Dissection of hypothalamic-pituitary-adrenal axis pathology in 1-month-abstinent alcohol-dependent men, part 1: adrenocortical and pituitary glucocorticoid responsiveness. Alcohol Clin Exp Res 2005;29:517–527.
40 Bernardy NC, King AC, Parsons OA, Lovallo WR: Altered cortisol response in sober alcoholics: an examination of contributing factors. Alcohol 1996;13: 493–498.
41 Stephens MA, Wand G: Stress and the HPA axis: role of glucocorticoids in alcohol dependence. Alcohol Res 2012;34:468–483.
42 Groote Veldman R, Meinders AE: On the mechanism of alcohol-induced pseudo-Cushing's syndrome. Endocr Rev 1996;17:262–268.
43 Leggio L, Malandrino N, Ferrulli A, Cardone S, Miceli A, Gasbarrini G, Capristo E, Addolorato G: Is cortisol involved in the alcohol-related fat mass impairment? A longitudinal clinical study. Alcohol Alcohol 2009;44:211–215.
44 Junghanns K, Backhaus J, Tietz U, Lange W, Bernzen J, Wetterling T, Rink L, Driessen M: Impaired serum cortisol stress response is a predictor of early relapse. Alcohol Alcohol 2003;38:189–193.
45 Besemer F, Pereira AM, Smit JW: Alcohol-induced Cushing syndrome. Hypercortisolism caused by alcohol abuse. Neth J Med 2011;69:318–323.
46 Meikle AW: Dexamethasone suppression tests: usefulness of simultaneous measurement of plasma cortisol and dexamethasone. Clin Endocrinol (Oxf) 1982;16:401–408.
47 Invitti C, Pecori Giraldi F, De Martin M, Cavagnini F: Diagnosis and management of Cushing's syndrome: results of an Italian multicentre study. Study Group of the Italian Society of Endocrinology on the Pathophysiology of the Hypothalamic-Pituitary-Adrenal Axis. J Clin Endocrinol Metab 1999;84:440–448.
48 Kreitschmann-Andermahr I, Psaras T, Tsiogka M, Starz D, Kleist B, Siegel S, Milian M, Kohlmann J, Menzel C, Führer-Sakel D, Honegger J, Sure U, Müller O, Buchfelder M: From first symptoms to final diagnosis of Cushing's disease: experiences of 176 patients. Eur J Endocrinol 2015;172:285–289.
49 Cavagnini F, Pecori Giraldi F: Epidemiology and follow-up of patients with Cushing's disease. Ann Endocrinol (Paris) 2001;62:168–179.
50 Pecori Giraldi F, Pivonello R, Ambrogio AG, De Martino MC, De Martin M, Scacchi M, Colao A, Toja PM, Lombardi G, Cavagnini F: The dexamethasone-suppressed corticotropin-releasing hormone stimulation test and the desmopressin test to distinguish Cushing's syndrome from pseudo-Cushing's states. Clin Endocrinol (Oxf) 2007;66:251–257.
51 Tirabassi G, Faloia E, Papa R, Furlani G, Boscaro M, Arnaldi G: Use of the desmopressin test in the differential diagnosis of pseudo-Cushing state form Cushing's disease. J Clin Endocrinol Metab 2010;95: 1115–1122.
52 Tabarin A, Perez P: Pros and cons of screening for occult Cushing syndrome. Nat Rev Endocrinol 2011; 7:445–455.
53 Newell-Price J, Trainer PJ, Besser GM, Grossman AB: The diagnosis and differential diagnosis of Cushing's syndrome and pseudo-Cushing's states. Endocr Rev 1998;19:647–672.
54 Yanovski JA, Cutler Jr. GB, Chrousos GP, Nieman LK: Corticotropin-releasing hormone stimulation following low-dose dexamethasone administration. JAMA 1993;269:2232–2238.
55 Erickson D, Natt N, Nippoldt TB, Young Jr. WF, Carpenter PC, Petterson T, Christianson T: Dexamethasone-suppressed corticotropin-releasing hormone stimulation test for diagnosis of mild hypercortisolism. J Clin Endocrinol Metab 2007;92: 2972–2976.
56 Alwani RA, Schmit Jongbloed LW, De Jong FH, van der Lely AJ, De Herder WW, Feelders RA: Differentiating between Cushing's disease and pseudo-Cushing's syndrome: comparison of four tests. Eur J Endocrinol 2014;170:477–486.
57 Martin NM, Dhillo WS, Banerjee A, Abdulali A, Jayasena CN, Donaldson M, Todd JF, Meeran K: Comparison of the dexamethasone-suppressed corticotrophin-releasing hormone test and low-dose dexamethasone suppression test in the diagnosis of Cushing's syndrome. J Clin Endocrinol Metab 2006; 91:2582–2586.

58 Reimondo G, Bovio S, Allasino B, De Francia S, Zaggia B, Micossi I, Termine A, De Martino F, Paccotti P, Di Carlo F, Angeli A, Terzolo M: The combined low-dose dexamethasone suppression corticotropin-releasing hormone test as a tool to rule out Cushing's syndrome. Eur J Endocrinol 2008;159: 569–576.
59 Batista D, Courkoutsakis NA, Riar J, Keil MF, Stratakis CA: Severe obesity confounds the interpretation of low dose dexamethasone test with the administration of ovine corticotrophin releasing hormone in childhood Cushing syndrome. J Clin Endocrinol Metab 2008;93:4323–4330.
60 Gatta B, Chabre O, Cortet C, Martinie M, Corcuff JB, Roger P, Tabarin A: Reevaluation of the combined dexamethasone suppression-corticotropin-releasing hormone test for differentiation of mild Cushing's disease from pseudo-Cushing's syndrome. J Clin Endocrinol Metab 2007;92:4290–4293.
61 Pecori Giraldi F, Ambrogio AG: Variability in laboratory parameters used for management of Cushing's syndrome. Endocrine 2015;50:580–589.
62 Malerbi DA, Bilharinho de Mendonça B, Liberman B, Toledo SPA, Corradini MC, Cunha-Neto MB, Villares Fragoso MCB, Wajchenberg BL: The desmopressin stimulation test in the differential diagnosis of Cushing's syndrome. Clin Endocrinol (Oxf) 1993;38:463–472.
63 Malerbi DA, Villares Fragoso MC, Vieira Filho AH, Brenlha EM, Bilharinho de Mendonça B: Cortisol and adrenocorticotropin response to desmopressin in women with Cushing's disease compared with depressive illness. J Clin Endocrinol Metab 1996;81: 2233–22.37
64 Tsagarakis S, Vasiliou V, Kokkoris P, Stavropoulos G, Thalassinos N: Assessment of cortisol and ACTH responses to the desmopressin test in patients with Cushing's syndrome and simple obesity. Clin Endocrinol (Oxf) 1999;51:473–477.
65 Moro M, Putignano P, Losa M, Invitti C, Maraschini C, Cavagnini F: The desmopressin test in the differential diagnosis between Cushing's disease and pseudo-Cushing states. J Clin Endocrinol Metab 2000;85: 3569–3574.
66 Rollin GA, Costenaro F, Gerchman F, Rodrigues TC, Czepielewski MA: Evaluation of the DDAVP test in the diagnosis of Cushing's disease. Clin Endocrinol (Oxf) 2015;82:793–800.
67 Tirabassi G, Papa R, Faloia E, Boscaro M, Arnaldi G: Corticotrophin-releasing hormone and desmopressin tests in the differential diagnosis between Cushing's disease and pseudo-Cushing state: a comparative study. Clin Endocrinol (Oxf) 2011;75:666–672.
68 Luque RM, Ibañez-Costa A, López-Sánchez LM, Jiménez-Reina L, Venegas-Moreno E, Gálvez MA, Villa-Osaba A, Madrazo-Atutxa AM, Japón MA, de la Riva A, Cano DA, Benito López P, Soto-Moreno A, Gahete MD, Leal Cerro A, Castaño JP: A cellular and molecular basis for selective desmopressin-induced ACTH release in Cushing disease patients: key role of AVPR1b receptor and potential therapeutic implications. J Clin Endocrinol Metab 2013;98: 4160–4169.
69 Pecori Giraldi F, Marini E, Torchiana E, Mortini P, Dubini A, Cavagnini F: Corticotrophin-releasing activity of desmopressin in Cushing's disease. Lack of correlation between in vivo and in vitro responsiveness. J Endocrinol 2003;177:373–379.
70 Pecori Giraldi F, Saccani A, Cavagnini F; Study Group of the Italian Society of Endocrinology on the Pathophysiology of the Hypothalamic-Pituitary-Adrenal Axis: Assessment of ACTH assay variability: a multicenter study. Eur J Endocrinol 2011;164:505–512.
71 Guignat L, Bertherat J: The diagnosis of Cushing's syndrome: an Endocrine Society Clinical Practice Guideline: commentary from a European perspective. Eur J Endocrinol 2010;163:9–13.
72 Pecori Giraldi F: Recent challenges in the diagnosis of Cushing's syndrome. Horm Res 2009;71(suppl 1):123–127.
73 Yanovski JA, Cutler GB Jr, Doppman JL, Miller DL, Chrousos GP, Oldfield EH, Nieman LK: The limited ability of inferior petrosal sinus sampling with corticotropin-releasing hormone to distinguish Cushing's disease from pseudo-Cushing states or normal physiology. J Clin Endocrinol Metab 1993;77:503–509.
74 Findling JW, Raff H: Cushing's syndrome: important issues in diagnosis and management. J Clin Endocrinol Metab 2006;91:3746–3753.
75 Pecori Giraldi F: PseudoCushing: why a clinical challenge? J Endocrinol Invest 2015;38:1137–1139.

Francesca Pecori Giraldi, MD
Istituto Auxologico Italiano
Piazzale Brescia 20
IT–20149 Milan (Italy)
E-Mail fpg@auxologico.it

Arvat E, Falorni A (eds): Cortisol Excess and Insufficiency.
Front Horm Res. Basel, Karger, 2016, vol 46, pp 15–27 (DOI: 10.1159/000443861)

Cushing's Syndrome: Where and How to Find It

Miguel Debono · John D. Newell-Price

Academic Unit of Endocrinology, University of Sheffield, Sheffield, UK

Abstract

The diagnosis of Cushing's syndrome is challenging to endocrinologists as patients often present with an insidious history, together with subtle external clinical features. Moreover, complications of endogenous hypercortisolism, such as visceral obesity, diabetes, hypertension and osteoporosis, are conditions commonly found in the population, and discerning whether these are truly a consequence of hypercortisolism is not straightforward. To avoid misdiagnosis, a careful investigative approach is essential. The investigation of Cushing's syndrome is a three-step process. Firstly, after exclusion of exogenous glucocorticoid use, the decision to initiate investigations should be based on whether there is a clinical index of suspicion of the disease. Specific signs of endogenous hypercortisolism raise the a priori probability of a truly positive test. Secondly, if the probability of hypercortisolism is high, one should carry out specific tests as indicated by Endocrine Society guidelines. Populations with non-distinguishing features of Cushing's syndrome should not be screened routinely as biochemical tests have a high false-positive rate if used indiscriminately. Thirdly, once hypercortisolism is confirmed, one should move to establish the cause. This usually entails distinguishing between adrenal or pituitary-related causes and the remoter possibility of the ectopic adrenocorticotropic hormone syndrome. It is crucial that the presence of Cushing's syndrome is established before any attempt at differential diagnosis.

Endogenous Cushing's syndrome results from the primary chronic autonomous and inappropriate secretion of excess cortisol. Since the first description by Harvey Cushing in the early 20th century, diagnosis and management has remained a challenge. Making the right decision at each step in the diagnostic work-up of patients with suspected Cushing's syndrome is vital, and since this condition is associated with a high-standardised mortality ratio, and increased risk of cardiovascular events and infections [1], delays in diagnosis should be avoided.

Cushing's syndrome is a rare disorder, and the annual incidence of Cushing's disease is estimated to be around 2.4 per million with a prevalence of 39.1 per million [2]; however, this may be an underestimate as mild cases may be missed by the unwary physician. Eighty-five percent of cases are caused by adrenocorticotropic hormone (ACTH)-dependent causes: Cushing's disease due to an ACTH-secreting corticotroph adenoma of the pituitary gland (70%), a non-pituitary tumour ectopically secreting ACTH (10%) or an unknown source of ACTH (5%). The other 15% are caused by ACTH-independent adrenal disorders: 10% adrenal adenomas, 5% adrenal carcinomas and a few rare conditions including macronodular adrenal hyperplasia, McCune-Albright syndrome and primary pigmented nodular adrenal disease [3].

The difficulty in the diagnosis of Cushing's syndrome is discriminating the condition from others where the hypothalamic-pituitary-adrenal (HPA) axis may secondarily be activated, including uncontrolled diabetes, severe obesity, alcohol dependence, depression/psychosis and glucocorticoid resistance [4]. Although patients presenting with clear-cut features may be easily recognised, mild disease may be harder to discriminate. Complications of cortisol excess such as osteoporosis, diabetes or hypertension are highly prevalent conditions in the ageing population, making diagnosis all the more difficult, but if several of these features are present in a younger individual, it increases the chances of Cushing's syndrome being present.

The investigation of Cushing's syndrome is a three-step process in which the following questions must be answered. Is there a clinical index of suspicion for Cushing's syndrome? Is there hypercortisolaemia? What is the cause? It is essential that these steps are followed in sequence and that no attempts at differential diagnosis are made before a clear diagnosis of Cushing's syndrome is established (fig. 1).

Is There a Clinical Index of Suspicion for Cushing's Syndrome?

Exclude Exogenous Cushing's Syndrome

The commonest cause of Cushing's syndrome is the excessive use of exogenous glucocorticoids from inhalers, topical, rectal, oral and parenteral formulations. Exclusion of exogenous Cushing's syndrome is, therefore, essential. A thorough drug history to identify the use of any glucocorticoid formulation, including over-the-counter drugs, should be taken. In general, features are similar to those found in patients with endogenous cortisol excess, but may develop more quickly and be clearly linked to a time shortly after the commencement of glucocorticoid formulations, especially at high doses [5]. The chance of developing clinical features of Cushing's syndrome due to exogenous glucocorticoids, and the severity of these, varies widely and depends on individual factors as well as pharmacokinetic and pharmacodynamic characteristics of the formulation used. Unless hydrocortisone is being administered, serum cortisol and plasma ACTH will be suppressed. Ideally the cortisol level should be measured by liquid chromatography tandem mass spectrometry (LC-MS/MS) to circumvent

1. **Is there a clinical index of suspicion for Cushing's syndrome?**
   - **Exclude exogenous Cushing's syndrome**
   - **Identify specific clinical features of Cushing's syndrome**
     - Easy bruising
     - Facial plethora
     - Proximal myopathy
     - Purple striae
     - Weight gain with decreasing growth velocity
   - **Avoid screening in these populations unless specific features are present or unusual presentation**
     - Obesity, diabetes, osteoporosis, hypertension, hyperandrogenism, dependent alcoholism, depression and psychosis

2. **Is there hypercortisolaemia?**
   - **1-mg ONDST**
   - **2-mg 48-hour LDDST**
   - **Midnight salivary or serum cortisol**
   - **24-hour urine free cortisol**

   If two tests are positive and a hyperactive HPA axis and physiological hypercortisolism are excluded, look for the cause

3. **What is the cause?**
   - **Adrenal Cushing's syndrome (ACTH-independent)**
     - Low ACTH <5 pg/ml
     - CT/MRI adrenals
       - Adrenal adenoma or carcinoma
       - AIMAH – investigate for aberrant receptors
       - No abnormality – PPNAD, factitious hydrocortisone use
     - Other syndrome – McCune-Albright syndrome

   - **Pituitary Cushing's syndrome (ACTH-dependent)**
     - High ACTH >15 pg/ml
     - Adenoma >6 mm on MRI pituitary
       - Positive CRH test
     - Adenoma <6 mm on MRI pituitary or not visible
       - BIPSS (C:P ACTH baseline >2 post-CRH >3; prolactin normalised ACTH IPS/P ratio >1.3)
       - No BIPSS available: >30% suppression on LDDST; >20% cortisol increase on CRH test

   - **Ectopic Cushing's syndrome (ACTH-dependent)**
     - High ACTH >15 pg/ml
     - CT/MRI neck/chest/abdomen/pelvis
     - Ga-68 DOTATATE PET-CT
     - Hypokalaemia
     - Tumour markers

Fig. 1. Investigating Cushing's syndrome: a three-step process. ONDST = Overnight dexamethasone suppression test; PPNAD = primary pigmented nodular adrenocortical disease; BIPSS = bilateral inferior petrosal sinus sampling; C:P = central:peripheral; IPS/P = inferior petrosal sinus/peripheral.

problems related to cross-reaction with other synthetic steroids. This technique also allows identification of the factitious use of other glucocorticoids. It should be borne in mind that inhibitors of CYP3A4 may cause huge increases in circulating glucocorticoids and hence Cushing's syndrome in situations where the dose and route of administration would not normally cause such problems. A good example is in patients taking the anti-retroviral drug ritonavir, where severe Cushing's syndrome is well described with even modest doses of the inhaled glucocorticoid flixotide [6].

Identify Specific Clinical Features of Excess Cortisol Secretion

The diagnosis of Cushing's syndrome demands a well-structured and organised approach involving a multidisciplinary team including endocrinologists, radiologists, chemical and histopathologists, surgeons, and endocrine nurses [3]. In most cases patients present with symptoms and signs that have been progressing for around 3–5 years. Clinical features are variable and in some cases cyclical. The features most typical of cortisol excess are those related to protein catabolism, namely thin skin, easy bruising and proximal muscle weakness [4]. A number of other features frequently found in Cushing's syndrome include purple striae, especially over the abdomen and are related to an increase in weight, moon facies and psychiatric disturbances [7]. Facial plethora, one of the oldest signs described in medicine and an indicator of average blood volume in the cheeks, is another important sign of active disease, and its decrease has been shown to be an indicator of Cushing's syndrome outcome after surgery [8]. Other features that should prompt investigation include features that are unusual for age, including osteoporosis, diabetes and hypertension in young adults, and obesity and decreased growth velocity in children. In addition, evidence of progression of signs and symptoms should be sought, ideally using past photographs for confirmation. Gender differences may exist, with males having a tendency towards higher systolic blood pressure and haemoglobin, worse liver function tests and a higher prevalence of fatty liver [9].

Are There Circumstances in Specific Patient Populations When We Should Screen for Cushing's Syndrome?

Cushing's syndrome may be considered in patient groups such as those suffering from obesity, diabetes, hypertension and osteoporosis. Widespread indiscriminate biochemical testing in patients with these conditions, where there is a low probability of Cushing's syndrome, will yield a high false-positive rate leading to unnecessary investigations and increasing patient anxiety. In contrast, in specific situations the diagnosis should be considered so as not to cause delays that may result in harm to patients. These populations are now discussed in further detail.

Obesity

Typically in Cushing's syndrome there is a redistribution of fat with predominant accumulation in the visceral compartment in both men and women, and less fat deposited in the subcutaneous compartment, as demonstrated by computed tomography [10]. The problem facing clinicians is that central obesity, the metabolic syndrome and Cushing's syndrome may have similar features, and testing the HPA axis in a patient with simple obesity may lead to false-positive results. Moreover, altered circadian secretion of cortisol has been demonstrated in obesity and this can make diagnosis harder, although dexamethasone testing appears more reliable in this setting

[11, 12]. In obesity there may also be more regeneration of cortisol from cortisone through the action of 11β-hydroxysteroid dehydrogenase type 1 [13]. These factors should be borne in mind when considering the diagnosis of Cushing's syndrome in obese patients. As an example, in a study of 369 overweight or obese subjects there was a high rate of false-positive tests irrespective of 5–6 signs or symptoms potentially attributable to Cushing's syndrome besides obesity [14]. This underscores the importance of not screening obese patients indiscriminately for Cushing's syndrome unless unusual or multiple and progressive features are present [4].

Diabetes

Type 2 diabetes is common in the general population and high levels of glucocorticoids are well known to cause insulin resistance and diabetes by increasing gluconeogenesis, stimulating glycogenolysis, inhibiting insulin secretion and enhancing insulin resistance. Impaired glucose tolerance or diabetes may be found in around 40–45% of patients with Cushing's disease [7]. Several studies have assessed the prevalence of Cushing's syndrome in patients with type 2 diabetes. Results have been conflicting. In 200 overweight patients with type 2 diabetes, 2% of the patients were deemed to be suffering from definitive occult Cushing's syndrome, whereas another 3.5% had mild occult disease, and 8 of these patients had adrenal tumours [15]. Conversely, in a prospective multicentre study in 813 patients with known type 2 diabetes mellitus, only 0.6% of patients were diagnosed with Cushing's syndrome, all 5 of which were adrenal dependent. The difficulty here is that the prevalence of adrenal masses secreting cortisol is high in this population, but whether these are the cause of the glucose intolerance or diabetes is not clear in general, although metabolic control was achieved in 4 of the patients who had an adrenalectomy [16]. In addition, a prospective study in which 201 consecutive patients attending a diabetes clinic, satisfying at least 2 out of 3 criteria (Hba1c >7%, BMI >25 and history of hypertension or BP >140/90 mm Hg), were screened for hypercortisolism, none were diagnosed with Cushing's syndrome [17]. These data do not support widespread screening of patients with type 2 diabetes, although they do suggest that the prevalence of hypercortisolism secondary to adrenal tumours may be higher than previously recognised. Therefore, on the basis of a low prevalence of Cushing's syndrome in patients with type 2 diabetes and a higher possibility of a hyperactive HPA axis in patients with hyperinsulinaemia, routine screening is not recommended and should be reserved for cases where unusual or multiple and progressive features are present [4].

Osteoporosis

The prevalence of osteoporosis in patients with Cushing's disease is high, affecting 32% of women and 47% of men with the condition [7]. The converse, however, does not hold true, and whilst some studies suggest increased rates of Cushing's syndrome in osteoporosis, these are all cross-sectional in nature and at risk of biased selection with enrichment for hypercortisolaemia. As an example, the prevalence of biochemical evidence of low-grade endogenous hypercortisolism in 219 subjects referred for the assessment of osteoporosis was 7/65 patients with osteoporotic vertebral fracture. Six patients with an osteoporotic vertebral fracture had adrenal tumours (4 unilateral; 2 bilateral), whereas the other patient had an ACTH-secreting pituitary adenoma [18]. Longitudinal studies are needed to confirm this finding before any recommendations are made to screen for Cushing's syndrome in the general osteoporotic population. On the other hand, if a young patient suffers a non-traumatic vertebral or rib fracture in the absence of another obvious cause, screening for Cushing's syndrome is justified.

Hypertension

Hypertension is common in patients with Cushing's syndrome, affecting around 70% of subjects [7]. In a prospective study of 1,020 patients suffering from hypertension in Japan, around 2% were diagnosed with Cushing's syndrome (6 Cushing's syndrome from adrenal adenoma, 10 pre-clinical Cushing's syndrome from adrenal tumour and 5 with Cushing's disease). At 1 year after surgery, 14/16 patients were cured from hypertension and the other 2 patients – one with Cushing's syndrome and the other with pre-clinical Cushing's – improved [19]. Although these data should make physicians vigilant to avoid missing patients with Cushing's syndrome presenting with hypertension, there is no indication to screen all patients with hypertension for Cushing's syndrome.

Adrenal Incidentaloma

A significant number of patients with adrenal incidentalomas have evidence of excess circulating low-grade cortisol but do not have any of the external clinical features of Cushing's. On the other hand, these patients with adrenal incidentalomas and excess cortisol secretion have increased cardiovascular risk, including high rates of hypertension, diabetes, impaired glucose tolerance, dyslipidaemia and visceral obesity [20, 21]. In addition, there is an increased rate of cardiovascular events and mortality from cardiovascular disease and infections [22, 23]. The challenge for endocrinologists is to identify individual patients with cortisol excess in whom these complications are secondary to an ACTH-independent cortisol-secreting tumour as opposed to a hyperactive HPA axis causing a false-positive test [24]. Therefore, until prospective, definitive interventional studies are carried out, patients with adrenal incidentaloma should be screened for Cushing's syndrome using dexamethasone testing, but any intervention requires careful individualisation to weigh up the risks and potential benefits.

Weight Gain and Growth Retardation in Children

Children suffering from Cushing's syndrome may present with different clinical signs compared to adults. Weight gain and growth retardation are common features in children and are found in 90 and 83% of patients, respectively [25]. Therefore, when children present with a decreasing height velocity and increased weight, a low threshold for investigation for hypercortisolism is recommended. Identifying the disease early is crucial since catch-up growth after remission is possible, in addition to remission of other complications and neurocognitive sequelae.

Other Causes of Hypercortisolism

Other disorders, such as psychotic depression or alcohol dependence, may be associated with hypercortisolism secondary to a hyperactive HPA axis, whereas intense chronic exercise, malnutrition and physical stress may cause physiological hypercortisolism [4]. Prior to embarking on testing for hypercortisolism, one should enquire about the presence of these conditions. Abstinence from alcohol will reverse or ameliorate excess cortisol secretion.

Is There Hypercortisolaemia?

Initial Testing

In a patient with a high pre-test probability for Cushing's syndrome, initial testing should be with either the 1-mg overnight dexamethasone suppression test, 24-hour urine cortisol, salivary or serum midnight cortisol, or the low-dose dexamethasone suppression test (LDDST) as recommended by Endocrine Society guidelines [4]. One positive test should be supported by another positive test. In cases where mild or episodic hypercortisolism is suspected, multiple tests should be performed before the diagnosis is excluded, and these should be repeated at an interval if discordant results are found between tests. If a patient is taking oral oestrogens, any assessment of serum cortisol should be performed 6 weeks after withdrawal. It is essential that Cushing's syndrome is established as a diagnosis before any attempt is made to find a cause.

The 1-mg Overnight Dexamethasone Suppression Test

Patients with Cushing's syndrome secrete cortisol autonomously and negative feedback is impaired, justifying the rationale for using this test. To enhance the sensitivity of this test, a post-dexamethasone cortisol cut-off of 50 nmol/l at 08.00–09.00 h is recommended, although this at the expense of a lower specificity depending on the population being screened. Around 5% of patients with proven Cushing's disease suppress serum cortisol to <50 nmol/l [26], and thus one cannot rely totally on this test to confirm the diagnosis. In populations with impaired negative feedback, such as obesity, there may be a high rate of false-positive tests, highlighting the difficulties an investigator may encounter when using this test indiscriminately [12]. Some patients may also be on drugs that induce CYP450 3A4, resulting in increased metabolism of dexamethasone and higher cortisol levels. In these situations, if clinically possible, the test should be performed after withdrawal of the drug, otherwise the use of other tests discussed below is recommended.

2-mg 48-Hour Low-Dose Dexamethasone Suppression Test

This test has similar sensitivity for Cushing's syndrome as the 1-mg test, but slightly higher specificity. The use of salivary cortisol post-LDDST has recently been studied in 27 patients with untreated Cushing's disease and 89 controls. With a 3.4-nmol/l cut-off, the sensitivity and specificity were 96.3 and 97.7%, respectively. In the same group, when measuring a serum cortisol post-LDDST, with a cut-off of 50 nmol/l, the sensitivity was 100% while specificity was 97.7%. The specificity was much better for saliva than serum in women on oral contraceptive pills (90.5 vs. 61.9%) [27]. The LDDST may be used in patients with borderline results of the overnight dexamethasone suppression test and in whom the diagnosis is debatable, and the use of saliva is an option in patients on oestrogens.

Midnight Salivary and Serum Cortisol

Cortisol has a well-defined circadian rhythm overlying ultradian pulsatility. In patients with Cushing's syndrome the circadian rhythm is blunted with a reduction in amplitude, higher mean cortisol levels and cortisol levels higher than 50 nmol/l between 23.00 and 03.00 h [28]. The use of salivary cortisol, a measure of the free fraction of cortisol in the circulation, is a practical and convenient way to measure late night cortisol levels at home to detect abnormalities in cortisol rhythm. The cut-off values used to define normality vary depending on assay used. In a meta-analysis of the use of salivary cortisol in the diagnosis of Cushing's syndrome including a total of 947 patients (339 with Cushing's syndrome), sensitivity was 92% and specificity was 96% [29]. Importantly, interpretation of salivary cortisol must take into consideration the threshold used, as lower cut-offs may result in false-positive tests especially in the elderly and patients with type 2 diabetes [30]. The use of LC-MS/MS to measure salivary cortisol eliminates cross-reaction of steroids, hence increasing specificity, which is an advantage over immunoassays [14]. A recent study has shown that late night salivary cortisol is superior to urine free cortisol, confirming the diagnosis of Cushing's syndrome even in patients with normal urine cortisol levels [31]. Although salivary cortisol may be used as a first-line test, other supporting tests are necessary. It is recommended that two samples are taken and the highest value be taken into consideration. Salivary cortisol also has advantages for the assessment of cyclical Cushing's syndrome, but should not be taken as evidence alone of hypercortisolaemia; other confirmatory tests are needed at the time that salivary cortisol levels are high.

Similarly, the use of a sleeping midnight serum cortisol >50 nmol/l has a sensitivity of 100% for the diagnosis of Cushing's syndrome [32], but is not practical in many institutions, and is not specific, being elevated in physical ill health. A higher cut-off of 207 nmol/l has been used when patients are awake. When 263 patients had an indwelling catheter and blood was drawn multiple times between 23.00 and 01.00 h, an 'awake' serum midnight cortisol >207 nmol/l was 96% sensitive and 100% specific, discriminating all patients with pseudo-Cushing (n = 23) and was more accurate than urine free cortisol [33]. This test is most useful to rule out Cushing's syndrome – if the level of sleeping midnight serum cortisol is <50 nmol/l then Cushing's syndrome is excluded.

Urine Free Cortisol

Twenty-four hour urine collections of cortisol are widely used for the diagnosis of Cushing's syndrome, but are less sensitive than dexamethasone and salivary cortisol testing [34]. Collections are cumbersome, frequently incomplete and if the eGFR is <60 ml/min there is a risk of false-negative results, whilst volumes >4 litres per 24 h may yield false positives. As it is a measure of free cortisol, reflecting serum cortisol levels after CBG saturation, mild hypercortisolism may not be detected, and values are normal in up to 15% of patients with known Cushing's disease. Furthermore, three samples are usually needed to compensate for variability, which is usually around 50%, and levels do not correlate with clinical features of hypercortisolism such as insulin resistance, blood pressure and BMI [35]. Diagnostic accuracy may improve with the use of LC-MS/MS as this technique excludes interference from other steroids, although this is at the expense of reducing sensitivity since some patients may excrete different cortisol metabolites that are detected by immunoassay. Therefore, assay-specific cut-offs to define Cushing's syndrome using these assays are essential. In a recent study, urine free cortisol >170 nmol/24 h had a sensitivity and specificity of 97 and 91%, and had a combined higher positive and lower negative likelihood ratio when compared to other first-line tests for detecting Cushing's syndrome [36]. Urine free cortisol may be used as a first-line test, but it is less sensitive for mild clinical hypercortisolism and screening of adrenal incidentaloma. It may be used in cyclical Cushing's and in pregnancy.

Other Tests
It is the opinion of the authors that other tests such as the dexamethasone-suppressed CRH test and desmopressin (1-deamino-8D-arginine vasopressin) tests are of little additional utility in the assessment of Cushing's syndrome, although they are used in some centres. When two of the above-mentioned tests are abnormal and a hyperactive HPA axis or physiological cause for hypercortisolism is excluded, Cushing's syndrome is confirmed.

What Is the Cause?

Once Cushing's syndrome is established, the first step is to measure plasma ACTH level on two occasions as sometimes the values in patients with Cushing's disease can be low. Samples need careful handling with collection on ice and immediate centrifugation to avoid falsely low values. Levels <5 pg/ml are highly suggestive of ACTH-independent Cushing's syndrome, whereas levels >15 pg/ml are usually related to ACTH-dependent Cushing's syndrome. Typically the values of ACTH in Cushing's disease are in the upper half, or just above, of the normal range. If plasma ACTH is suppressed, CT or MRI of the adrenals will reveal an adrenal adenoma or adrenal cancer in most cases. If ACTH-independent macronodular adrenal hyperplasia (AIMAH) is found, consideration should be given to the presence of aberrant receptors to vasopressin, gastric inhibitory peptide, serotonin, β-agonists and LH/HCG, which, when stimulated, result in excess cortisol secretion. Recent reports have demonstrated an inherited mutation in the armadillo repeat-containing 5 *(ARMC5)* gene in some patients with AIMAH and family members with unsuspected AIMAH [37], and thus consideration to family screening may be justified. If there is no apparent abnormality on imaging, then the diagnosis may be primary pigmented nodular adrenal disease or factitious ingestion of hydrocortisone or cortisone acetate if cross-reactivity with other synthetic glucocorticoids has been excluded.

The differential diagnosis of ACTH-dependent Cushing's syndrome is more complex, and focuses on differentiating between pituitary Cushing's syndrome and ectopic ACTH secretion. In general, the ectopic ACTH syndrome is associated with more severe hypercortisolaemia, but this is not uniform and neuroendocrine tumours of non-pituitary origin, for example in the lung, can result in a clinical picture identical to Cushing's disease. In women with ACTH-dependent Cushing's syndrome, the pre-test probability of Cushing's disease is 90% and in men 66%, thus any test should improve on these probabilities to have added value. Unless there is a clear macroadenoma of the pituitary gland, reliance should be placed on biochemical testing because of the 10% prevalence of pituitary incidentaloma in the general population [38].

In cases where a pituitary adenoma is clearly present on MRI (>6 mm) and there is a positive response to CRH [ACTH response 35–50% at 15 and 30 min and a cortisol increase 14–20% at 30 and 45 min after ovine CRH administration (100 μg; intravenous)], and there has been suppression on either high-dose dexamethasone testing or on the LDDST, these combined data are highly suggestive of pituitary Cushing's, and some centres will not go on to perform bilateral inferior petrosal sinus sampling. In all other circumstances, bilateral inferior petrosal sinus sampling (when available) is recommended, and in many centres is the investigation of choice. A baseline central to periphery ACTH ratio >2 and a level >3 post-CRH at a time of hypercortisolaemia favour the presence of pituitary-dependent ACTH syndrome.

One of the main problems with this test is unsuccessful catheterisation, especially in cases of anomalous venous drainage or poor technique. Even with correct catheter placement, 5% of patients with Cushing's disease may have a false-negative gradient, whilst false-positive gradients, in the context of ectopic ACTH syndrome, are very uncommon. Normalising the ACTH gradient to the prolactin values may be used to improve sensitivity when no gradient is detected: a level <0.7 favouring ectopic ACTH and one >1.3 favouring Cushing's disease, but this still leaves a few patients in a 'grey zone' [39]. Bilateral inferior petrosal sinus sampling can help guide surgeons towards the site of the adenoma in the pituitary, but as lateralisation using this technique lacks accuracy, exploration of all the gland is highly recommended when an adenoma is not found at the predicted site [40].

The high-dose dexamethasone suppression test is no longer recommended as it has a sensitivity for Cushing's disease of 80%, which is less than the pre-test probability, at least in women [41] and does not offer more information than the LDDST.

In ectopic ACTH syndrome, basal plasma ACTH levels may be normal in around 32% of patients and around 10% may respond to dexamethasone testing or CRH [42]. The cause for ectopic ACTH secretion may be overt (clear tumour found on initial imaging), covert (tumour found on detailed subsequent imaging or follow-up) or occult (tumour never found), with patients most commonly presenting with weakness, weight gain and hypertension. Axial imaging with CT or MRI will locate about 75% of ACTH-secreting tumours and are the first recommended tests to diagnose ectopic ACTH. Octreotide scans may detect around 49% of tumours [42], whilst Ga-68 DOTATATE PET-CT is likely to have a higher sensitivity [43]. Current functional imaging modalities are unlikely to disclose an occult lesion not visualised on CT or MRI, and hypercortisolaemia causes downregulation of somatostatin 2 receptors, the target for the ligand used in these scans – a situation that may reverse by reducing the effect of high circulating cortisol [44]. A high rate of hypokalaemia is present due to saturation of 11β-hydroxysteroid dehydrogenase type 2 and excess cortisol acting at the mineralocorticoid receptor. Tumour markers such as 24-hour urine 5HIAA or calcitonin in carcinoids or medullary thyroid cancer, respectively, may be elevated; however, these markers may also be high in other neuroendocrine tumours. A high chromogranin A (when not due to other causes such as renal failure and use of proton pump inhibitors) in patients with a normal pituitary MRI is also highly suggestive of ectopic ACTH.

Conclusions

Cushing's syndrome is a complex disorder. Identifying this condition is challenging due to a lack of completely specific signs and tests that identify autonomous cortisol excess. The diagnosis is best considered in the presence of multiple clinical features most specific for cortisol excess, especially if these have a history that they are progressively worsening. Furthermore, populations such as those with diabetes, obesity or osteoporosis should not be screened routinely for the presence of Cushing's syndrome. Novel approaches to improve the accuracy and precision of diagnosis of Cushing's syndrome are needed, including identification of biomarkers for glucocorticoid excess.

References

1 Ntali G, Asimakopoulou A, Siamatras T, Komninos J, Vassiliadi D, Tzanela M, Tsagarakis S, Grossman AB, Wass JA, Karavitaki N: Mortality in Cushing's syndrome: systematic analysis of a large series with prolonged follow-up. Eur J Endocrinol 2013;169:715–723.

2 Etxabe J, Vazquez JA: Morbidity and mortality in Cushing's disease: an epidemiological approach. Clin Endocrinol (Oxf) 1994;40:479–484.

3 Newell-Price J Bertagna X, Grossman AB, Nieman LK: Cushing's syndrome. Lancet 2006;367:1605–1617.

4 Nieman LK, Biller BM, Findling JW, Newell-Price J, Savage MO, Stewart PM, Montori VM: The diagnosis of Cushing's syndrome: an Endocrine Society Clinical Practice Guideline. J Clin Endocrinol Metab 2008;93:1526–1540.

5 Hopkins RL, Leinung MC: Exogenous Cushing's syndrome and glucocorticoid withdrawal. Endocrinol Metab Clin North Am 2005;34:371–384, ix.

6 Mahlab-Guri K, Asher I, Gradstein S, Zung A, Radian-Sade R, Elbirt D, Sthoeger Z: Inhaled fluticasone causes iatrogenic Cushing's syndrome in patients treated with Ritonavir. J Asthma 2001;48:860–863.

7 Pecori Giraldi F, Moro M, Cavagnini F: Gender-related differences in the presentation and course of Cushing's disease. J Clin Endocrinol Metab 2003;88: 1554–1558.

8 Afshari A, Ardeshirpour Y, Beth Lodish M, Gourgari E, Sinaii N, Keil M, Belyavskaya E, Lyssikatos C, Chowdhry FA, Chernomordik V, Anderson AA, Mazzuchi TA, Gandjbakhche A, Stratakis CA: Facial plethora: modern technology for quantifying an ancient clinical sign and its use in Cushing syndrome. J Clin Endocrinol Metab 2015;100:3928–3933.

9 Liu X, Zhu X, Zeng M, Zhuang Y, Zhou Y, Zhang Z, Yang Y, Wang Y, Ye H, Li Y: Gender-specific differences in clinical profile and biochemical parameters in patients with cushing's disease: a single center experience. Int J Endocrinol 2015;2015:949620.

10 Rockall AG, Sohaib SA, Evans D, Kaltsas G, Isidori AM, Monson JP, Besser GM, Grossman AB, Reznek RH: Computed tomography assessment of fat distribution in male and female patients with Cushing's syndrome. Eur J Endocrinol 2003;149:561–567.

11 Rosmond R, Dallman MF, Bjorntorp P: Stress-related cortisol secretion in men: relationships with abdominal obesity and endocrine, metabolic and hemodynamic abnormalities. J Clin Endocrinol Metab 1998;83:1853–1859.

12 Ness-Abramof R, Nabriski D, Apovian CM, Niven M, Weiss E, Shapiro MS, Shenkman L: Overnight dexamethasone suppression test: a reliable screen for Cushing's syndrome in the obese. Obes Res 2002;10: 1217–1221.

13 Rask E, Olsson T, Soderberg S, Andrew R, Livingstone DE, Johnson O, Walker BR: Tissue-specific dysregulation of cortisol metabolism in human obesity. J Clin Endocrinol Metab 2001;86:1418–1421.

14 Baid R, Rubino D, Sinaii N, Ramsey S, Frank A, Nieman LK: Specificity of screening tests for Cushing's syndrome in an overweight and obese population. J Clin Endocrinol Metab 2009;94:3857–3864.

15 Catargi B, Rigalleau V, Poussin A, Ronci-Chaix N, Bex V, Vergnot V, Gin H, Roger P, Tabarin A: Occult Cushing's syndrome in type-2 diabetes. J Clin Endocrinol Metab 2003;88:5808–5813.

16 Terzolo M, Reimondo G, Chiodini I, Castello R, Giordano R, Ciccarelli E, Limone P, Crivellaro C, Martinelli I, Montini M, Disoteo O, Ambrosi B, Lanzi R, Arosio M, Senni S, Balestrieri A, Solaroli E, Madeo B, De Giovanni R, Strollo F, Battista R, Scorsone A, Giagulli A, Collura D, Scillitani A, Cozzi R, Faustini-Fustini M, Pia A, Rinaldi R, Allasino B, Peraga G, Tassone F, Garofalo P, Papini E, Borretta G: Screening of Cushing's syndrome in outpatients with type 2 diabetes: results of a prospective multicentric study in Italy. J Clin Endocrinol Metab 2012; 97:3467–3475.

17 Mullan K, Black N, Thiraviaraj N, Bell PM, Burgess C, Hunter SJ, McCance DR, Leslie H, Sheridan B, Atkinson AB: Is there value in routine screening for Cushing's syndrome in patients with diabetes? J Clin Endocrinol Metab 2010;95:2262–2265.

18 Chiodini I, Mascia ML, Muscarella S, Battista C, Minisola S, Arosio M, Santini SA, Guglielmi G, Carnevale V, Scillitani A: Subclinical hypercortisolism among outpatients referred for osteoporosis. Ann Intern Med 2007;147:541–548.

19 Omura M, Saito J, Yamaguchi K, Kakuta Y, Nishikawa T: Prospective study on the prevalence of secondary hypertension among hypertensive patients visiting a general outpatient clinic in Japan. Hypertens Res 2004;27:193–202.

20 Tauchmanova L, Rossi R, Biondi B, Pulcrano M, Nuzzo V, Palmieri EA, Fazio S, Lombardi G: Patients with subclinical Cushing's syndrome due to adrenal adenoma have increased cardiovascular risk. J Clin Endocrinol Metab 2002;87:4872–4878.

21 Debono M, Prema A, Hughes TJ, Bull M, Ross RJ, Newell-Price J: Visceral fat accumulation and post-dexamethasone serum cortisol levels in patients with adrenal incidentaloma. J Clin Endocrinol Metab 2013;98:2383–2391.

22 Di Dalmazi G, Vicennati V, Garelli S, Casadio E, Rinaldi E, Giampalma E, Mosconi C, Golfieri R, Paccapelo A, Pagotto U, Pasquali R: Cardiovascular events and mortality in patients with adrenal incidentalomas that are either non-secreting or associated with intermediate phenotype or subclinical Cushing's syndrome: a 15-year retrospective study. Lancet Diabetes Endocrinol 2014;2:396–405.

23 Debono M, Bradburn M, Bull M, Harrison B, Ross RJ, Newell-Price J: Cortisol as a marker for increased mortality in patients with incidental adrenocortical adenomas. J Clin Endocrinol Metab 2014;99:4462–4470.

24 Cawood TJ, Hunt PJ, O'Shea D, Cole D, Soule S: Recommended evaluation of adrenal incidentalomas is costly, has high false-positive rates and confers a risk of fatal cancer that is similar to the risk of the adrenal lesion becoming malignant; time for a rethink? Eur J Endocrinol 2009;161:513–527.

25 Magiakou MA, Mastorakos G, Oldfield EH, Gomez MT, Doppman JL, Cutler GB Jr, Nieman LK, Chrousos GP: Cushing's syndrome in children and adolescents. Presentation, diagnosis, and therapy. N Engl J Med 1994;331:629–636.

26 Findling JW, Raff H, Aron DC: The low-dose dexamethasone suppression test: a reevaluation in patients with Cushing's syndrome. J Clin Endocrinol Metab 2004;89:1222–1226.

27 Manetti L, Rossi G, Grasso L, Raffaelli V, Scattina I, Del Sarto S, Cosottini M, Iannelli A, Gasperi M, Bogazzi F, Martino E: Usefulness of salivary cortisol in the diagnosis of hypercortisolism: comparison with serum and urinary cortisol. Eur J Endocrinol 2013; 168:315–321.

28 Boyar RM, Witkin M, Carruth A, Ramsey J: Circadian cortisol secretory rhythms in Cushing's disease. J Clin Endocrinol Metab 1979;48:760–765.
29 Carroll T, Raff H, Findling JW: Late-night salivary cortisol for the diagnosis of Cushing syndrome: a meta-analysis. Endocr Pract 2009;15:335–342.
30 Liu H, Bravata DM, Cabaccan J, Raff H, Ryzen E: Elevated late-night salivary cortisol levels in elderly male type 2 diabetic veterans. Clin Endocrinol (Oxf) 2005;63:642–649.
31 Elias PC, Martinez EZ, Barone BF, Mermejo LM, Castro M, Moreira AC: Late-night salivary cortisol has a better performance than urinary free cortisol in the diagnosis of Cushing's syndrome. J Clin Endocrinol Metab 2014;99:2045–2051.
32 Newell-Price J, Trainer P, Perry L, Wass J, Grossman A, Besser M: A single sleeping midnight cortisol has 100% sensitivity for the diagnosis of Cushing's syndrome. Clin Endocrinol (Oxf) 1995;43:545–550.
33 Papanicolaou DA, Yanovski JA, Cutler GB Jr, Chrousos GP, Nieman LK: A single midnight serum cortisol measurement distinguishes Cushing's syndrome from pseudo-Cushing states. J Clin Endocrinol Metab 1998;83:1163–1167.
34 Elamin MB, Murad MH, Mullan R, Erickson R, Harris K, Nadeem S, Ennis R, Erwin PJ, Montori PV: Accuracy of diagnostic tests for Cushing's syndrome: a systematic review and metaanalyses. J Clin Endocrinol Metab 2008:93;1553–1562.
35 Petersenn S, Newell-Price J, Findling JW, Gu F, Maldonado M, Sen K, Salgado RA, Colao A, Biller BM: High variability in baseline urinary free cortisol values in patients with Cushing's disease. Clin Endocrinol (Oxf) 2014;80:261–269.
36 Ceccato F, Barbot M, Zilio M, Frigo AC, Albiger N, Camozzi V, Antonelli G, Plebani M, Mantero F, Boscaro M, Scaroni C: Screening tests for Cushing's syndrome: urinary free cortisol role measured by LC-MS/MS. J Clin Endocrinol Metab 2015;100:3856–3861.
37 Assie G, Libe R, Espiard S, Rizk-Rabin M, Guimier M, Luscap W, Barreau O, Lefevre L, Sibony M, Guignat L, Rodriguez S, Perlemoine K, Rene-Corail F, Letourneur F, Trabulsi B, Poussier A, Chabbert-Buffet N, Borson-Chazot F, Groussin L, Bertagna X, Stratakis CA, Ragazzon B, Bertherat J: ARMC5 mutations in macronodular adrenal hyperplasia with Cushing's syndrome. N Engl J Med 2013;369:2105–2114.
38 Hall WA, Luciano MG, Doppman JL, Patronas NJ, Oldfield EH: Pituitary magnetic resonance imaging in normal human volunteers: occult adenomas in the general population. Ann Intern Med 1994;120:817–820.
39 Sharma ST, Raff H, Nieman LK: Prolactin as a marker of successful catheterization during IPSS in patients with ACTH-dependent Cushing's syndrome. J Clin Endocrinol Metab 2011;96:3687–3694.
40 Wind JJ, Lonser RR, Nieman LK, DeVroom HL, Chang R, Oldfield EH: The lateralization accuracy of inferior petrosal sinus sampling in 501 patients with Cushing's disease. J Clin Endocrinol Metab 2013;98:2285–2293.
41 Invitti C, Pecori Giraldi F, de Martin M, Cavagnini F: Diagnosis and management of Cushing's syndrome: results of an Italian multicentre study. Study Group of the Italian Society of Endocrinology on the Pathophysiology of the Hypothalamic-Pituitary-Adrenal Axis. J Clin Endocrinol Metab 1999;84:440–448.
42 Ilias I, Torpy DJ, Pacak K, Mullen N, Wesley RA, Nieman LK: Cushing's syndrome due to ectopic corticotropin secretion: twenty years' experience at the National Institutes of Health. J Clin Endocrinol Metab 2005;90:4955–4962.
43 Ozkan ZG, Kuyumcu S, Balkose D, Ozkan B, Aksakal N, Yilmaz E, Sanli Y, Turkmen C, Aral F, Adalet I: The value of somatostatin receptor imaging with In-111 octreotide and/or Ga-68 DOTATATE in localizing ectopic ACTH producing tumors. Mol Imaging Radionucl Ther 2013;22:49–55.
44 de Bruin C, Hofland LH, Nieman LK, van Koetsveld PM, Waaijers AM, Sprij-Mooij DM, van Essen M, Lamberts SW, de Herder WW, Feelders RA: Mifepristone effects on tumor somatostatin receptor expression in two patients with Cushing's syndrome due to ectopic adrenocorticotropin secretion. J Clin Endocrinol Metab 2012;97:455–462.

Prof. John D. Newell-Price, MA, PhD, FRCP
Academic Unit of Endocrinology, University of Sheffield
Beech Hill Road
Sheffield S10 2RX (UK)
E-Mail j.newellprice@sheffield.ac.uk

Arvat E, Falorni A (eds): Cortisol Excess and Insufficiency.
Front Horm Res. Basel, Karger, 2016, vol 46, pp 28–38 (DOI: 10.1159/000443862)

Subclinical Hypercortisolism: How to Deal with It?

Iacopo Chiodini · Valentina Morelli

Unit of Endocrinology and Metabolic Diseases, Department of Clinical Sciences and Community Health, Fondazione IRCCS Cà Granda, Ospedale Maggiore Policlinico di Milano, University of Milan, Milan, Italy

Abstract

Subclinical hypercortisolism (SH) is a condition of mild cortisol excess, found in the 5–30% of patients with adrenal incidentalomas, defined as silent adrenal masses diagnosed throughout radiological examinations performed for unrelated diseases. Generally, the diagnosis of SH is supported by the presence of high cortisol levels after a 1-mg dexamethasone suppression test, low adrenocorticotropic hormone levels, altered cortisol circadian rhythm and 24-hour urinary free cortisol levels higher than the upper reference value. Less frequently, diagnosis is made by other tests. Unfortunately, up to now a consensus on SH diagnostic criteria is lacking. Although SH is characterized by the absence of the classical features of Cushing's syndrome by definition, it has been associated with the presence of different metabolic complications (mainly type 2 diabetes mellitus, arterial hypertension, central obesity and dyslipidemia), cardiovascular diseases, osteoporosis and vertebral fractures, altered coagulation parameters, worsening of quality of life, and increased mortality. The management of SH, as well as the improvement of metabolic parameters and other complications after surgical treatment, is still a matter of debate.

The presence of preclinical Cushing's syndrome (CS), defined as pathological cortisol secretion in the absence of specific signs and symptoms of hypercortisolism, is often detected in patients with incidentally diagnosed adrenal tumors (adrenal incidentaloma), which was first described in 1992 [1].

The term 'subclinical hypercortisolism' (SH) was later preferred to describe this condition, as the progression to an overt excessive cortisol secretion in these patients appeared to be rare [2]. In recent years the clinical impact of SH has been extensively studied mainly in patients with the adrenocorticotropic hormone (ACTH)-independent form, especially in adrenal incidentaloma, as (although possible) ACTH-dependent (pituitary or ectopic) SH is considered uncommon [3].

Diagnosis

The absence of the typical clinical signs and symptoms, the low reliability of the available hormonal assays, and the variability of cortisol secretion in these patients often make SH diagnosis difficult. Moreover, the diagnostic complexity depends also on individual cortisol sensitivity and tissue cortisol availability, respectively due to the presence of polymorphisms of the glucocorticoid receptor and to the activity of the 11β-hydroxysteroid dehydrogenase enzymes [2].

The first-line test for the detection of SH, recommended by the NIH [4], is the evaluation of cortisol levels after a 1-mg dexamethasone suppression test (1mg-DST) with a threshold of 5 μg/dl. However, diagnosing SH using this cutoff has shown low sensitivity, with the consequent risk of missing diagnosis. On the other hand, a cutoff of 1.8 μg/dl has poor specificity and could lead to false positives. To overcome this problem, a cutoff of 3 μg/dl has been proposed by some authors, but a consensus has not been achieved [2].

Two-day 2mg-DST should be preferred to 1mg-DST in patients with type 2 diabetes mellitus (T2DM), psychiatric disorders or alcoholism [2].

In these patients, basal ACTH levels are frequently low, with a blunted ACTH response to corticotropin-releasing hormone stimulation, suggesting an adrenal origin of SH [5]. However, normal ACTH levels are often observed in patients with ACTH-independent CS, limiting the diagnostic utility of this parameter. Moreover, in this context, corticotropin-releasing hormone stimulation does not seem to add any advantage to the basal ACTH level evaluation. On the other hand, in the presence of SH without suppressed ACTH levels, the corticotropin-releasing hormone test may be useful in order to exclude ACTH-dependent hypercortisolism [2]. Although high 24-hour urinary free cortisol (UFC; at least two measurements) is considered by the Endocrine Society as a test with high diagnostic accuracy for the initial diagnosis of CS [6], this alteration is scarcely reported among adrenal incidentaloma patients, even in the presence of SH. The use of UFC in SH identification is probably limited by the low sensitivity of the common assays in this setting. This limit could be overcome in the future by the widespread availability of new high-sensitive techniques such as gas chromatography-mass spectrometry (GC-MS) or liquid-chromatography tandem mass spectrometry (LC-MS/MS).

Altered cortisol circadian rhythm and, in particular, high midnight serum cortisol have often been reported in adrenal incidentaloma patients [2]. Recently, midnight salivary cortisol has been proposed instead of midnight serum cortisol as a sensitive and easy-to-perform marker for the diagnosis of CS. At the same time, independently from the detection method, midnight salivary cortisol has shown poor sensitivity in the identification of SH, which does not allow its use as a screening test [7].

Other parameters, such as low DHEAS levels or high 24-hour urinary 17-hydroxycorticosteroids, have been suggested as screening tests, but their utility is lim-

Table 1. Prevalence of SH in patients with adrenal incidentalomas reported by the most recent and largest (>200 patients) endocrine series

	Patients, n	SH, %	SH criteria
Morelli et al. [9], 2014	206	11.6	1mg-DST >5 μg/dl or ≥2 of: low ACTH, high UFC, 1mg-DST cortisol >3 μg/dl
Kim et al. [10], 2013	348	6.0	UFC
Babińska et al. [11], 2012	463	6.7	1mg-DST cortisol >5 μg/dl
Di Dalmazi et al. [12], 2012	348	5.5	1mg-DST cortisol >5 μg/dl
Comlekci et al. [13], 2010	376	10.9	1mg-DST cortisol >2.8 μg/dl and ≥1 of: ACTH, UFC, MSeC >7.5 μg/dl
Chiodini et al. [14], 2009	287	29.6	≥2 of: ACTH, UFC, 1mg-DST cortisol >3 μg/dl

The different criteria applied for SH diagnosis are also indicated. MSeC = Midnight serum cortisol levels.

ited by the fact that DHEAS is frequently altered in advanced age, and 24-hour urinary 17-hydroxycorticosteroid as well as the levels of some other cortisol precursors and metabolites in urine are still being discussed [2]. Adrenal scintigraphy has also been proposed to diagnose SH, but its routine application is not currently recommended [2].

To increase diagnostic accuracy, the combination of cortisol after 1mg-DST and ACTH and UFC levels has been proposed with different cutoffs to assess adrenal function in adrenal incidentaloma patients. In particular, one study [8] has been specifically designed to investigate which parameter(s) of hypothalamic-pituitary-adrenal function could be the best index of the presence of SH, based on the relationship with chronic complications. According to this study, the combination of cortisol after 1mg-DST >3 μg/dl, elevated UFC and ACTH <10 pg/ml seemed to be the best predictors of SH (accuracy = 75.8%) [8].

Prevalence

The prevalence of SH largely depends on the criteria used for its diagnosis. Considering the largest series of adrenal incidentaloma patients published in the last years, SH prevalence varies from 5.5 to 29.6% (table 1). Considering the prevalence of adrenal incidentaloma in adult series (4–7%), the overall SH prevalence can be estimated to be around 0.2–2% [5]. Considering populations at risk (i.e. patients with osteoporosis, hypertension and diabetes), undiagnosed SH has been estimated in up to 4.8, 8 and 9.4%, of the patients, respectively [3, 15, 16]. To date, no guidelines are available to define when and how to screen patients at risk for SH.

Table 2. Prevalence of complications in patients with SH reported in the most recent and largest (>20 cases) series

	Patients, n	Age, years	T2DM, %	Hypertension, %	Dyslipidemia, %	Obesity, %
Debono et al. [18], 2014	111	69	24	64	47	–
Morelli et al. [9], 2014	39	62±11	33.3	66.7	53.8	33.3
Morelli et al. [19], 2013	41	62±12	26.1	56.7	31.7	–
Chiodini et al. [20], 2009	22	66±11	45.5	72.7	–	–
Tauchmanovà et al. [21], 2002	28	56±11	35.7	60.7	71.4	–

Clinical Presentation and Complications

Although characterized by the absence of the classical features of CS, SH has been associated with the presence of various metabolic complications (namely T2DM, hypertension, visceral obesity and dyslipidemia) and with osteoporosis and vertebral fractures.

Metabolic Syndrome

The association between SH and the classical features of metabolic syndrome was first hypothesized in 1992 when Reincke et al. [1] observed a high prevalence of hypertension, obesity and T2DM in adrenal incidentaloma patients with mild cortisol hypersecretion.

It is known that chronic glucocorticoid excess has detrimental effects on glucose metabolism. Similarly to patients with CS, SH has also been associated with insulin resistance. Interestingly, it has also been hypothesized that adrenal incidentaloma could be itself a manifestation of metabolic syndrome. A role of hyperinsulinemia in the development of adrenal tumors has been suggested based on the possible proliferative effect of insulin on adrenal cells and cortisol secretion, although the exact pathogenic mechanisms remain to be clarified [17].

The prevalence of the various metabolic complications reported in the largest series of SH patients are summarized in table 2. Differences could be secondary to the different diagnostic procedures (i.e. fasting glucose vs. oral glucose tolerance test) and cutoffs applied. Some studies have also reported an increased prevalence of metabolic complications in patients with SH as compared with age- and sex-matched patients with nonfunctioning adenomas or healthy controls.

Osteoporosis and Vertebral Fractures

The detrimental effect of glucocorticoids on bone is both direct, as cortisol reduces bone apposition and increases its resorption, and indirect, as cortisol impairs the calcium absorption/secretion and gonadal function. Osteoporosis and bone fractures

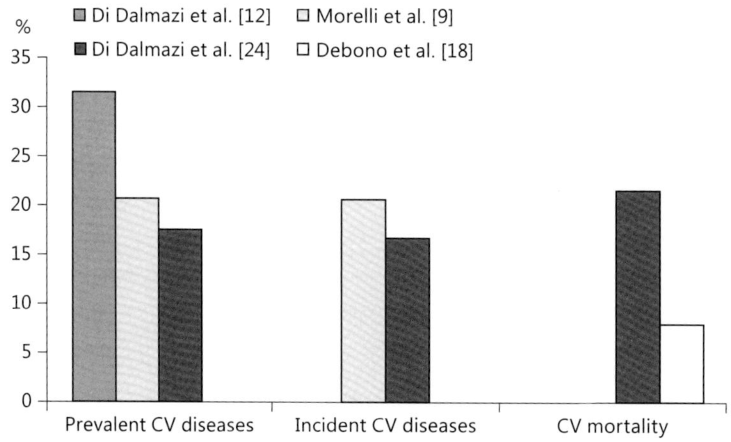

Fig. 1. Prevalence of cardiovascular (CV) diseases (coronary heart disease and stroke) and CV mortality in four different adrenal incidentaloma populations of patients with SH, although the definition of SH varied according to the different studies.

have been reported in up to 70% of patients with CS. Fortunately, in the majority of patients, bone mineral density increases and the risk of fractures normalizes after resolution of CS, although sometimes it takes several years. Similarly, the majority of recent cross-sectional studies suggest that SH is associated with an increased prevalence of osteoporosis. In particular, a longitudinal study specifically investigating the rate of spinal and femoral bone loss in female patients with adrenal incidentaloma [14] demonstrated that among patients with SH, those with higher levels of cortisol present a more severe loss rate of lumbar trabecular bone loss as compared with those with lower cortisol levels. Moreover, SH has been associated with an increased prevalence and incidence of vertebral fractures independently from bone mineral density, suggesting a possible reduction of bone quality in these patients [14]. The evaluation of bone quality and microarchitecture by the spinal deformity index (a tool evaluating both the number and severity of fractures) and the trabecular bone score [22, 23] confirmed that, among patients with adrenal incidentaloma, those with SH have higher spinal deformity index and worsen over time, while trabecular bone score is altered and inversely correlates with cortisol levels after 1mg-DST.

Cardiovascular Events and Mortality

Several studies have demonstrated that patients with SH are at increased risk of cardiovascular events (CVE; namely coronary heart disease and stroke) [9, 12, 18, 24] (fig. 1). In particular, the study by Morelli et al. [9] shows that SH is an independent risk factor for the occurrence of new CVE over time, with an annual rate of CVE events of 3.1%, which is similar to the incidence reported in populations at risk (i.e. patients with T2DM, hypertension and dyslipidemia). This result has been confirmed by subsequent studies. Furthermore, Di Dalmazi et al. [24], in a study specifically evaluating the mortality rate of adrenal incidentaloma patients after long-term follow-up, found that the survival rate for all-cause mortality was lower in adrenal incidentaloma patients with either a stable intermediate phenotype (defined as cortisol levels after 1mg-DST of 1.8–5 μg/dl) or SH (defined as cortisol levels after 1mg-DST >5 μg/dl) compared to those with stable nonsecreting masses (57 vs. 91%). Interestingly, the factors associated with increased mortality were age and mean cortisol levels after 1mg-DST, but not previous coronary heart disease. Similarly, as compared with patients with stable nonsecreting adrenal incidentaloma, unadjusted survival for cardiovascular-specific mortality was lower in patients with either a stable intermediate phenotype or SH, and in those with worsened secreting patterns. The frequency of death attributable to cancer did not differ between groups. These results have been subsequently confirmed by Debono et al. [18] who reported, in patients with adrenal incidentaloma, an increased mortality in those with SH; moreover, postdexamethasone cortisol levels >1.8 μg/dl were demonstrated to be a risk factor. Based on all these data, patients with SH deserve a careful follow-up of cardiovascular risk factors.

Two possible factors potentially involved in the pathogenesis of cardiovascular damage are growth hormone deficiency (GHD) and alterations of the coagulation pathway. Indeed, the evaluation of GH secretion in adrenal incidentaloma patients appears to be important since GHD has been associated with altered body composition, insulin resistance, and adverse lipid and cardiovascular risk profiles in adults. Therefore, GHD may contribute to many SH-related complications, although data on GH secretion in SH patients are scarce and discordant. A recent case-control study [25] suggests that SH is associated with a blunted GH secretion that increases after the recovery; moreover, GHD has been related to osteoporosis and to the deterioration of quality of life (QoL). Finally, compared to controls, patients with SH present significantly higher fibrinogen levels, with about 53.6% of the patients having at least one abnormal hemostatic parameter [20]. Disturbances in the endogenous anticoagulation system (protein C, free protein S activity and thrombomodulin concentration) have also been described, suggesting an impact of mild hypercortisolism on the coagulation system [26].

Impaired QoL

Only one study has evaluated the impact of SH on QoL by various questionnaires, demonstrating the impairment of some dimensions, namely mobility, performance of usual activities and an increase of anxiety/depression (using EQ-5D), physical functioning, physical role, general health, vitality, social functioning and emotional role (using SF-36), and physical fatigue (as assessed by MFI-20). The psychological aspects of the disease, such as patient worries about their condition, fear of having a tumor and anxiety for the future, probably impair QoL. At the same time, QoL scores of SH patients were not significantly different from those of other adrenal incidentaloma patients. The creation of an ad hoc questionnaire to investigate QoL in patients with SH could probably be more reliable than the use of generic ones [27].

The Role of Glucocorticoid Receptor Polymorphism
Besides the degree of hypercortisolism, the sensitivity to glucocorticoids may also play a role in determining the individual predisposition to develop complications in patients with SH. It is well known that N363S and *Bcl*I glucocorticoid receptor gene polymorphisms are associated with increased sensitivity to glucocorticoids. In patients carrying the sensitive variants of these polymorphisms, previous studies have demonstrated a higher prevalence of metabolic syndrome and bone complications. Recently, some authors have hypothesized a possible role of these sensitive variants in the pathogenesis of adrenal incidentaloma. Moreover, in a study performed in patients with endogenous glucocorticoid excess, a role of the *Bcl*I polymorphism in modifying the skeletal sensitivity to glucocorticoids was demonstrated. In particular, in patients affected by adrenal incidentaloma, it has been hypothesized that the contemporary presence of homozygous *Bcl*I and heterozygous N363S polymorphism of the glucocorticoid receptor could play an important role in the development of hypertension and vertebral fractures, alone or in combination. However, these findings were not confirmed by subsequent research, and were limited by the small size of the patient samples [28].

Clinical and Biochemical Follow-Up

Guidelines on the management of patients with SH are lacking. In adrenal incidentaloma patients with SH, the increased risk of metabolic derangement and CVE has to be taken into account for disease management. Although the value of periodic hormonal screening in adrenal incidentaloma patients without SH is uncertain, 1mg-DST should be repeated in those who develop clinical signs of hormone excess or experience worsening of metabolic status and cardiovascular risk profile, despite optimal medical treatment [2]. Patients who are not candidates for surgery should be followed up clinically to detect, treat and control cardiovascular risk factors. Surgical treatment should be considered for SH patients when medical treatment fails or there is progression of clinical features [2].

Surgical Treatment

Data regarding metabolic profile after surgical treatment of SH are conflicting. Some studies have described an improvement of some factors – in particular improvement in body weight, blood pressure and fasting glucose levels – after adrenalectomy,

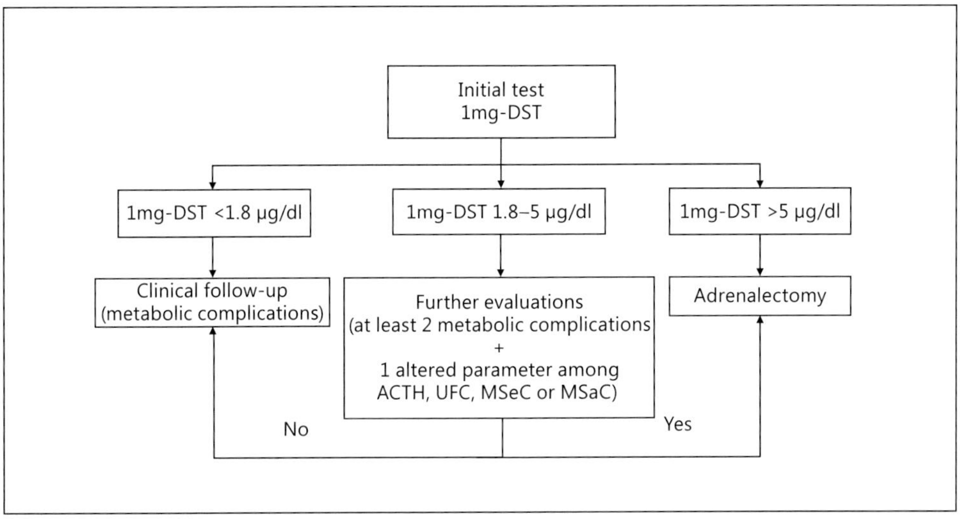

Fig. 2. Proposed flow chart for the management of patients with adrenal incidentalomas. MSeC = Midnight serum cortisol; MSaC = midnight salivary cortisol.

whereas others have given more conflicting results [2]. This discordance is possibly due to the small sample sizes and the lack of control groups in most studies, as well as different designs (i.e. retrospective vs. prospective). In addition, the diagnostic criteria are largely different, making the results of the various studies hard to compare. It is possible that in these patients surgery could avert the occurrence of CVE, thus improving the survival rate. Given the difficulties in diagnosing SH and the scarce, often contrasting, data on therapeutic outcomes, the treatment of choice (i.e. conservative with medical treatment of SH complications or surgical removal of the adrenal mass) remains a subject of debate for the majority of the patients with adrenal incidentaloma. The only available study specifically designed to clarify this point showed that, independently from the presence before surgery of SH metabolic complications, patients with 1mg-DST levels <2 µg/dl were likely to have no advantage from surgery, while in those with 1mg-DST levels >5 µg/dl the surgical excision of the adrenal mass was of benefit. In patients with 1mg-DST cortisol levels between 2 and 5 µg/dl, further biochemical investigations may be useful (e.g. morning ACTH and midnight serum cortisol levels). In the presence of an additional biochemical alteration and of at least 2 metabolic complications, surgery should be performed [29]. Based on our experience and on the basis of data provided by the abovementioned study, a possible approach in adrenal incidentaloma patients with suspected SH is reported in figure 2.

Another important issue is the need, after the surgical removal of an adrenal incidentaloma, for steroid replacement therapy. The prevalence of postsurgical adrenal insufficiency in patients with and without SH who underwent unilateral adrenalectomy for adrenal incidentaloma varies depending on the criteria used to diagnose SH and postsurgical hypocortisolism. Some authors suggest giving replacement therapy only to patients with SH, while others recommend steroid coverage in all. A recent literature review of 28 studies showed that the likelihood and severity of persistent suppression of HPA axis after adrenalectomy is related to the severity of functional presurgical adrenal impairment. Data analysis showed that replacement therapy can be withdrawn after 6.5 months in the majority of SH patients. Moreover, the authors underline the importance of assessing the integrity of the HPA axis by adequate tests (i.e. ACTH test), and that a substitutive dose of hydrocortisone of 12–15 mg/m^2/day is enough to prevent adrenal crisis and to allow a recovery of the HPA axis [30].

Future Perspectives

New techniques aimed at improving the reliability of hormonal assays and quantifying the role of glucocorticoid sensitivity on the response to the different tests are certainly needed. Moreover, a prospective randomized trial on a large sample of adrenal incidentaloma patients, treated with surgery or with a conservative approach, could help to define the indications, advantages and side effects of the various treatments in relation to the clinical and biochemical patient profile. In particular, the development of safe medical treatments aimed at controlling cortisol secretion in SH patients who are not candidates for surgery could be of help in the management of this subtle but not harmless disease.

References

1 Reincke M, Nieke J, Krestin GP, Saeger W, Allolio B, Winkelmann W: Preclinical Cushing's syndrome in adrenal 'incidentalomas': comparison with adrenal Cushing's syndrome. J Clin Endocrinol Metab 1992; 75:826–832.

2 Chiodini I: Diagnosis and treatment of subclinical hypercortisolism. J Clin Endocrinol Metab 2011;96: 1223–1236.

3 Chiodini I, Mascia ML, Muscarella S, Battista C, Minisola S, Arosio M, Santini SA, Guglielmi G, Carnevale V, Scillitani A: Subclinical hypercortisolism among outpatients referred for osteoporosis. Ann Intern Med 2007;147:541–548.

4 NIH state-of-the-science statement on management of the clinically inapparent adrenal mass ('incidentaloma'). NIH Consens State Sci Statements 2002;19: 1–25.

5 Reincke M: Subclinical Cushing's syndrome. Endocrinol Metab Clin North Am 2000;29:43–56.

6 Nieman LK, Biller BM, Findling JW, Newell-Price J, Savage MO, Stewart PM, Montori VM: The diagnosis of Cushing's syndrome: an Endocrine Society Clinical Practice Guideline. J Clin Endocrinol Metab 2008;93:1526–1540.

7 Palmieri S, Morelli V, Polledri E, Fustinoni S, Mercadante R, Olgiati L, Eller Vainicher C, Cairoli E, Zhukouskaya VV, Beck-Peccoz P, Chiodini I: The role of salivary cortisol measured by liquid chromatography-tandem mass spectrometry in the diagnosis of subclinical hypercortisolism. Eur J Endocrinol 2013;168:289–296.

8 Morelli V, Masserini B, Salcuni AS, Eller-Vainicher C, Savoca C, Viti R, Coletti F, Guglielmi G, Battista C, Iorio L, Beck-Peccoz P, Ambrosi B, Arosio M, Scillitani A, Chiodini I: Subclinical hypercortisolism: correlation between biochemical diagnostic criteria and clinical aspects. Clin Endocrinol 2010;73:161–166.

9 Morelli V, Reimondo G, Giordano R, Della Casa S, Policola C, Palmieri S, Salcuni AS, Dolci A, Mendola M, Arosio M, Ambrosi B, Scillitani A, Ghigo E, Beck-Peccoz P, Terzolo M, Chiodini I: Long-term follow-up in adrenal incidentalomas: an Italian multicenter study. J Clin Endocrinol Metab 2014;99:827–834

10 Kim J, Bae KH, Choi YK, Jeong JY, Park KG, Kim JG, Lee IK: Clinical characteristics for 348 patients with adrenal incidentaloma. Endocrinol Metab 2013;28: 20–25.

11 Babińska A, Siekierska-Hellmann M, Błaut K, Lewczuk A, Wiśniewski P, Gnacińska M, Obołończyk L, Swiątkowska-Stodulska R, Sworczak K: Hormonal activity in clinically silent adrenal incidentalomas. Arch Med Sci 2012;8:97–103.

12 Di Dalmazi G, Vicennati V, Rinaldi E, Morselli-Labate AM, Giampalma E, Mosconi C, Pagotto U, Pasquali R: Progressively increased patterns of subclinical cortisol hypersecretion in adrenal incidentalomas differently predict major metabolic and cardiovascular outcomes: a large cross-sectional study. Eur J Endocrinol 2012;166:669–677.

13 Comlekci A, Yener S, Ertilav S, Secil M, Akinci B, Demir T, Kebapcilar L, Bayraktar F, Yesil S, Eraslan S: Adrenal incidentaloma, clinical, metabolic, follow-up aspects: single centre experience. Endocrine 2010;37:40–46.

14 Chiodini I, Morelli V, Masserini B, Salcuni AS, Eller-Vainicher C, Viti R, Coletti F, Guglielmi G, Battista C, Carnevale V, Iorio L, Beck-Peccoz P, Arosio M, Ambrosi B, Scillitani A: Bone mineral density, prevalence of vertebral fractures, and bone quality in patients with adrenal incidentalomas with and without subclinical hypercortisolism: an Italian multicenter study. J Clin Endocrinol Metab 2009;94:3207–3214.

15 Terzolo M, Reimondo G, Chiodini I, Castello R, Giordano R, Ciccarelli E, Limone P, Crivellaro C, Martinelli I, Montini M, Disoteo O, Ambrosi B, Lanzi R, Arosio M, Senni S, Balestrieri A, Solaroli E, Madeo B, De Giovanni R, Strollo F, Battista R, Scorsone A, Giagulli VA, Collura D, Scillitani A, Cozzi R, Faustini-Fustini M, Pia A, Rinaldi R, Allasino B, Peraga G, Tassone F, Garofalo P, Papini E, Borretta G: Screening of Cushing's syndrome in outpatients with type 2 diabetes: results of a prospective multicentric study in Italy. J Clin Endocrinol Metab 2012; 97:3467–3475.

16 Martins LC, Conceição FL, Muxfeldt ES, Salles GF: Prevalence and associated factors of subclinical hypercortisolism in patients with resistant hypertension. J Hypertens 2012;30:967–973.

17 Giordano R, Guaraldi F, Berardelli R, Karamouzis I, D'Angelo V, Marinazzo E, Picu A, Ghigo E, Arvat E: Glucose metabolism in patients with subclinical Cushing's syndrome. Endocrine 2012;41:415–423.

18 Debono M, Bradburn M, Bull M, Harrison B, Ross RJ, Newell-Price J: Cortisol as a marker for increased mortality in patients with incidental adrenocortical adenomas. J Clin Endocrinol Metab 2014;99:4462–4470.

19 Morelli V, Palmieri S, Salcuni AS, Eller-Vainicher C, Cairoli E, ZhukouskayaV, Scillitani A, Beck-Peccoz P, Chiodini I: Bilateral and unilateral adrenal incidentalomas: biochemical and clinical characteristics. Eur J Endocrinol 2013;168:235–241.

20 Chiodini I, Viti R, Coletti F, Guglielmi G, Battista C, Ermetici F, Morelli V, Salcuni A, Carnevale V, Urbano F, Muscarella S, Ambrosi B, Arosio M, Beck-Peccoz P, Scillitani A: Eugonadal male patients with adrenal incidentalomas and subclinical hypercortisolism have increased rate of vertebral fractures. Clin Endocrinol 2009;70:208–213.

21 Tauchmanovà L, Rossi R, Biondi B, Pulcrano M, Nuzzo V, Palmieri EA, Fazio S, Lombardi G: Patients with subclinical Cushing's syndrome due to adrenal adenoma have increased cardiovascular risk. J Clin Endocrinol Metab 2002;87:4872–4878.

22 Morelli V, Eller-Vainicher C, Salcuni AS, Coletti F, Iorio L, Muscogiuri G, Della Casa S, Arosio M, Ambrosi B, Beck-Peccoz P, Chiodini I: Risk of new vertebral fractures in patients with adrenal incidentaloma with and without subclinical hypercortisolism: a multicenter longitudinal study. J Bone Miner Res 2011;26:1816–1821.

23 Eller-Vainicher C, Morelli V, Ulivieri FM, Palmieri S, Zhukouskaya VV, Cairoli E, Pino R, Naccarato A, Scillitani A, Beck-Peccoz P, Chiodini I: Bone quality, as measured by trabecular bone score in patients with adrenal incidentalomas with and without subclinical hypercortisolism. J Bone Miner Res 2012;27: 2223–2230.

24 Di Dalmazi G, Vicennati V, Garelli S, Casadio E, Rinaldi E, Giampalma E, Mosconi C, Golfieri R, Paccapelo A, Pagotto U, Pasquali R: Cardiovascular events and mortality in patients with adrenal incidentalomas that are either non-secreting or associated with intermediate phenotype or subclinical Cushing's syndrome: a 15-year retrospective study. Lancet Diabetes Endocrinol 2014;2:396–405.

25 Palmieri S, Morelli V, Salcuni AS, Eller-Vainicher C, Cairoli E, Zhukouskaya VV, Beck-Peccoz P, Scillitani A, Chiodini I: GH secretion reserve in subclinical hypercortisolism. Pituitary 2014;17:470–476.

26 Swiatkowska-Stodulska R, Kaniuka-Jakubowska S, Wisniewski P, Skibowska-Bielinska A, Sworczak K: The estimation of selected endogenous anticoagulation system parameters in patients with subclinical Cushing's syndrome. Eur J Endocrinol 2011;165: 865–871.

27 Kastelan D, Dzubur F, Dusek T, Poljicanin T, Crncevic-Orlic Z, Kraljevic I, Solak M, Bencevic T, Aganovic I, Knezevic N, Kastelan Z, Korsic M: Health-related quality of life and fatigue in patients with adrenal incidentaloma. Endocrine 2011;40:84–89.

28 Tzanela M, Mantzou E, Saltiki K, Tampourlou M, Kalogeris N, Hadjidakis D, Tsagarakis S, Alevizaki M: Clinical and biochemical impact of BCL1 polymorphic genotype of the glucocorticoid receptor gene in patients with adrenal incidentalomas. J Endocrinol Invest 2012;35:395–400.

29 Eller-Vainicher C, Morelli V, Salcuni AS, Battista C, Torlontano M, Coletti F, Iorio L, Cairoli E, Beck-Peccoz P, Arosio M, Ambrosi B, Scillitani A, Chiodini I: Accuracy of several parameters of hypothalamic-pituitary-adrenal axis activity in predicting before surgery the metabolic effects of the removal of an adrenal incidentaloma. Eur J Endocrinol 2010; 163:925–935.

30 Di Dalmazi G, Berr CM, Fassnacht M, Beuschlein F, Reincke M: Adrenal function after adrenalectomy for subclinical hypercortisolism and Cushing's syndrome: a systematic review of the literature. J Clin Endocrinol Metab 2014;99:2637–2645.

Iacopo Chiodini, MD
Unit of Endocrinology and Metabolic Diseases, Department of Clinical Sciences and Communuty Health, Fondazione IRCCS Cà Granda, Ospedale Maggiore Policlinico di Milano
University of Milan
Padiglione Granelli, Via Francesco Sforza 35
IT–20122 Milan (Italy)
E-Mail iacopo.chiodini@unimi.it

Arvat E, Falorni A (eds): Cortisol Excess and Insufficiency.
Front Horm Res. Basel, Karger, 2016, vol 46, pp 39–53 (DOI: 10.1159/000443863)

Etiopathogeny of Primary Adrenal Hypercortisolism

Fritz-Line Vélayoudom-Céphise[a, b] · Magali Haissaguerre[a, c, d] · Antoine Tabarin[a, c, d]

[a]Department of Endocrinology, USN Haut-Lévêque, University Hospital of Bordeaux, Pessac, [b]Research Group Clinical Epidemiology and Medicine ECM/LAMIA EA 4540, University of Antilles and Guyane, Guadeloupe, [c]University of Bordeaux 2 – Victor-Segalen, and [d]INSERM U862, Neurocentre Magendie, Bordeaux, France

Abstract

Primary adrenal hypercortisolism is mainly due to cortisol-producing adrenocortical adenomas, bilateral micronodular or macronodular disease, and adrenal carcinomas. Important advances in the pathophysiology of primary adrenal hypercortisolism have been made in the last few years, partly through the use of new molecular biology tools. Most adrenal abnormalities leading to increased cortisol production involve somatic or germinal mutations of genes encoding elements of the cyclic AMP/protein kinase A signaling pathway, as shown in adrenal adenomas in 2014. One peculiar condition is primary macronodular adrenal hyperplasia (PMAH), which has given rise to new pathophysiological concepts such as regulation of cortisol secretion by illegitimate ligands through aberrant expression of G protein-coupled transmembrane receptors in adrenal nodules and stimulation of cortisol production by local adrenocorticotropic hormone production through autocrine/paracrine mechanisms. These findings provide a basis for the development of targeted therapies as an alternative to surgery. The recent identification of germinal mutations of *ARMC5* in PMAH raises the possibility that this is much more frequently an inherited disease than previously suspected. It also offers the possibility of earlier diagnosis of PMAH by genetic screening and, hopefully, of earlier intervention to prevent the onset of hypercortisolism and its complications. The pathophysiology of Cushing's syndrome associated with a subset of adrenal adenomas, including subclinical cortisol-secreting incidentalomas and adrenal carcinomas, remains to be determined.

The etiologies of endogenous Cushing's syndrome (CS) are classified according to dependence on adrenocorticotropic hormone (ACTH) secreted by anterior pituitary cells. Primary adrenal hypercortisolism (PAH) corresponds to the ACTH-independent form and represents 20–30% of the cases of endogenous CS [1]. PAH is mainly caused by cortisol-producing adrenocortical adenomas (ACAs) and, less frequently, by bilateral adrenal disease, the latter including micronodular and macronodular adrenal hyperplasias/dysplasias – such as primary pigmented nodular adrenocortical disease (PPNAD) and primary adrenocorticotropin-independent macronodular adrenocortical hyperplasia (PMAH). Very rare, PAH is secondary to adrenal carcinoma [1]. Important advances in our understanding of the etiopathogeny of PAH have been made during the last 2 years.

The cAMP/PKA Signaling Pathway

Most of the molecular abnormalities implicated to date in the pathogenesis of ACTH-independent CS or PAH involve elements of the cyclic AMP/protein kinase A (cAMP/PKA) signaling pathway in the adrenal cortex. ACTH activates the cAMP/PKA signaling pathway by binding to the melanocortin-2 receptor (MC2R), a member of the G protein-coupled transmembrane receptor (GPCR) family. G proteins are composed of α-, β- and γ-subunits. The α-subunit activates adenylate cyclase, which stimulates the production of cAMP from ATP. PKA is a heterotetrameric protein composed of two catalytic (C) and two regulatory (R) subunits. Two cAMP molecules bind to each R subunit of PKA, thus releasing the C subunits that translocate to the nucleus where they phosphorylate various PKA substrates, particularly CREB (cAMP response element-binding protein), a ubiquitous ultimate effector of PKA action. CREB binds to CRE (the cAMP response element) after phosphorylation on Ser133 by PKA, and stimulates transcription of target genes involved in cortisol biosynthesis and cell growth (fig. 1) [2]. In humans, three genes encode the catalytic subunits of PKA *(PRKACA, -CB* and *-CG)* and four genes encode the regulatory subunits *(PRKAR1A, PRKAR1B, PRKAR2A* and *PRKAR2B)* [2].

ACTH-Independent Cushing's Syndrome and Micronodular Adrenal Disease

PPNAD is characterized by small or normal-sized adrenal glands containing multiple pigmented adrenocortical micronodules with an atrophic and disorganized internodular cortex. Adrenal cells within micronodules are characterized by a granular eosinophilic cytoplasm containing lipofuscin, due to intracellular organelle damage and autophagocytosis. Aside from this typical anatomical phenotype, unilateral or bilateral macronodules have been described in 20–30% of PPNAD cases [3].

CS secondary to PPNAD occurs in the 2nd decade of life in more than 50% of cases; rare cases have been described during early childhood [3]. Hypercortisolism may manifest as mild, atypical ('subclinical') CS, be cyclic or episodic with alternating secretory and nonsecretory phases, or gradually develop over time [4]. PPNAD can occur sporadically (isolated PPNAD), while it is associated with other tumors in the

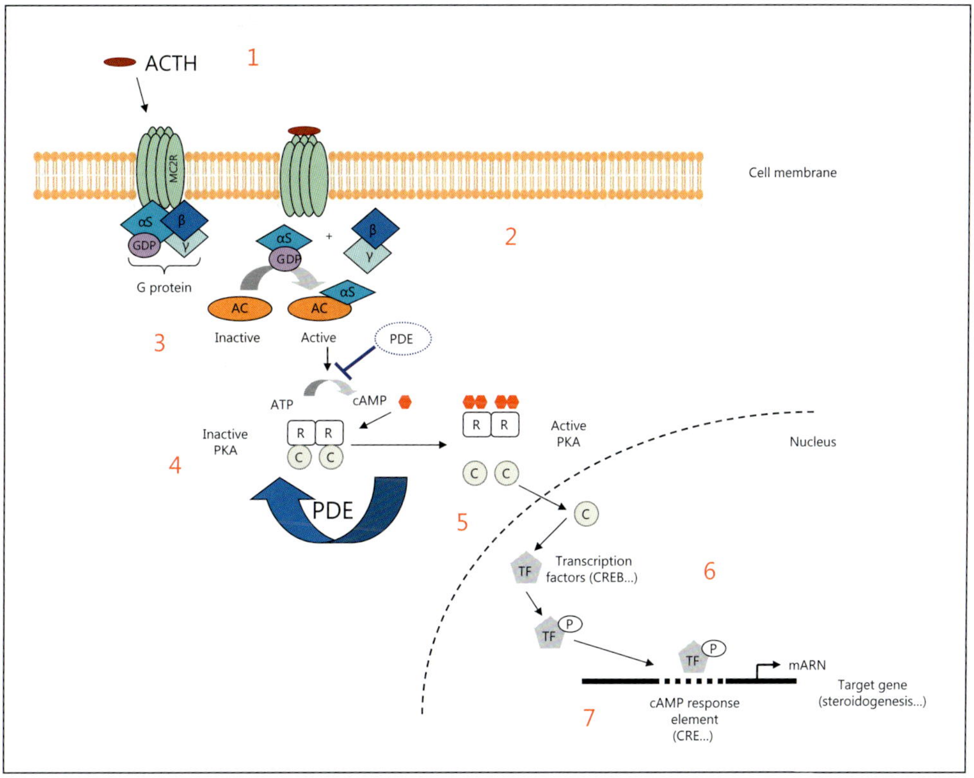

Fig. 1. The cAMP/PKA signaling pathways. AC = Adenylate cyclase; TF = transcription factors; PDE = phosphodiesterases.

inherited Carney complex in 60% of the cases [5]. PPNAD is inherited in an autosomal dominant manner and is caused by heterozygous inactivating germline mutations of the PKA regulatory RIα subunit tumor suppressor gene (*PRKAR1A*). Most mutations responsible for PPNAD generate premature stop codons or frameshifts leading to an overall reduction in RIα protein synthesis [3].

cAMP activation augments PKA activity and activates the catalytic subunits of PKA (fig. 2). In mice, *PRKAR1A* knockout leads to the upregulation of D-type cyclin expression, suggesting that inactivating mutations may also cause adrenal tumorigenesis [6]. No clear genotype-phenotype correlation has been described in PPNAD, although large deletions of *PRKAR1A* may lead to severe CS [5]. Among patients with Carney complex, those with *PRKAR1A* mutations have a more severe phenotype and PPNAD mainly affects females [5]. *PRKAR1A* mutations have also been described in sporadic cases of isolated PPNAD [5].

A peculiar characteristic of PPNAD is the paradoxical increase in plasma or urinary cortisol after administration of large doses of dexamethasone [7]. This unique feature, present in about 70% of cases, is associated with increased glucocorticoid re-

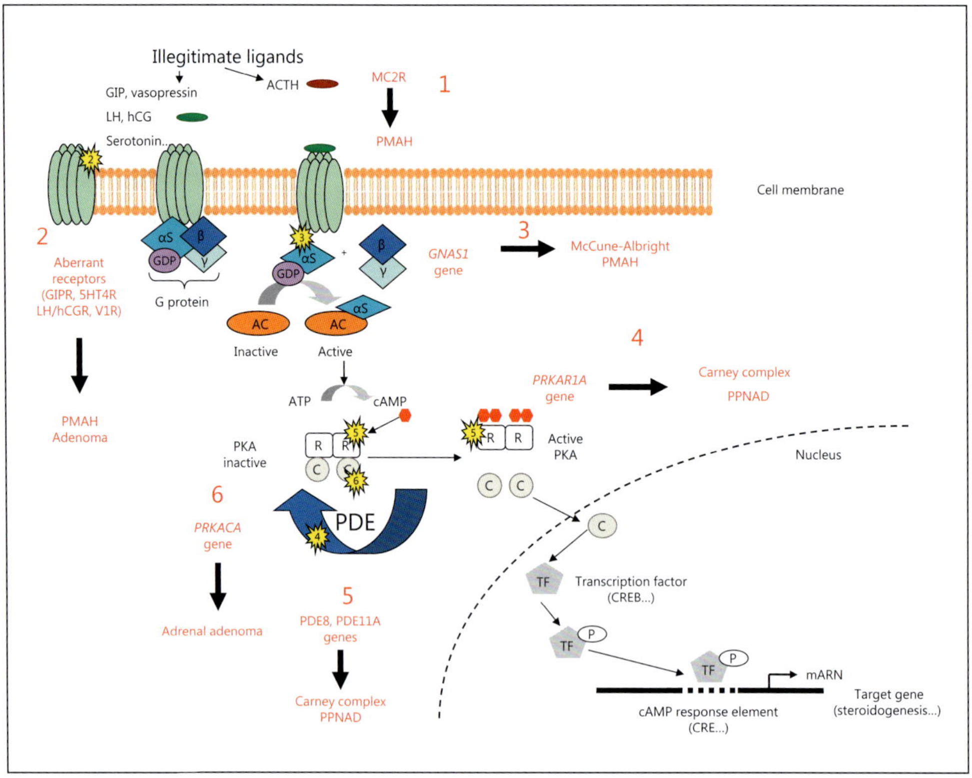

Fig. 2. Main alterations of the cAMP/PKA signaling pathways responsible for PAH. 5HT4R = Serotonin receptor; V1R = vasopressin receptor; GNAS = guanine nucleotide-binding protein, α-stimulating activity polypeptide; PRKAR1A = PKA regulatory RIα subunit; PRKACA = catalytic subunits of PKA; PDE = phosphodiesterases.

ceptor expression in cortical cells of PPNAD nodules. The significance of this finding is a subject of debate, but it has been suggested that genomic upregulation of PKA catalytic subunits by glucocorticoid receptors creates a local amplification loop in PPNAD cells [7].

CS has been described at an early age, especially in females with isolated micronodular adrenocortical disease. A single nucleotide polymorphism-based genome-wide association study of kindreds with CS related to isolated micronodular adrenocortical disease and negative for *PRKRA1A* mutations identified inactivating mutations of the *PDE11A* and *PDE8B* genes that encode phosphodiesterases involved in cAMP degradation (fig. 2). *PDE11A* is located in chromosome region 2q31.2 and *PDE8* at locus 5q13 [3]. Phosphodiesterase gene mutations disrupt cAMP hydrolysis, inducing high cellular cAMP levels, as confirmed in vitro in adrenal cells transfected with *PDE11A* or *PDE8B* mutants. Contrary to patients with classical PPNAD, pigmentation is rarely found in patients with *PDE11A* mutations [3].

Primary Macronodular Adrenal Hyperplasia

PMAH is characterized by bilateral, multiple and markedly enlarged adrenal nodules. Primary bilateral macronodular adrenal hyperplasia (PBMAH) occurs independently from circulating ACTH, contrary to bilateral adrenal hyperplasia secondary to chronic adrenal cortex stimulation by ACTH, as seen in long-standing Cushing's disease. The pathophysiology of PBMAH includes aberrant regulation by illegitimate receptors, intratumoral ACTH production and various genetic alterations.

PMAH: A Model of Aberrant Regulation

CS associated with PBMAH is classically diagnosed during the 5th to 6th decade of life and is generally associated with mild hypercortisolism, which explains why PBMAH is often diagnosed incidentally during abdominal imaging. The seminal work of Lacroix et al. [8] unveiled the mechanisms leading to CS in patients with PBMAH through aberrant stimulation of the cAMP/PKA cascade in adrenocortical cells by illegitimate GPCRs (aberrant adrenal expression of ectopic receptors or increased activity/expression of eutopic peptide receptors). Upon activation by their ligands, GPCRs reproduce the cellular responses observed after MC2R activation by ACTH, including PKA activation and increased cortisol secretion, independently of pituitary ACTH [9]. Thus, cortisol secretion becomes driven by a hormone that escapes cortisol-mediated negative feedback (fig. 3).

This pathophysiological framework accounts for about 80% of cases of PBMAH associated with overt or 'subclinical' CS [9, 10]. The first description of CS linked to aberrant GPCRs expression was 'food-dependent' CS, an entity characterized by low fasting plasma cortisol concentrations that increase after meals due to activation of adrenal nodular cells by GIP (glucose-dependent insulinotropic polypeptide), a gut hormone that augments postprandial insulin secretion [8].

Aberrant expression of a wide variety of ectopic GPCRs and increased activity/expression of eutopic peptide receptors have been described. In several series, more than 85% of patients with PBMAH were found to have at least one and usually several aberrant responses, the most frequent being those induced by vasopressin and serotonin 5-hydroxytryptamine 4 agonists [9, 10]. Increased activity of the 'eutopic' V1-vasopressin receptor leads to increased cortisol secretion in the upright posture or following other stimuli of endogenous vasopressin, such as hypertonic saline. Following aberrant adrenal expression of β-adrenergic receptors, cortisol release increases with the stimulation of endogenous catecholamines by upright posture, insulin-induced hypoglycemia, exercise and isoproterenol infusion, whereas propranolol blocks this effect and reduces cortisol secretion.

Aberrant expression of LH/hCG receptors has been held responsible for CS, which is transient during pregnancy but persists after menopause due to the sustained increase in LH secretion. Administration of the long-acting gonadotropin-releasing hormone agonist leuprolide acetate suppresses endogenous LH and normalizes cor-

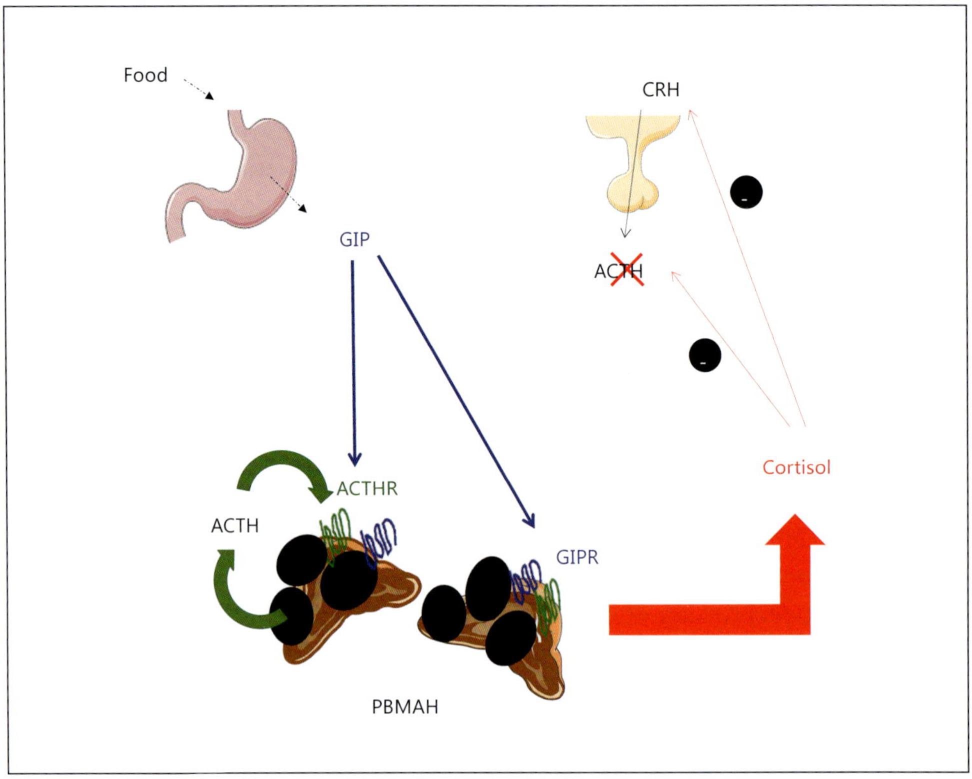

Fig. 3. Pathophysiological model of 'food-dependent' CS in PBMAH. Cortisol production is stimulated by an illegitimate ligand (GIP) through the aberrant expression of its receptor that is coupled to the cAMP/PKA pathway. While pituitary production of ACTH is suppressed, GIP may trigger the local production of ACTH within the adrenal nodules to amplify the cortisol response through autocrine/paracrine mechanisms.

tisol production [9]. Strong overexpression of serotonin 5-hydroxytryptamine 4 receptors is associated with increased cortisol secretion following stimulation with cisapride or metoclopramide [11]. Increases in plasma cortisol release in the upright posture in patients with PBMAH have also been linked to abnormal responses to endogenous angiotensin and can be inhibited by an angiotensin I receptor antagonist [9].

In a study designed to identify new GPCRs by using cDNA chips to screen mRNAs from 18 PBMAH patients, several previously undescribed GPCR genes were found to be strongly expressed – these included the α2A adrenergic receptor (13 of the 18 patients), which is not expressed in the normal adrenal cortex, and (less frequently) receptors for motilin and γ-aminobutyric acid [12]. The ADRA2A agonist clonidine enhances both basal and stimulated cortisol production, while clonidine-induced cortisol stimulation is blocked by the ADRA2A antagonist yohimbine [12].

It is unclear whether aberrant GPCRs expression causes PBMAH or is simply an epiphenomenon resulting from cell proliferation and dedifferentiation. However, in a model of genetically modified adrenocortical cells transplanted into adrenalectomized immunodeficient mice, forced expression of the GIP receptor or LH receptor genes in adrenocortical cells resulted in tissue hyperplasia and features of CS [13]. Thus, aberrant GPCR expression appears to be sufficient to trigger adrenocortical tumorigenesis, at least in experimental animals.

From a practical standpoint, physiological tests (posture, fasting, feeding) and pharmacological challenges (gonadotropin-releasing hormone and AVP perfusion, administration of 5HT4 receptor agonists and antagonists) can be used to screen PBMAH patients for aberrant GPCRs. Ideally, these aberrant GPCRs could be targeted pharmacologically to control hypercortisolism and thus avoid bilateral adrenalectomy, but treatments of this type have so far proven effective in only a handful of patients.

ACTH-Independent Macronodular Hyperplasia: A Misnomer?

Hypercortisolism associated with PBMAH was previously considered to be ACTH-independent, thus explaining the widespread use of the term 'adrenal-independent macronodular hyperplasia' (AIMAH). However, in 2003 a French team reported local ACTH production by hyperplastic cells of AIMAH patients with CS [14]. This intriguing observation, together with other work by the same team, suggested that autocrine or paracrine phenomena might be involved in the pathophysiology of hypercortisolism in AIMAH [5]. Ten years later the French team resolved this enigma [15]. Indeed, they detected pro-opiomelanocortin and prohormone convertase 1 expression in the majority of adrenal samples from 30 patients with PBMAH, while ACTH immunostaining was found in clusters of steroidogenic cells in PMAH tissues. No ACTH staining was found in the normal adrenal cortex or in cortisol-secreting adenomas. ACTH-positive cells also expressed insulin-like 3 factor, a marker of Leydig cells that is not expressed in normal adrenal tissue. As adrenocortical and gonadal stem cells both derive from the mesonephros, it is conceivable that gonadal-like cells may arise in the adrenal glands through abnormal differentiation of certain steroidogenic cell progenitors or by defective migration of gonadal stem cells during embryogenesis [15].

Perifusion of PMAH nodules revealed pulsatile ACTH secretion correlating tightly with their cortisol secretion. This ectopic adrenal ACTH secretion was not regulated by corticotropin-releasing hormone or dexamethasone, but cortisol secretion was abolished by MC2R inhibitors. Local ACTH secretion by adrenal nodules was further confirmed in vivo by the demonstration of high ACTH concentrations in adrenal vein samples from 2 patients and suppressed concentration in antecubital vein samples. Together, these results suggest that local ACTH production occurred in PMAH nodules in vivo and that it participated in the elevated cortisol secretion in an autocrine or paracrine fashion [15].

Interestingly, during perifusion studies with GIP, serotonin and hCG, adrenal nodules that contained aberrant GPCRs for these ligands released both ACTH and cortisol. MC2R inhibitors reduced stimulated cortisol secretion by 40%, suggesting that cortisol production was controlled both by aberrant GPCRs and ACTH produced within the adrenocortical nodules themselves, and also that local ACTH production amplified the cortisol response to activation of aberrant receptors [15].

Cortisol secretion thus involves adrenal ACTH production, challenging the ACTH independence of so-called 'AIMAH', which should thus be renamed 'PMAH'. Theoretically, MC2R antagonists could be used to treat CS associated with PBMAH, despite the inhibition of pituitary ACTH production. Further studies are needed to determine the importance of paracrine adrenal ACTH production in cortisol regulation.

Genetic Aspects of Macronodular Adrenal Hyperplasia associated with CS

Several abnormal molecular mechanisms have been identified in PMAH, indicating that this is a heterogeneous disease which might occur in conjunction with other syndromes.

PMAH has been described in some carriers of somatic mutations of the guanine nucleotide-binding protein, α-stimulating activity polypeptide *(GNAS1)* gene that encodes the activating α-subunit of G proteins (Gαs). These mutations occur during early embryogenesis and have a mosaic tissue distribution. In adrenal cells, they induce constitutive activation of Gsα, leading to high adenylate cyclase activity, increased cAMP levels and stimulation of steroidogenesis, while the internodular adrenal cortex, where the Gαs mutation is not present, becomes atrophic. *GNAS1* mutations have also occasionally been described in PMAH patients with CS but no other clinical signs of MAS [16].

Rare familial cases of PMAH associated with inactivating germline mutations of *PDE11A,* which promote cAMP accumulation, have been reported [15, 16]. In a recent study, comparative genomic hybridization of samples from 35 patients with cortisol-secreting PMAH and overt CS identified 5 patients with germline duplications of *PRKACA* (encoding the main catalytic subunit of PKA), resulting in increased PKA activity [17].

Germline mutations of *MEN1* (multiple endocrine neoplasia type 1) [18] and rare inactivating germline mutations of the tumor suppressor gene *APC* (adenomatous polyposis coli) and the *FH* gene (fumarate hydratase), responsible for HLRCC (hereditary leiomyomatosis and renal cell cancer) [16], have been described in patients with ACTH-independent CS associated with PBMAH, as well as in patients with unilateral nodules. Activating mutations of the ACTH receptor (*MC2R*) gene have rarely been described in adrenal tumors, including PMAH.

ARMC5 Mutations in PMAH: A Model of Inherited Multiple-Step Adrenal Tumorigenesis

Until recently, most cases of PMAH were thought to be sporadic. However, the bilateral nature of MAH and reports of familial cases of PMAH with aberrant GPCR expression, compatible with autosomal dominant transmission, have raised the possibility that PMAH may be caused by genetic alterations, such as somatic mutations in

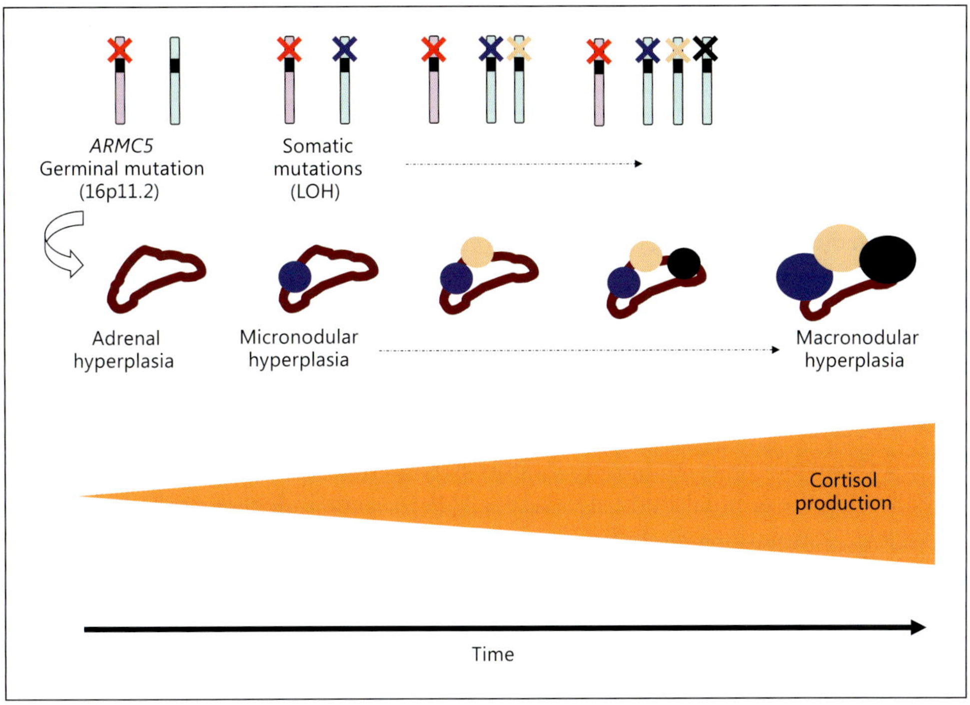

Fig. 4. Hypothetical natural history of PMAH related to *ARMC5* mutations. Both *ARMC5* alleles carried mutations, one germline and the other somatic. This pattern of mutation is consistent with the 'two-hit' model of tumor suppressor gene mutation, in which a germline inactivating mutation is followed by a second mutation that stimulates cell proliferation and leads to tumor development.

progenitor adrenal cells during embryogenesis or germline mutations [9]. Based on the hypothesis that most inherited endocrine tumors are secondary to mutation of tumor suppressing genes, Assié et al. [19] performed whole-genome sequencing, microsatellite marker analysis and single nucleotide polymorphism analysis in adrenal tissues and circulating DNA from 33 patients with apparently sporadic PMAH associated with CS. A recurrent copy-neutral loss of heterozygosity was identified in chromosome region 16p11.2, suggesting the presence of a tumor suppressor gene. Whole-genome sequencing of paired leukocyte and tumor DNA identified inactivating mutations of the armadillo repeat containing 5 gene (*ARMC5*). Finally, Sanger sequencing of the entire cohort identified *ARMC5* mutations in 55% of the patients. Importantly, in every case, both *ARMC5* alleles carried mutations, one germline and the other somatic. Only the germline mutation was present in internodular hyperplasia, while different somatic *ARMC5* mutations or deletions were found in each adrenal nodule examined. This pattern of mutation is consistent with the 'two-hit' model of tumor suppressor gene mutation, in which a germline inactivating mutation is followed by a second mutation that stimulates cell proliferation and leads to tumor development [19] (fig. 4).

Transcriptome-based classification of PMAH tissues by Assié et al. [19] indicated that *ARMC5* mutations influenced gene expression, as all cases with mutations clustered together. Preliminary functional studies of *ARMC5* are consistent with tumor suppressive features. Cell transfection studies show that ARMC5 expression in adrenal carcinoma cell lines promotes cell death and apoptosis [19]. Moreover, inactivation of *ARMC5* by short interfering RNA rendered these cells resistant to apoptosis. Unexpectedly, *ARMC5* inactivation also reduced the expression of genes encoding steroidogenic enzymes and MC2R, suggesting that steroidogenesis is relatively inefficient in individual cells and that a large increase in adrenal size and cell mass is required to produce overt hypercortisolism [19]. Interestingly, in two independent studies, *ARMC5*-mutated index patients had a more severe phenotype of CS including younger age at diagnosis, increased intensity of hypercortisolism and increased size of the adrenal glands as compared to non-carriers of *ARMC5* mutations [19, 20].

Following the seminal study of Assié et al. [19], several independent groups identified *ARMC5* mutations, including novel germline variants, in PMAH families [21–23]. Familial studies involving genetic screening revealed that PMAH might be more frequently inherited than previously suspected. For example, 11 apparently asymptomatic first-degree relatives of 7 probands from Assié's study [19] were screened for *ARMC5* mutations and 54% were found to have a germline mutation. Of note, systematic screening studies of affected families revealed the superiority of genomic screening over clinical evaluation [21, 22, 24]. Indeed, the clinical expression of the disease among *ARMC5*-mutated patients appears to be variable, resulting in different phenotypes with some affected individuals exhibiting few if any signs of CS or only a few small, unilateral adrenal nodules. These findings are consistent with a disease that progresses slowly along with the occurrence of new *ARMC5* somatic mutations in the adrenal cortex, which in turn is compatible with a clinical onset that often occurs after the 5th decade. From a practical perspective, early detection of PMAH by genetic screening of relatives of carriers of *ARMC5* mutations offers the possibility of early diagnosis and, hopefully, early intervention to prevent Cushing's families syndrome and its complications. Further studies are needed to determine the ability of familial screening to improve long-term clinical outcomes by enabling earlier treatment.

These studies also raise the issue of the real frequency of *ARMC5* mutations among unrelated patients with apparently sporadic PMAH. An American study revealed *ARMC5* germline mutations in 41% of 34 patients with apparently sporadic PMAH [24]. Inactivating mutations of *ARMC5* were identified in 5 (24%) of 21 Brazilian patients with apparently sporadic PMAH [22]. Lastly, in a multicenter French study, damaging *ARMC5* mutations were found in 26% of 98 unrelated index cases [20]. Thus, these results demonstrate that *ARMC5* mutations are frequently involved not only in familial PMAH, but also in apparently sporadic PMAH and suggest that genetic screening should be performed regardless of the familial history, thereby offering the possibility of genetic screening for relatives of affected individuals. Elsewhere, it should be noted that somatic mutations of genes involved in regulating cell proliferation and chromatin modification have also been described in PMAH tissues of patients with CS. A recent study of PMAH tissue samples from 7 Chinese patients with CS identified mutations of *DOT1L* (histone H3 lysine 79 methyltransferase gene), the histone deacetylase *HDAC9* gene and the *PRUNE2* gene [25]. These data suggest that deregulated chromatin modification might also contribute to adrenal nodule growth in PMAH.

As the tumor suppressor gene *ARMC5* is expressed in many organs, another concern is the possible proliferative impact of *ARMC5* mutations on other tissues. Interestingly, meningiomas have been previously described in 43% of an affected Brazilian family of PMAH [22]. The recent identification of an additional damaging somatic *ARMC5* mutation in an intracranial meningioma of a patient from a large family with *ARMC5*-related PMAH confirms a role for *ARMC5* in extra-adrenal tumorigenesis [23]. Thus, patients carrying an *ARMC5* germline mutation should be carefully monitored for other tumors to define the full spectrum of *ARMC5*-related neoplasias.

As hypercortisolism linked to illegitimate GPCRs expression is frequent in PMAH, more work is needed to understand the relation between *ARMC5* mutations and GPCR expression. Some PMAH patients with *ARMC5* mutations have an aberrant cortisol response to the upright stance or metoclopramide challenge, suggesting illegitimate expression of V1 of the serotonin 5HT4 receptor in adrenal nodules. In contrast, no patients with food-dependent CS have been found to carry *ARMC5* mutations [19, 21]. Thus, the relationship between *ARMC5* mutations and illegitimate GPCR expression needs further clarification, and other culprit genes in subclasses of PMAH patients should be sought.

Cushing's Syndrome and Adrenocortical Adenomas

ACAs are the most frequent cause of adrenal CS, but their pathogenesis was only recently unveiled. Screening studies identified aberrant responses to illegitimate ligands, as described in PMAH, in a subset of ACA patients, but their role in the pathogenesis of hypercortisolism remains unclear [9]. A transcriptome study of 22 ACAs revealed two groups of adenomas with different levels of cortisol secretion, suggesting that the disease is genetically heterogeneous [26]. As all benign adrenal tumors that cause hypercortisolism and whose pathophysiology is known (i.e. PPNAD, Carney syndrome, McCune-Albright syndrome) are associated with cAMP-PKA pathway alterations, the same pathway might be altered in a subset of ACAs.

In 2014, a hotspot mutation in the *PRKACA* gene encoding the catalytic subunits of PKA (PKAC) was described in cortisol-producing ACAs almost simultaneously by three independent groups [17, 27, 28]. In the work of Beuschlein et al. [17], exome sequencing of tumor samples identified a recurring somatic hotspot mutation of *PRKACA* in 37% of 59 patients with overt CS and cortisol-producing ACAs, while no mutation was found in adrenal tissue from patients with subclinical CS (mild hypercortisolism) or in patients with other secretory adrenal tumors. No mutation was found in leukocyte DNA of affected patients, indicating the somatic and heterozygous nature of the mutations [17, 29]. Similarly, Cao et al. [25], then Goh et al. [27], reported a recurring hotspot mutation at position 617, resulting in leucine to arginine substitution at amino acid 206 (Leu206Arg or L206R) in, respectively, 69 and 55% of cortisol-producing ACAs. The crystal structure of PKA revealed that the Leu206 residue is located at the interface between the C subunit and the inhibitory region of the R subunit of PKA, named the P+1 loop of PKAC responsible for its catalytic activity [25, 28]. The *L206R* mutation could thus disrupt binding of the C and R subunits, resulting in constitutive cAMP-independent PKA activation. These results suggest that *L206R* is a gain-of-function mutation [17]. Several functional studies have since confirmed this and have also demonstrated the pathogenetic role of this mutation in hypercortisolism. Using fluorescence resonance energy transfer microscopy, Beuschlein et al. [17] confirmed that transfection of cells with the L206R mutant led to constitutive PKA activation through a loss of the interaction between the two PKA subunits. Biochemical approaches have revealed that Leu206Arg PRKACA displays impaired PRKAR1A binding, resulting in increased phosphorylation of downstream targets. Likewise, immunohistochemical studies have shown higher expression of phosphorylated CREB in mutant ACAs than in non-mutant ACAs [27]. After RNA sequencing of L206R mutant ACAs, bioinformatic analysis of gene expression showed increased expression of more than 200 genes involved in steroidogenesis and adrenal cell growth, such as those encoding StAR (steroidogenic acute regulatory protein) and MC2R. Increased expression and phosphorylation of StAR have also been shown in mutant ACAs by means of RT-PCR and Western blot [25].

L206R mutation of ACAs is associated with a more severe clinical phenotype, including earlier age at diagnosis and higher cortisol levels than in non-*PRKACA*-mutated patients, even though the adenomas are smaller, suggesting increased steroidogenic activity of individual mutant cells [17, 27, 28]. In vitro, PRKACA inhibitors inhibit constitutive PKA activity in L206R mutant cells, indicating therapeutic potential in this setting [28]. The pathophysiology of a subset of cortisol-secreting adenomas, including 'subclinical' forms (which are far more frequent), remains to be determined.

Adrenocortical Carcinoma and Cushing's Syndrome

ACTH-independent CS is present in 60–70% of patients with adrenocortical carcinomas (ACCs) and is associated with a worse prognosis, possibly due to the consequences of hypercortisolism or to a distinct behavior of secretory ACCs [30]. As shown by in vivo metabolomic analysis of steroid secretion, hypercortisolism in ACC is characterized by a global disruption of steroidogenesis, including increased production of mineralocorticoids and androgen precursors [31], a finding consistent with immunoreactivity studies of steroidogenic enzymes (CYP11A1, CYP17, 3β-HSD, CYP21A2) in ACCs [32].

ACCs are associated with various somatic genetic alterations that disrupt multiple intracellular signaling pathways, and this could theoretically account for the increased steroidogenesis. There are no specific studies on the molecular mechanisms of hypercortisolism in patients with ACCs.

Conclusions

Important advances in the pathophysiology of PAH were recently enabled by the development of new molecular genetic tools. A variety of mechanisms appear to be involved, mainly affecting the cAMP/PKA-signaling pathway and including intra-adrenal paracrine and autocrine loops. Elsewhere, the recent discovery of *ARMC5* mutations disputes the notion of 'sporadic' PMAH. Knowledge of the natural history of this disease is expected to improve in the near future. In addition to their purely mechanistic implications, these recent discoveries raise new therapeutic perspectives, including genetic screening and the development of targeted therapies for PAH that could avoid surgery and reduce morbidity related to CS.

References

1 Newell-Price J, Bertagna X, Grossman AB, Nieman LK: Cushing's syndrome. Lancet 2006;367:1605–1617.

2 Stratakis CA, Cho-Chung YS: Protein kinase A and human disease. Trends Endocrinol Metab 2002;13:50–52.

3 Horvath A, Stratakis CA: Unraveling the molecular basis of micronodular adrenal hyperplasia. Curr Opin Endocrinol Diabetes Obes 2008;15:227–233.

4 Gunther DF, Bourdeau I, Matyakhina L, Cassarino D, Kleiner DE, Griffin K, Courkoutsakis N, Abu-Asab M, Tsokos M, Keil M, Carney JA, Stratakis CA: Cyclical Cushing syndrome presenting in infancy: an early form of primary pigmented nodular adrenocortical disease, or a new entity? J Clin Endocrinol Metab 2004;89:3173–3182.

5 Bertherat J, Horvath A, Groussin L, Grabar S, Boikos S, Cazabat L, Libe R, René-Corail F, Stergiopoulos S, Bourdeau I, Bei T, Clauser E, Calender A, Kirschner LS, Bertagna X, Carney JA, Stratakis CA: Mutations in regulatory subunit type 1A of cyclic adenosine 5′-monophosphate-dependent protein kinase (PRKAR1A): phenotype analysis in 353 patients and 80 different genotypes. J Clin Endocrinol Metab 2009;94:2085–2091.

6 Basso F, Rocchetti F, Rodriguez S, Nesterova M, Cormier F, Stratakis CA, Ragazzon B, Bertherat J, Rizk-Rabin M: Comparison of the effects of PRKAR1A and PRKAR2B depletion on signaling pathways, cell growth, and cell cycle control of adrenocortical cells. Horm Metab Res 2014;46:883–888.

7 Louiset E, Stratakis CA, Perraudin V, Griffin KJ, Libe R, Cabrol S, Fève B, Young J, Groussin L, Bertherat J, Lefebvre H: The paradoxical increase in cortisol secretion induced by dexamethasone in primary pigmented nodular adrenocortical disease involves a glucocorticoid receptor-mediated effect of dexamethasone on protein kinase A catalytic subunits. J Clin Endocrinol Metab 2009;94:2406–2413.

8 Lacroix A, Bolte E, Tremblay J, Dupre J, Poitras P, Fournier H, Garon J, Garrel D, Bayard F, Taillefer R, et al: Gastric inhibitory polypeptide-dependent cortisol hypersecretion – a new cause of Cushing's syndrome. N Engl J Med 1992;327:974–980.

9 Lacroix A, Bourdeau I, Lampron A, Mazzuco TL, Tremblay J, Hamet P: Aberrant G-protein coupled receptor expression in relation to adrenocortical overfunction. Clin Endocrinol (Oxf) 2010;73:1–15.

10 Libe R, Coste J, Guignat L, Tissier F, Lefebvre H, Barrande G, Ajzenberg C, Tauveron I, Clauser E, Dousset B, Bertagna X, Bertherat J, Groussin L: Aberrant cortisol regulations in bilateral macronodular adrenal hyperplasia: a frequent finding in a prospective study of 32 patients with overt or subclinical Cushing's syndrome. Eur J Endocrinol 2010;163:129–138.

11 Reznik Y, Lefebvre H, Rohmer V, Charbonnel B, Tabarin A, Rodien P, Lecomte P, Bardet S, Coffin C, Mahoudeau J; REHOS Study Group: Aberrant adrenal sensitivity to multiple ligands in unilateral incidentaloma with subclinical autonomous cortisol hypersecretion: a prospective clinical study. Clin Endocrinol (Oxf) 2004;61:311–319.

12 Assie G, Louiset E, Sturm N, Rene-Corail F, Groussin L, Bertherat J, Thomas M, Lefebvre H, Feige JJ, Clauser E, Chabre O, Cherradi N: Systematic analysis of G protein-coupled receptor gene expression in adrenocorticotropin-independent macronodular adrenocortical hyperplasia identifies novel targets for pharmacological control of adrenal Cushing's syndrome. J Clin Endocrinol Metab 2010;95:E253–E262.

13 Mazzuco TL, Chabre O, Sturm N, Feige JJ, Thomas M: Ectopic expression of the gastric inhibitory polypeptide receptor gene is a sufficient genetic event to induce benign adrenocortical tumor in a xenotransplantation model. Endocrinology 2006;147:782–790.

14 Lefebvre H, Duparc C, Chartrel N, Jegou S, Pellerin A, Laquerriere A, Ivell R, Vaudry H, Kuhn JM: Intraadrenal adrenocorticotropin production in a case of bilateral macronodular adrenal hyperplasia causing Cushing's syndrome. J Clin Endocrinol Metab 2003;88:3035–3042.

15 Louiset E, Duparc C, Young J, Renouf S, Tetsi Nomigni M, Boutelet I, Libé R, Bram Z, Groussin L, Caron P, Tabarin A, Grunenberger F, Christin-Maitre S, Bertagna X, Kuhn JM, Anouar Y, Bertherat J, Lefebvre H: Intraadrenal corticotropin in bilateral macronodular adrenal hyperplasia. N Engl J Med 2013; 369:2115–2125.

16 Hsiao HP, Kirschner LS, Bourdeau I, Keil MF, Boikos SA, Verma S, Boikos SA, Verma S, Robinson-White AJ, Nesterova M, Lacroix A, Stratakis CA: Clinical and genetic heterogeneity, overlap with other tumor syndromes, and atypical glucocorticoid hormone secretion in adrenocorticotropin-independent macronodular adrenal hyperplasia compared with other adrenocortical tumors. J Clin Endocrinol Metab 2009;94:2930–2937.

17 Beuschlein F, Fassnacht M, Assie G, Calebiro D, Stratakis CA, Osswald A, Ronchi CL, Wieland T, Sbiera S, Faucz FR, Schaak K, Schmittfull A, Schwarzmayr T, Barreau O, Vezzosi D, Rizk-Rabin M, Zabel U, Szarek E, Salpea P, Forlino A, Vetro A, Zuffardi O, Kisker C, Diener S, Meitinger T, Lohse MJ, Reincke M, Bertherat J, Strom TM, Allolio B: Constitutive activation of PKA catalytic subunit in adrenal Cushing's syndrome. N Engl J Med 2014;370:1019–1028.

18 Gatta-Cherifi B, Chabre O, Murat A, Niccoli P, Cardot-Bauters C, Rohmer V, Young J, Delemer B, Du Boullay H, Verger MF, Kuhn JM, Sadoul JL, Ruszniewski P, Beckers A, Monsaingeon M, Baudin E, Goudet P, Tabarin A: Adrenal involvement in MEN1. Analysis of 715 cases from the Groupe d'etude des Tumeurs Endocrines database. Eur J Endocrinol 2012;166:269–279.

19 Assié G, Libe R, Espiard S, Rizk-Rabin M, Guimier A, Luscap W, Barreau O, Lefèvre L, Sibony M, Guignat L, Rodriguez S, Perlemoine K, René-Corail F, Letourneur F, Trabulsi B, Poussier A, Chabbert-Buffet N, Borson-Chazot F, Groussin L, Bertagna X, Stratakis CA, Ragazzon B, Bertherat J: ARMC5 mutations in macronodular adrenal hyperplasia with Cushing's syndrome. N Engl J Med 2013;369:2105–2114.

20 Espiard S, Drougat L, Libe R, Assie G, Perlemoine K, Guignat L, Barrande G, Brucker-Davis F, Doullay F, Lopez S, Sonnet E, Torremocha F, Pinsard D, Chabbert-Buffet N, Raffin-Sanson ML, Groussin L, Borson-Chazot F, Coste J, Bertagna X, Stratakis CA, Beuschlein F, Ragazzon B, Bertherat J: ARMC5 mutations in a large cohort of primary macronodular adrenal hyperplasia: clinical and functional consequences. J Clin Endocrinol Metab 2015;100:E926–E935.

21 Gagliardi L, Schreiber AW, Hahn CN, Feng J, Cranston T, Boon H, Hotu C, Oftedal BE, Cutfield R, Adelson DL, Braund WJ, Gordon RD, Rees DA, Grossman AB, Torpy DJ, Scott HS: ARMC5 mutations are common in familial bilateral macronodular adrenal hyperplasia. J Clin Endocrinol Metab 2014; 99:E1784–E1792.

22 Alencar GA, Lerario AM, Nishi MY, Mariani BM, Almeida MQ, Tremblay J, Hamet P, Bourdeau I, Zerbini MC, Pereira MA, Gomes GC, Rocha Mde S, Chambo JL, Lacroix A, Mendonca BB, Fragoso MC: ARMC5 mutations are a frequent cause of primary macronodular adrenal hyperplasia. J Clin Endocrinol Metab 2014;99:E1501–E1509.

23 Elbelt U, Trovato A, Kloth M, Gentz E, Finke R, Spranger J, Galas D, Weber S, Wolf C, König K, Arlt W, Büttner R, May P, Allolio B, Schneider JG: Molecular and clinical evidence for an ARMC5 tumor syndrome: concurrent inactivating germline and somatic mutations are associated with both primary macronodular adrenal hyperplasia and meningioma. J Clin Endocrinol Metab 2015;100:E119–E128.

24 Faucz FR, Zilbermint M, Lodish MB, Szarek E, Trivellin G, Sinaii N, Berthon A, Libé R, Assié G, Espiard S, Drougat L, Ragazzon B, Bertherat J,Stratakis CA: Macronodular adrenal hyperplasia due to mutations in an armadillo repeat containing 5 (ARMC5) gene: a clinical and genetic investigation. J Clin Endocrinol Metab 2014;99:E1113–E1119.

25 Cao Y, He M, Gao Z, Peng Y, Li Y, Li L, Zhou W, Li X, Zhong X, Lei Y, Su T, Wang H, Jiang Y, Yang L, Wei W, Yang X, Jiang X, Liu L, He J, Ye J, Wei Q, Li Y, Wang W, Wang J, Ning G: Activating hotspot L205R mutation in PRKACA and adrenal Cushing's syndrome. Science 2014;344:913–917.

26 Wilmot Roussel H, Vezzosi D, Rizk-Rabin M, Barreau O, Ragazzon B, Rene-Corail F, de Reynies A, Bertherat J, Assié G: Identification of gene expression profiles associated with cortisol secretion in adrenocortical adenomas. J Clin Endocrinol Metab 2013;98:E1109–E1121.

27 Goh G, Scholl UI, Healy JM, Choi M, Prasad ML, Nelson-Williams C, Kunstman JW, Korah R, Suttorp AC, Dietrich D, Haase M, Willenberg HS, Stålberg P, Hellman P, Akerström G, Björklund P, Carling T, Lifton RP: Recurrent activating mutation in PRKACA in cortisol-producing adrenal tumors. Nat Genet 2014;46:613–617.

28 Sato Y, Maekawa S, Ishii R, Sanada M, Morikawa T, Shiraishi Y, Yoshida K, Nagata Y, Sato-Otsubo A, Yoshizato T, Suzuki H, Shiozawa Y, Kataoka K, Kon A, Aoki K, Chiba K, Tanaka H, Kume H, Miyano S, Fukayama M, Nureki O, Homma Y, Ogawa S: Recurrent somatic mutations underlie corticotropin-independent Cushing's syndrome. Science 2014;344:917–920.

29 Di Dalmazi G, Kisker C, Calebiro D, Mannelli M, Canu L, Arnaldi G, Quinkler M, Rayes N, Tabarin A, Laure Jullié M, Mantero F, Rubin B, Waldmann J, Bartsch DK, Pasquali R, Lohse M, Allolio B, Fassnacht M, Beuschlein F, Reincke M: Novel somatic mutations in the catalytic subunit of the protein kinase A as a cause of adrenal Cushing's syndrome: a European multicentric study. J Clin Endocrinol Metab 2014;99:E2093–E2100.

30 Berruti A, Baudin E, Gelderblom H, Haak HR, Porpiglia F, Fassnacht M, Pentheroudakis G; ESMO Guidelines Working Group: Adrenal cancer: ESMO Clinical Practice Guidelines for diagnosis, treatment and follow-up. Ann Oncol 2012;23(suppl 7):vii131–vii138.

31 Arlt W, Biehl M, Taylor AE, Hahner S, Libe R, Hughes BA, Schneider P, Smith DJ, Stiekema H, Krone N, Porfiri E, Opocher G, Bertherat J, Mantero F, Allolio B, Terzolo M, Nightingale P, Shackleton CH, Bertagna X, Fassnacht M, Stewart PM: Urine steroid metabolomics as a biomarker tool for detecting malignancy in adrenal tumors. J Clin Endocrinol Metab 2011;96:3775–3784.

32 Sasano H, Suzuki T, Nagura H, Nishikawa T: Steroidogenesis in human adrenocortical carcinoma: biochemical activities, immunohistochemistry, and in situ hybridization of steroidogenic enzymes and histopathologic study in nine cases. Hum Pathol 1993;24:397–404.

Prof. Antoine Tabarin
Service d'Endocrinologie, Diabétologie et Maladies Métaboliques, Hôpital Haut-Lévêque,
Centre Hospitalier Universitaire de Bordeaux
Avenue de Magellan
FR–33600 Pessac (France)
E-Mail antoine.tabarin@chu-bordeaux.fr

Arvat E, Falorni A (eds): Cortisol Excess and Insufficiency.
Front Horm Res. Basel, Karger, 2016, vol 46, pp 54–65 (DOI: 10.1159/000443864)

Metabolic Alterations and Cardiovascular Outcomes of Cortisol Excess

Rosario Pivonello · Maria Cristina De Martino · Davide Iacuaniello · Chiara Simeoli · Giovanna Muscogiuri · Francesco Carlomagno · Monica De Leo · Alessia Cozzolino · Annamaria Colao

Division of Endocrinology, Department of Clinical Medicine and Surgery, University Federico II di Napoli, Naples, Italy

Abstract

Cushing's syndrome (CS) is a severe chronic and systemic condition caused by endogenous or exogenous excess of glucocorticoids, associated with increased morbidity and mortality. Patients with active CS suffer from many metabolic alterations, including visceral obesity, systemic arterial hypertension, impairment of glucose metabolism and dyslipidemia. Additionally, in these patients several cardiovascular abnormalities, i.e. atherosclerosis, clotting disorders, left ventricular hypertrophy, concentric remodeling and diastolic dysfunction have been documented. These alterations, which persist even long after hypercortisolism remission, account for the increased cardiovascular risk and greatly contribute to the increased mortality observed in patients with CS. The current review aims to discuss the main adverse effects of CS on metabolism and cardiovascular risk, focusing on the active and remission phases of disease, and underlining the importance of long-term monitoring and treatment of these complications during active disease, as well as in the long-term follow-up after CS remission.

Cushing's syndrome (CS) is defined as a chronic and systemic condition caused by endogenous or exogenous excess of glucocorticoids (GCs). Endogenous CS is a rare disease, with an estimated incidence of about 0.7–2.3/million per year, which may be related to an adrenocorticotropic hormone (ACTH)-secreting pituitary tumor – pituitary-dependent CS or Cushing's disease (CD), representing approximately 70% of cases – or to an ACTH-secreting extrapituitary tumor – ectopic CS, representing approximately 5–10% of cases. In addition, adrenal diseases, including unilateral benign

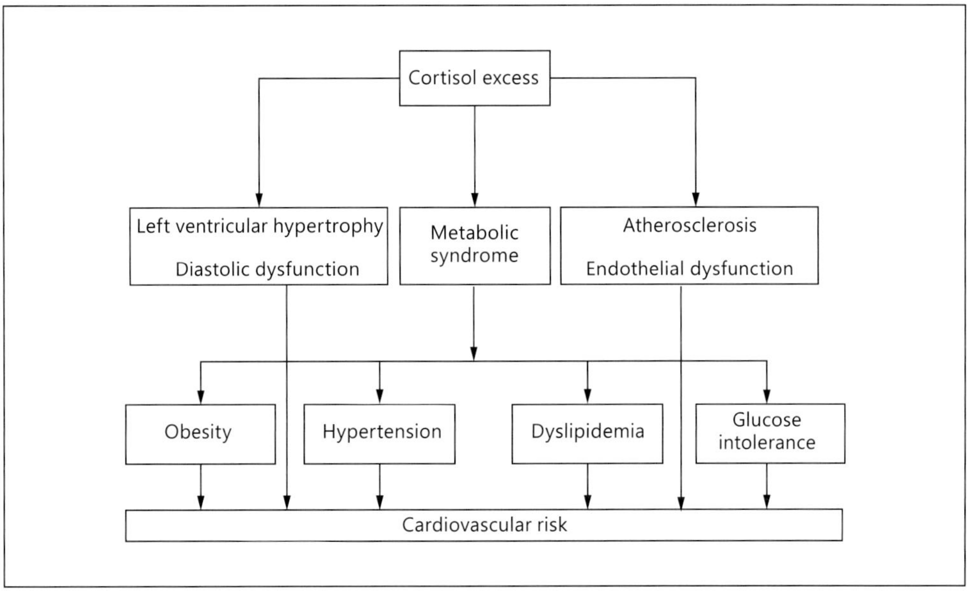

Fig. 1. Schematic representation of the effect of GC excess on the development of metabolic and cardiac alterations responsible for increased cardiovascular risk.

or malignant adrenal tumors, bilateral adrenal hyperplasia or dysplasia, may be responsible for ACTH-independent cortisol hypersecretion or adrenal-dependent CS (approx. 20–25% of cases) [1–6].

GC excess exerts multiple and complex effects on metabolism, inducing visceral obesity, systemic arterial hypertension, insulin resistance with impairment of glucose tolerance and dyslipidemia. These complications configure a condition of metabolic syndrome [7] that plays an important role in increasing cardiovascular risk, mostly during the active phase of disease, and the mortality rate in CS (fig. 1). A recent meta-analysis reported a standardized mortality ratio (SMR) of 1.84 in patients with CD, with a particularly high SMR in the subset of patients with persistent disease (SMR: 3.73), and lower SMR in those with initial remission (SMR: 1.23) [8]. Higher SMRs have been reported in patients with CS related to malignant tumors, such as adrenal cancer or a malignant ACTH-secreting tumor [9]. This implies that the prompt cure of the disease, or at least a rapid resolution of hypercortisolism, becomes of major importance to decrease the long-term morbidity and mortality associated with CS. However, remission of CS usually decreases but does not completely resolve these systemic complications [10]. Previous studies have reported the persistence of abnormal metabolic and cardiovascular risk parameters in CS as compared to controls, even long after hormonal remission [10–13].

The current review aims to discuss the main adverse effects of CS on metabolism and cardiovascular risk, focusing on the active and remission phases of disease.

Metabolic and Cardiovascular Alterations in Patients with Active Cushing's Syndrome

CS is characterized by a series of metabolic and cardiovascular alterations that increases cardiovascular risk and causes severe atherosclerotic damage which develops in parallel with acquired metabolic syndrome [7].

Metabolic Alterations

Patients with CS often present clinical features that are typical of the metabolic syndrome, a severe clinical condition characterized by visceral obesity associated with systemic blood hypertension, glucose and lipid abnormalities, and which leads to increased cardiovascular risk [14].

Visceral Obesity

Visceral or abdominal obesity is a common feature of CS, affecting up to 100% of patients [7]. GCs exert multiple effects on adipose tissue, acting on up to 20% of genes expressed in adipocytes [15, 16]; whether the preferential increase in abdominal adipose storage in CS is due to an increase in adipogenesis or hypertrophy of existing adipocytes is not known [17, 18] and data in humans are scant [19]. GCs are required for the full differentiation of adipocytes and they act in a dose-dependent manner [20, 21]; their actions on adipogenesis are explained by the stimulation of the differentiation of preadipocytes into adypocytes, the induction of C/EBPβ, a key adipogenic transcription factor, and the suppression of the expression of factors (Pref-1 and Runx2) known to inhibit adipogenesis [22–25]. Furthermore, higher cortisol synthesis [26] and expression of a GC receptor in abdominal adipose tissue, as compared with subcutaneous adipose tissue, may contribute to the preferential expansion of abdominal adipose storage [27–29]. However, whether the effects of GCs are mediated by a GC receptor or mineralocorticoid receptor is not clear [30–32]. On the other hand, GCs induce the expression and stimulate the activity of lipoprotein lipase and the expression of enzymes involved in triglyceride synthesis. These effects are greater in abdominal than subcutaneous adipose tissue, contributing to the hypertrophy of abdominal adipocytes [33, 34]. Moreover, GCs impair brown adipose tissue function and promote a 'brown' to 'white' phenotypic conversion [19, 35, 36]. However, it should be noted that GCs have differential effects in peripheral adipose tissue, where they display a shrinking action and they induce a free fatty acid mobilization contributing to the typical adipose tissue distribution in CS [37, 38].

The increased levels of leptin and resistin, as well as the release of proinflammatory cytokines, such as tumor necrosis factor-α and interleukin-6, can also contribute to the increased cardiovascular risk in CS [39]. Adipokines secreted by adipose tissue have effects on inflammation, atherosclerosis and insulin resistance, and could be an important link between adiposity and cardiovascular disease [13].

Systemic Arterial Hypertension

Hypertension is a common finding in CS, affecting 70–85% of adults and 50–78% of children and adolescents [40–42], and is characterized by a typical nondipping pattern [41], probably related, at least in part, to the lack of circadian rhythm of cortisol secretion. Several mechanisms are involved in the pathogenesis of hypertension in CS, including mineralocorticoid effects of cortisol, activation of the renin angiotensin system, increased sensitivity to β-receptor agonists and alteration of vasoregulatory system enhancing vasoconstriction (e.g. increased levels of endothelin-1 and erythropoietin) and reducing vasodilation (e.g. reduced nitric oxide synthase activity and prostacyclin production) [42].

Among these mechanisms, the mineralocorticoid effects of cortisol have been traditionally considered the major players of hypertension secondary to hypercortisolism. These effects are mediated predominantly by mineralocorticoid receptors. It has been postulated that in hypertension the decreased renal conversion of cortisol to cortisone could increase the mineralocorticoid action. The high cortisol levels in CS overwhelm the ability of 11β-hydroxysteroid dehydrogenase type 2 to convert cortisol in cortisone, leading to the spillover of cortisol to the mineralocorticoid receptor. The result is a pathologic state that mimics aldosterone excess and causes hypokalemia, increased renal tubular sodium reabsorption, intravascular volume expansion and hypertension [41].

The renin angiotensin system may take part in the pathogenesis of GC-induced hypertension through upregulation of central and peripheral angiotensin II receptors. It has been reported that GCs increase the hepatic synthesis of angiotensinogen and the tissue expression of angiotensin II receptor type 1A [43, 44]. Although GC excess increases circulating levels of the vasodilator atrial natriuretic peptide [45], its biologic activity is decreased [46]. GCs also decrease the production of nitric oxide synthase that may increase blood pressure by decreasing the nitric oxide and consequently peripheral vasodilatation [47, 48]. In addition, patients with CS have been reported to have high levels of endothelin-1, a potent vasoconstrictor [49]. Sleep apnea and insulin resistance may also contribute [42].

Impairment of Glucose Metabolism

The impairment of glucose metabolism is also frequent in CS (10–30 and 20–50% of the patients present impaired glucose tolerance and diabetes, respectively) [37, 50]. GC excess contributes to hyperglycemia, increasing gluconeogenesis and determining insulin resistance. Particularly, GCs induce liver gene expression of key enzymes involved in gluconeogenesis, resulting in increased liver glucose release. GCs directly interfere with the insulin receptor-signaling pathway, impairing insulin sensitivity both in the liver and in the skeletal muscles. Therefore, they decrease skeletal muscle glucose uptake and reduce glycogen synthesis in both liver and skeletal muscles. Additionally, GCs stimulate proteolysis and lipolysis, increasing levels of amino acids and fatty acids, respectively, which contribute to impair insulin sensitivity by an indirect mechanism [37].

Table 1. Prevalence and main pathogenetic mechanisms underlying common metabolic alterations associated with CS

Alteration	Prevalence	Main pathogenetic mechanisms
Abdominal obesity	up to 100%	– promotion of preadipocytes differentiation – stimulation of adipogenesis – stimulation of lipoprotein-lipase – promotion of a 'brown' to 'white' phenotypic conversion of adipose tissue – shrinking action in peripheral adipose tissue – mobilization of free fatty acids in peripheral adipose tissue
Hypertension	70–85%	– mineralocorticoid effects of cortisol – activation of the renin angiotensin system – increased sensitivity to β-receptor agonists – increased vasoconstriction – impaired vasodilation
Diabetes Impaired glucose tolerance	20–50% 10–30%	– increased gluconeogenesis – impaired insulin sensitivity
Dyslipidemia	20–71%	– multifactorial pathogenesis

Dyslipidemia

Dyslipidemia in patients with CS has been poorly investigated and a variable prevalence has been described (20–71%). Common findings are elevated total and low-density lipoprotein cholesterol levels, reduced high-density lipoprotein cholesterol levels and elevated triglyceride levels [11, 12, 51–53]. Direct and indirect cortisol action on lipolysis, free fatty acid production and turnover, very-low-density lipoprotein cholesterol synthesis, and fatty accumulation in the liver may contribute to the multifactorial pathogenesis of dyslipidemia in CS [38].

Finally, growth hormone (GH) deficiency might impair metabolic profile in patients with both active and remitting CD, although this phenomenon has been better investigated in patients after hypercortisolism resolution [54, 55]. Table 1 summarizes the prevalence and main pathogenetic mechanisms of the most common metabolic alterations in CS.

Cardiovascular Alterations

The most common cardiovascular alterations associated with CS include vascular and cardiac abnormalities, and coagulopathies, all significantly contributing to increase the mortality rate of CS patients as compared to the general population [6, 56, 57].

Vascular Disorders

Systemic atherosclerosis is considered the main vascular alteration associated with CS. Carotid intima-media thickness (IMT), a strong predictor of systemic atherosclerosis, was found to be significantly higher in patients with active CD as compared with sex-, age- and BMI-matched controls, and was associated with premature development of carotid atherosclerosis plaques [11]. Common carotid, carotid bulb and aorta IMT were significantly higher in CS patients compared with controls matched for sex, age and some cardiovascular risk factors (i.e. smoking habit, BMI, blood pressure, glucose and lipid levels) [58]. Moreover, it has been demonstrated that in CD patients the distensibility coefficient at the level of common carotid arteries is lower than in sex- and age-matched controls, suggesting the presence of an increased stiffness of carotid artery walls in these patients [11]. The presence of functional vascular alterations has also been suggested by the assessment of endothelium-dependent flow-mediated vasodilation that was reported to be impaired in patients with CS as compared with controls [59]. Additionally, coronary flow reserve – a measure of microvascular function – has been observed to be pathologically reduced in a number of CS patients without clinical symptoms of ischemic heart disease and in the absence of detectable epicardial coronary artery lesions [60].

Clotting Disorders

Coagulopathies and consequent increased incidence of thromboembolic complications have been reported in patients with CS (1–3). These alterations are associated with cortisol excess that induces prothrombotic changes in blood by several complex mechanisms. The hypercoagulable state in CS is due to an increase in plasma-clotting factors, especially factor VIII, IX and von Willebrand factor (vWF) complex [61–65]. Besides higher plasmatic levels of vWF, the presence of unusually large vWF multimers, which are known to have increased hemostatic capacity, has been reported in active CS patients [65, 66]. The fibrinolytic system has also been found to be impaired in CS as observed by a decrease in tissue plasminogen activator antigen, and an increase in PAI-1 [67], plasmin-antiplasmin complex, plasminogen activity, tissue-type plasminogen activator antigen and α_2-antiplasmin activity. Furthermore, the increased levels of factor XII activity and kallikrein described in patients with active CS could contribute to the altered fibrinolytic function. CS has been reported to be associated with hyperhomocysteinemia, a well-known risk factor for cardiovascular disease predisposing to a prothrombotic state [68]. Hypotaurinemia, reported in CS, could further contribute to increase the cardiovascular risk [69].

Cardiac Disorders

Few studies have explored the presence of cardiac structural and functional abnormalities in CS. Data suggest that patients with CS have an increased prevalence of left ventricular hypertrophy, concentric remodeling and diastolic dysfunction (1–3). Particularly, a number of studies have reported an increased left ventricular mass index and the presence of higher relative wall thickness in CS as compared with controls matched for sex and age, as well as for some comorbidities in some of the studies [70–74]. No clinically relevant systolic dysfunction has been reported [70–74], while a limited number of studies have shown the presence of subclinical systolic dysfunction [70, 73, 74], together with a reduced E/A ratio, indicating the presence of diastolic dysfunction in CS [70–72, 74]. Increased myocardial fibrosis, detected by echocardiography, was also reported in patients with CS [75], but this finding was not confirmed by another study based on cardiac magnetic resonance [76].

Metabolic and Cardiovascular Alterations after Cushing's Syndrome Remission

In patients in remission from CS, the persistence of many metabolic and cardiovascular alterations has been described [10].

Metabolic Alterations

The impact of hypercortisolism treatment on metabolism has been predominantly evaluated in patients with CD. The persistence of metabolic syndrome 1 year after hypercortisolism remission was demonstrated in 25 patients with CD as BMI, waist circumference, systolic and diastolic blood pressure, fasting blood glucose and insulin, serum triglycerides, total cholesterol, and low-density lipoprotein and high-density lipoprotein cholesterol improved, although not significantly nor completely in the vast majority of patients. Particularly, in this study abdominal obesity persisted in 62.5%, hypertension in 55.6%, glucose intolerance in 60%, hypercholesterolemia 77% and hypertriglyceridemia in 60% of the patients [11]. Moreover, the metabolic condition of these patients was significantly different to that of the normal population, but close to that of a population with similar BMI, suggesting that the persistence of abdominal obesity is a key player in the persistence of metabolic alterations after short-term hypercortisolism remission [10, 11].

The metabolic parameters after long-term (>5 years) remission from CD have been explored in 15 patients. Abdominal obesity was present in 73%, blood hypertension in 40%, impairment of glucose tolerance or diabetes mellitus in 60% and dyslipidemia in 30%, showing an increased prevalence of metabolic syndrome compared with either age-matched controls or BMI-matched controls [12]. Interestingly, the persistence of hypertension after the remission of hypercortisolism appears to be related to the duration and the degree of hypertension during the active CS phase, suggesting the importance of blood pressure control to reduce cardiovascular risk [77].

In patients in remission from CS, the persistence of increased leptin and resistin levels, as well as of proinflammatory cytokines (i.e. tumor necrosis factor-α and interleukin-6) has also been reported [39]. Similarly, despite long-term cure, patients who have suffered from CS have shown a persistent accumulation of central fat, with the consequent unfavorable adipokine profile, leading to a state of low-grade inflammation and insulin resistance [13].

GH deficiency might contribute to the persistence of cardiovascular risk after hypercortisolism resolution. The prevalence of metabolic syndrome, cardiovascular and cerebrovascular risk has been explored in patients who had previously suffered from

CD versus nonfunctioning pituitary adenoma, treated with GH and followed for 3 years. This study did not show a significant difference in prevalence of the metabolic syndrome and diabetes mellitus at baseline or after 3 years of GH replacement between the two groups, whereas higher prevalence of cardiovascular and cerebrovascular disease was observed in patients with previous CD, both at baseline and after the 3-year follow-up [55]. Another study evaluated the effect of 2-year GH replacement treatment in 15 patients with a previous history of CD as compared with 15 patients with a previous history of nonfunctioning pituitary adenoma, demonstrating that GH treatment helped in reducing diastolic blood pressure in patients with CD, presenting higher values at baseline, thus suggesting that GH replacement treatment might partially help improve cardiovascular risk in patients in remission from CD, although further studies are required to better address this point [54].

Cardiovascular Alterations

Previous studies have reported that patients in remission from CS showed the persistence of abnormal cardiovascular alterations compared to controls, even long after hormonal remission [10–13]. In a group of 25 CD patients, studied during the active phase and prospectively followed for 1 year after hypercortisolism remission, mean IMT significantly decreased and the distensibility coefficient increased, while the prevalence of atherosclerotic plaques remained unchanged (32%). In patients with 1-year remission, mean IMT and the distensibility coefficient remained abnormal compared to sex- and age-matched controls, but not compared to BMI-matched controls [11]. Additionally, both in the active and remission phases, CD patients showed an increased prevalence of atherosclerotic plaques as compared with controls [11]. After long-term disease remission, a higher carotid IMT, a lower distensibility coefficient and a higher prevalence of atherosclerotic plaques were found in patients with CS as compared to sex- and age-matched or BMI-matched controls [12], suggesting a long-term persistence, or even worsening, of increased cardiovascular risk [10].

An immune system rebound following the normalization of cortisol levels has also been hypothesized as an explanation of the worsening of atherosclerosis over time in subjects in remission from CS [7, 10].

Regarding altered coagulation and fibrinolytic parameters observed in CS, there were no univocal results with a significant difference between patients with active versus CS in remission at the different follow-ups, except for the increase of factor VIII, IX and vWF [61, 64, 68].

Additionally, in CS patients evaluated after at least a 5-year remission, both hyperhomocysteinemia and hypotaurinemia, observed during the active state of disease, appear to be reversible [69].

Very little is known about the evolution of cardiac structural and functional abnormalities in patients with CS after hypercortisolism resolution. Regarding the left ventricular geometry, the relative wall thickness was found reduced in a study comparing CS patients after remission at different time points (median: 46.4 months) with active

CS patients [73]. Additionally, some indices of subclinical systolic dysfunction (i.e. global circumferential strain and global longitudinal strain) were found to be higher in short- and long-term (median: 2 weeks and 12 months, respectively) follow-up compared with active disease patients [74], suggesting at least a partial recovery of the systolic function after hypercortisolism remission.

Myocardial fibrosis, assessed by echocardiography, also appeared to be diminished in CS patients after 1-year remission compared with patients with active disease [75].

Conclusions

Several studies have demonstrated the importance of appropriate evaluation and management of cardiovascular risk factors – including visceral obesity, systemic arterial hypertension, glucose intolerance or diabetes, dyslipidemia, endothelial dysfunction and the prothrombotic state – in patients with CS, not only during the active phase, but also in long-term follow-up. Indeed, disease remission is associated with a significant improvement of metabolic parameters, although the recovery is incomplete in the great majority of the cases. Therefore, both during the active and remission phases of CS, the goals of therapy should include not only the assessment and control of cortisol secretion, but also the long-term follow-up and the optimal management of metabolic and cardiovascular alterations.

References

1 Arnaldi G, Angeli A, Atkinson AB, Bertagna X, Cavagnini F, Chrousos GP, Fava GA, Findling JW, Gaillard RC, Grossman AB, Kola B, Lacroix A,Mancini T, Mantero F, Newell-Price J, Nieman LK, Sonino N, Vance ML, Giustina A, Boscaro M: Diagnosis and complications of Cushing's syndrome: a consensus statement. J Clin Endocrinol Metab 2003;88:5593–5602.

2 Pivonello R, De Martino MC, De Leo M, Lombardi G, Colao A: Cushing's syndrome. Endocrinol Metab Clin North Am 2008;37:135–149, ix.

3 Newell-Price J, Bertagna X, Grossman AB, Nieman LK: Cushing's syndrome. Lancet 2006;367:1605–1617.

4 Valassi E, Santos A, Yaneva M, Tóth M, Strasburger CJ, Chanson P, Wass JA, Chabre O, Pfeifer M, Feelders RA, Tsagarakis S, Trainer PJ, Franz H, Zopf K, Zacharieva S, Lamberts SW, Tabarin A, Webb SM; ERCUSYN Study Group: The European Registry on Cushing's syndrome: 2-year experience. Baseline demographic and clinical characteristics. Eur J Endocrinol 2011;165:383–392.

5 Steffensen C, Bak AM, Rubeck KZ, Jorgensen JO: Epidemiology of Cushing's syndrome. Neuroendocrinology 2010;92(suppl 1):1–5.

6 Lindholm J, Juul S, Jørgensen JO, Astrup J, Bjerre P, Feldt-Rasmussen U, Hagen C, Jørgensen J, Kosteljanetz M, Kristensen L, Laurberg P, Schmidt K, Weeke J: Incidence and late prognosis of Cushing's syndrome: a population-based study. J Clin Endocrinol Metab 2001;86:117–123.

7 Pivonello R, Faggiano A, Lombardi G, Colao A: The metabolic syndrome and cardiovascular risk in Cushing's syndrome. Endocrinol Metab Clin North Am 2005;34:327–339, viii.

8 Graversen D, Vestergaard P, Stochholm K, Gravholt CH, Jorgensen JO: Mortality in Cushing's syndrome: a systematic review and meta-analysis. Eur J Intern Med 2012;23:278–282.

9 Yaneva M, Kalinov K, Zacharieva S: Mortality in Cushing's syndrome: data from 386 patients from a single tertiary referral center. Eur J Endocrinol 2013; 169:621–627.

10 Pivonello R, De Martino MC, De Leo M, Tauchmanovà L, Faggiano A, Lombardi G, Colao A: Cushing's syndrome: aftermath of the cure. Arq Bras Endocrinol Metabol 2007;51:1381–1391.

11 Faggiano A, Pivonello R, Spiezia S, De Martino MC, Filippella M, Di Somma C, Lombardi G, Colao A: Cardiovascular risk factors and common carotid artery caliber and stiffness in patients with Cushing's disease during active disease and 1 year after disease remission. J Clin Endocrinol Metab 2003;88:2527–2533.

12 Colao A, Pivonello R, Spiezia S, Faggiano A, Ferone D, Filippella M, Marzullo P, Cerbone G, Siciliani M, Lombardi G: Persistence of increased cardiovascular risk in patients with Cushing's disease after five years of successful cure. J Clin Endocrinol Metab 1999;84: 2664–2672.

13 Barahona MJ, Sucunza N, Resmini E, Fernández-Real JM, Ricart W, Moreno-Navarrete JM, Puig T, Farrerons J, Webb SM: Persistent body fat mass and inflammatory marker increases after long-term cure of Cushing's syndrome. J Clin Endocrinol Metab 2009; 94:3365–3371.

14 Alberti KG, Zimmet P, Shaw J: Metabolic syndrome – a new world-wide definition. A consensus statement from the International Diabetes Federation. Diabet Med 2006;23:469–480.

15 Lee MJ, Gong DW, Burkey BF, Fried SK: Pathways regulated by glucocorticoids in omental and subcutaneous human adipose tissues: a microarray study. Am J Physiol Endocrinol Metab 2011;300:E571–E580.

16 Yu CY, Mayba O, Lee JV, Tran J, Harris C, Speed TP, Wang JC: Genome-wide analysis of glucocorticoid receptor binding regions in adipocytes reveal gene network involved in triglyceride homeostasis. PLoS One 2010;5:e15188.

17 Geer EB, Shen W, Gallagher D, Punyanitya M, Looker HC, Post KD, Freda PU: MRI assessment of lean and adipose tissue distribution in female patients with Cushing's disease. Clin Endocrinol (Oxf) 2010; 73:469–475.

18 Wajchenberg BL, Bosco A, Marone MM, Levin S, Rocha M, Lerário AC, Nery M, Goldman J, Liberman B: Estimation of body fat and lean tissue distribution by dual energy X-ray absorptiometry and abdominal body fat evaluation by computed tomography in Cushing's disease. J Clin Endocrinol Metab 1995;80:2791–2794.

19 Lee MJ, Pramyothin P, Karastergiou K, Fried SK: Deconstructing the roles of glucocorticoids in adipose tissue biology and the development of central obesity. Biochim Biophys Acta 2014;1842:473–481.

20 Campbell JE, Peckett AJ, D'Souza AM, Hawke TJ, Riddell MC: Adipogenic and lipolytic effects of chronic glucocorticoid exposure. Am J Physiol Cell Physiol 2011;300:C198–C209.

21 Rebuffe-Scrive M, Walsh UA, McEwen B, Rodin J: Effect of chronic stress and exogenous glucocorticoids on regional fat distribution and metabolism. Physiol Behav 1992;52:583–590.

22 Tomlinson JJ, Boudreau A, Wu D, Atlas E, Hache RJ: Modulation of early human preadipocyte differentiation by glucocorticoids. Endocrinology 2006;147: 5284–5293.

23 Wiper-Bergeron N, Salem HA, Tomlinson JJ, Wu D, Hache RJ: Glucocorticoid-stimulated preadipocyte differentiation is mediated through acetylation of C/EBPbeta by GCN5. Proc Natl Acad Sci USA 2007; 104:2703–2708.

24 Zhang YY, Li X, Qian SW, Guo L, Huang HY, He Q, Liu Y, Ma CG, Tang QQ: Down-regulation of type I Runx2 mediated by dexamethasone is required for 3T3-L1 adipogenesis. Mol Endocrinol 2012;26:798–808.

25 Sul HS: Minireview: Pref-1: role in adipogenesis and mesenchymal cell fate. Mol Endocrinol 2009;23: 1717–1725.

26 Bujalska IJ, Kumar S, Hewison M, Stewart PM: Differentiation of adipose stromal cells: the roles of glucocorticoids and 11beta-hydroxysteroid dehydrogenase. Endocrinology 1999;140:3188–3196.

27 Miller LK, Kral JG, Strain GW, Zumoff B: Differential binding of dexamethasone to ammonium sulfate precipitates of human adipose tissue cytosols. Steroids 1987;49:507–522.

28 Pedersen SB, Jonler M, Richelsen B: Characterization of regional and gender differences in glucocorticoid receptors and lipoprotein lipase activity in human adipose tissue. J Clin Endocrinol Metab 1994; 78:1354–1359.

29 Veilleux A, Laberge PY, Morency J, Noel S, Luu-The V, Tchernof A: Expression of genes related to glucocorticoid action in human subcutaneous and omental adipose tissue. J Steroid Biochem Mol Biol 2010; 122:28–34.

30 Caprio M, Antelmi A, Chetrite G, Muscat A, Mammi C, Marzolla V, Fabbri A, Zennaro MC, Fève B: Antiadipogenic effects of the mineralocorticoid receptor antagonist drospirenone: potential implications for the treatment of metabolic syndrome. Endocrinology 2011;152:113–125.

31 Caprio M, Feve B, Claes A, Viengchareun S, Lombes M, Zennaro MC: Pivotal role of the mineralocorticoid receptor in corticosteroid-induced adipogenesis. FASEB J 2007;21:2185–2194.

32 Hoppmann J, Perwitz N, Meier B, Fasshauer M, Hadaschik D, Lehnert H, Klein J: The balance between gluco- and mineralo-corticoid action critically determines inflammatory adipocyte responses. J Endocrinol 2010;204:153–164.

33 Appel B, Fried SK: Effects of insulin and dexamethasone on lipoprotein lipase in human adipose tissue. Am J Physiol 1992;262:E695–E699.

34 Fried SK, Russell CD, Grauso NL, Brolin RE: Lipoprotein lipase regulation by insulin and glucocorticoid in subcutaneous and omental adipose tissues of obese women and men. J Clin Invest 1993;92:2191–2198.

35 Viengchareun S, Penfornis P, Zennaro MC, Lombes M: Mineralocorticoid and glucocorticoid receptors inhibit UCP expression and function in brown adipocytes. Am J Physiol Endocrinol Metab 2001;280:E640–E649.
36 Soumano K, Desbiens S, Rabelo R, Bakopanos E, Camirand A, Silva JE: Glucocorticoids inhibit the transcriptional response of the uncoupling protein-1 gene to adrenergic stimulation in a brown adipose cell line. Mol Cell Endocrinol 2000;165:7–15.
37 Pivonello R, De Leo M, Vitale P, Cozzolino A, Simeoli C, De Martino MC, Lombardi G, Colao A: Pathophysiology of diabetes mellitus in Cushing's syndrome. Neuroendocrinology 2010;92(suppl 1):77–81.
38 Arnaldi G, Scandali VM, Trementino L, Cardinaletti M, Appolloni G, Boscaro M: Pathophysiology of dyslipidemia in Cushing's syndrome. Neuroendocrinology 2010;92(suppl 1):86–90.
39 Valassi E, Biller BM, Klibanski A, Misra M: Adipokines and cardiovascular risk in Cushing's syndrome. Neuroendocrinology 2012;95:187–206.
40 Magiakou MA, Smyrnaki P, Chrousos GP: Hypertension in Cushing's syndrome. Best Pract Res Clin Endocrinol Metab 2006;20:467–482.
41 Pecori Giraldi F, Toja PM, De Martin M, Maronati A, Scacchi M, Omboni S, Cavagnini F, Parati G: Circadian blood pressure profile in patients with active Cushing's disease and after long-term cure. Horm Metab Res 2007;39:908–914.
42 Isidori AM, Graziadio C, Paragliola RM, Cozzolino A, Ambrogio AG, Colao A, Corsello SM, Pivonello R; ABC Study Group: The hypertension of Cushing's syndrome: controversies in the pathophysiology and focus on cardiovascular complications. J Hypertens 2015;33:44–60.
43 Saruta T, Suzuki H, Handa M, Igarashi Y, Kondo K, Senba S: Multiple factors contribute to the pathogenesis of hypertension in Cushing's syndrome. J Clin Endocrinol Metab 1986;62:275–279.
44 Shibata H, Suzuki H, Maruyama T, Saruta T: Gene expression of angiotensin II receptor in blood cells of Cushing's syndrome. Hypertension 1995;26:1003–1010.
45 Yamaji T, Ishibashi M, Yamada A, Takaku F, Itabashi A, Katayama S, Ishii J, Takami M, Fukushima T: Plasma levels of atrial natriuretic hormone in Cushing's syndrome. J Clin Endocrinol Metab 1988;67:348–352.
46 Yasunari K, Kohno M, Murakawa K, Yokokawa K, Takeda T: Glucocorticoids and atrial natriuretic factor receptors on vascular smooth muscle. Hypertension 1990;16:581–586.
47 Radomski MW, Palmer RM, Moncada S: Glucocorticoids inhibit the expression of an inducible, but not the constitutive, nitric oxide synthase in vascular endothelial cells. Proc Natl Acad Sci USA 1990;87:10043–10047.
48 Wallerath T, Witte K, Schäfer SC, Schwarz PM, Prellwitz W, Wohlfart P, Kleinert H, Lehr HA, Lemmer B, Förstermann U: Down-regulation of the expression of endothelial NO synthase is likely to contribute to glucocorticoid-mediated hypertension. Proc Natl Acad Sci USA 1999;96:13357–13362.
49 Kirilov G, Tomova A, Dakovska L, Kumanov P, Shinkov A, Alexandrov AS: Elevated plasma endothelin as an additional cardiovascular risk factor in patients with Cushing's syndrome. Eur J Endocrinol 2003;149:549–553.
50 Munir A, Newell-Price J: Management of diabetes mellitus in Cushing's syndrome. Neuroendocrinology 2010;92(suppl 1):82–85.
51 Chanson P, Salenave S: Metabolic syndrome in Cushing's syndrome. Neuroendocrinology 2010;92(suppl 1):96–101.
52 De Leo M, Pivonello R, Auriemma RS, Cozzolino A, Vitale P, Simeoli C, De Martino MC, Lombardi G, Colao A: Cardiovascular disease in Cushing's syndrome: heart versus vasculature. Neuroendocrinology 2010;92(suppl 1):50–54.
53 Mancini T, Kola B, Mantero F, Boscaro M, Arnaldi G: High cardiovascular risk in patients with Cushing's syndrome according to 1999 WHO/ISH guidelines. Clin Endocrinol (Oxf) 2004;61:768–777.
54 Johannsson G, Sunnerhagen KS, Svensson J: Baseline characteristics and the effects of two years of growth hormone replacement therapy in adults with growth hormone deficiency previously treated for Cushing's disease. Clin Endocrinol (Oxf) 2004;60:550–559.
55 Webb SM, Mo D, Lamberts SW, Melmed S, Cavagnini F, Pecori Giraldi F, Strasburger CJ, Zimmermann AG, Woodmansee WW; International HypoCCS Advisory Board: Metabolic, cardiovascular, and cerebrovascular outcomes in growth hormone-deficient subjects with previous Cushing's disease or non-functioning pituitary adenoma. J Clin Endocrinol Metab 2010;95:630–638.
56 Etxabe J, Vazquez JA: Morbidity and mortality in Cushing's disease: an epidemiological approach. Clin Endocrinol (Oxf) 1994;40:479–484.
57 Clayton RN, Raskauskiene D, Reulen RC, Jones PW: Mortality and morbidity in Cushing's disease over 50 years in Stoke-on-Trent, UK: audit and meta-analysis of literature. J Clin Endocrinol Metab 2011;96:632–642.
58 Albiger N, Testa RM, Almoto B, Ferrari M, Bilora F, Petrobelli F, Pagnan A, Mantero F, Scaroni C: Patients with Cushing's syndrome have increased intimal media thickness at different vascular levels: comparison with a population matched for similar cardiovascular risk factors. Horm Metab Res 2006;38:405–410.

59 Baykan M, Erem C, Gedikli O, Hacihasanoglu A, Erdogan T, Kocak M, Kaplan S, Korkmaz L, Celik S: Impairment of flow-mediated vasodilatation of brachial artery in patients with Cushing's syndrome. Endocrine 2007;31:300–304.

60 Fallo F, Famoso G, Capizzi D, Sonino N, Dassie F, Maffei P, Martini C, Paoletta A, Iliceto S, Tona F: Coronary microvascular function in patients with Cushing's syndrome. Endocrine 2013;43:206–213.

61 Fatti LM, Bottasso B, Invitti C, Coppola R, Cavagnini F, Mannucci PM: Markers of activation of coagulation and fibrinolysis in patients with Cushing's syndrome. J Endocrinol Invest 2000;23:145–150.

62 Van Zaane B, Nur E, Squizzato A, Dekkers OM, Twickler MT, Fliers E, Gerdes VE, Büller HR, Brandjes DP: Hypercoagulable state in Cushing's syndrome: a systematic review. J Clin Endocrinol Metab 2009;94:2743–2750.

63 Patrassi GM, Dal Bo Zanon R, Boscaro M, Martinelli S, Girolami A: Further studies on the hypercoagulable state of patients with Cushing's syndrome. Thromb Haemost 1985;54:518–520.

64 Dal Bo Zanon R, Fornasiero L, Boscaro M, Cappellato G, Fabris F, Girolami A: Increased factor VIII associated activities in Cushing's syndrome: a probable hypercoagulable state. Thromb Haemost 1982; 47:116–117.

65 Casonato A, Pontara E, Boscaro M, Sonino N, Sartorello F, Ferasin S, Girolami A: Abnormalities of von Willebrand factor are also part of the prothrombotic state of Cushing's syndrome. Blood Coagul Fibrinolysis 1999;10:145–151.

66 Federici AB, Bader R, Pagani S, Colibretti ML, De Marco L, Mannucci PM: Binding of von Willebrand factor to glycoproteins Ib and IIb/IIIa complex: affinity is related to multimeric size. Br J Haematol 1989;73:93–99.

67 Patrassi GM, Sartori MT, Viero ML, Scarano L, Boscaro M, Girolami A: The fibrinolytic potential in patients with Cushing's disease: a clue to their hypercoagulable state. Blood Coagul Fibrinolysis 1992;3: 789–793.

68 Terzolo M, Allasino B, Bosio S, Brusa E, Daffara F, Ventura M, Aroasio E, Sacchetto G, Reimondo G, Angeli A, Camaschella C: Hyperhomocysteinemia in patients with Cushing's syndrome. J Clin Endocrinol Metab 2004;89:3745–3751.

69 Faggiano A, Melis D, Alfieri R, De Martino M, Filippella M, Milone F, Lombardi G, Colao A, Pivonello R: Sulfur amino acids in Cushing's disease: insight in homocysteine and taurine levels in patients with active and cured disease. J Clin Endocrinol Metab 2005;90:6616–6622.

70 Muiesan ML, Lupia M, Salvetti M, Grigoletto C, Sonino N, Boscaro M, Rosei EA, Mantero F, Fallo F: Left ventricular structural and functional characteristics in Cushing's syndrome. J Am Coll Cardiol 2003;41:2275–2279.

71 Baykan M, Erem C, Gedikli O, Kaplan S, Kiriş A, Durmuş I, Celik S: Assessment of left ventricular diastolic function and Tei index by tissue Doppler imaging in patients with Cushing's syndrome. Echocardiography 2008;25:182–190.

72 Bayram NA, Ersoy R, Aydin C, Gul K, Keles T, Topaloglu O, Durmaz T, Bozkurt E, Cakir B: Assessment of left ventricular functions by tissue Doppler echocardiography in patients with Cushing's disease. J Endocrinol Invest 2009;32:248–252.

73 Toja PM, Branzi G, Ciambellotti F, Radaelli P, De Martin M, Lonati LM, Scacchi M, Parati G, Cavagnini F, Pecori Giraldi F: Clinical relevance of cardiac structure and function abnormalities in patients with Cushing's syndrome before and after cure. Clin Endocrinol (Oxf) 2012;76:332–338.

74 Pereira AM, Delgado V, Romijn JA, Smit JW, Bax JJ, Feelders RA: Cardiac dysfunction is reversed upon successful treatment of Cushing's syndrome. Eur J Endocrinol 2010;162:331–340.

75 Yiu KH, Marsan NA, Delgado V, Biermasz NR, Holman ER, Smit JW, Feelders RA, Bax JJ, Pereira AM: Increased myocardial fibrosis and left ventricular dysfunction in Cushing's syndrome. Eur J Endocrinol 2012;166:27–34.

76 Kamenicky P, Redheuil A, Roux C, Salenave S, Kachenoura N, Raissouni Z, Macron L, Guignat L, Jublanc C, Azarine A, Brailly S, Young J, Mousseaux E, Chanson P: Cardiac structure and function in Cushing's syndrome: a cardiac magnetic resonance imaging study. J Clin Endocrinol Metab 2014; 99:E2144–E2153.

77 Suzuki T, Shibata H, Ando T, Kurihara I, Kobayashi S, Hayashi K, Hayashi M, Kawabe H, Saito I, Murai M, Saruta T: Risk factors associated with persistent postoperative hypertension in Cushing's syndrome. Endocr Res 2000;26:791–795.

Prof. Rosario Pivonello, MD, PhD
Division of Endocrinology, Department of Clinical Medicine and Surgery
University Federico II di Napoli
Via Sergio Pansini 5
IT–80131 Naples (Italy)
E-Mail rosario.pivonello@unina.it

Arvat E, Falorni A (eds): Cortisol Excess and Insufficiency.
Front Horm Res. Basel, Karger, 2016, vol 46, pp 66–73 (DOI: 10.1159/000443866)

Skeletal Fragility in Endogenous Hypercortisolism

Gherardo Mazziotti[a] · Adriano Delgado[a, b] · Filippo Maffezzoni[a] · Annamaria Formenti[a] · Andrea Giustina[a]

[a]Endocrinology, University of Brescia, Brescia, Italy; [b]Endocrine Service, Hospital Santo Tomas, Panama City, Panama

Abstract

Skeletal fragility is a frequent complication of endogenous hypercortisolism, and fragility fractures may be the first clinical manifestation of the disease. Fractures involve more frequently the vertebrae and may occur in 30–50% of the patients exposed to glucocorticoid excess, in close relationship with severity and duration of hypercortisolism. Although improvement of bone mineral density was reported after resolution of hypercortisolism, there are patients with persistently high fracture risk after the cure of hypercortisolism, and other patients in whom the resolution of hypercortisolism may take a long time, implying a multistep therapeutic approach. Since vertebral fractures tend to occur early during the natural history of disease, a skeletal-specific approach should be undertaken in these patients; however, the cost-effectiveness of this approach is still largely unknown since data on effectiveness and safety of bone-active drugs in endogenous hypercortisolism are scarce.

Glucocorticoid-induced osteoporosis (GIO) is the most common form of secondary osteoporosis [1]. Although exogenous Cushing's syndrome is the most common form, endogenous hypercortisolism is also relevant to clinical practice and can also produce deleterious effects on bone. All degrees of hypercortisolism, clinical and subclinical, can affect bone remodeling and thus predispose to fragility fractures [2]. As a matter of fact, fragility fractures may be the first clinical manifestation of Cushing's syndrome [3]. Fractures involve more frequently the vertebrae and may occur in 30–50% of the patients with endogenous hypercortisolism, in close relationship with the severity and/or duration of disease [4].

Pathophysiological Aspects

Following glucocorticoid exposure, there is a rapid, early phase of bone loss due to excessive bone resorption, followed by a more chronic and progressive phase in which bone mass declines due to impaired bone formation [1]. The early increase in bone resorption is caused by stimulation of the receptor activator of the NF-κB ligand (RANK-L) and concomitant inhibition of its soluble decoy receptor, osteoprotegerin, in stromal and osteoblastic cells [1]. Glucocorticoids also enhance the expression of colony-stimulating factor-1 and upregulate receptor subunits for osteoclastogenic cytokines of the gp130 family [1]. While all these actions lead to enhanced bone resorption, the central pathophysiological mechanism of GIO is reduced bone formation due to inhibition of Wnt/β-catenin and bone morphogenetic protein-2 signaling and induction of peroxisome proliferator activated receptor-γ_2 [5]. Glucocorticoids may also affect the number and function of osteocytes, inducing apoptosis, and reduce the mineral matrix with an increase in lacunar size [1]. These effects of glucocorticoids on osteoblasts and osteocytes might account for a disproportionate loss of bone strength in relation to bone mass (see next section). In addition to the direct actions of glucocorticoids on bone-specific cells, other skeletal effects are mediated by neuroendocrine changes, such as functional growth hormone (GH) deficiency, hypogonadism and possible qualitative abnormalities of PTH secretion [6–8]. Moreover, glucocorticoids cause negative calcium balance by inhibiting intestinal absorption and tubular renal reabsorption [1]. As a consequence of the catabolic action of glucocorticoids on protein metabolism, patients exposed to glucocorticoid excess present a classical myopathy with muscle weakness typically affecting the pelvic area. This serious complication may lead to falls and contribute to fractures. It is also postulated that myopathy and muscle weakness may contribute to bone loss by removing the stimulating activity on the bone exerted by strong muscle contraction [1].

All the aforementioned mechanisms are shared by endogenous and exogenous hypercortisolism, although some differences may exist between the two conditions [9]. Differently from exogenous glucocorticoid excess, in endogenous hypercortisolism, the early and transient phase of high bone turnover is not usually evident since the diagnosis of disease is often delayed with respect to onset of hypercortisolism. When endogenous hypercortisolism is diagnosed, the skeletal phenotype is usually characterized by low bone turnover with only a slight and uncoupled increase in bone resorption, as it classically occurs during chronic treatment with glucocorticoids [9]. Another factor to be taken into account in patients with endogenous hypercortisolism is the magnitude of androgen secretion, which is greater in ACTH-dependent hypercortisolism than in ACTH-independent cortisol excess, which may explain, at least in part, the relatively less severe skeletal damage occurring in patients with Cushing's disease as compared to primary adrenal disease [10].

Individual susceptibility to glucocorticoid excess varies considerably, possibly because of differences in the number and affinity of glucocorticoid receptors, as suggested by differences in bone mineral density (BMD) and fracture rate in relation to polymorphisms of the glucocorticoid receptor gene [11, 12]. The activity of 11β-hydroxysteroid dehydrogenase enzyme system, which in turn converts the glucocorticoids' active and inactive forms, may also influence the variability of skeletal fragility caused by exposure to glucocorticoid excess [13, 14]. Two 11β-hydroxysteroid dehydrogenase enzymes have been described: 11β-hydroxysteroid dehydrogenase type I, which is primarily a glucocorticoid activator, converting cortisone to cortisol, and 11β-hydroxysteroid dehydrogenase type II, an inhibitor enzyme expressed in mineralocorticoid target tissues. These are widely expressed in glucocorticoid target tissues, including bone, and their reciprocal activities are influenced by either genetic polymorphisms [14] or neuroendocrine factors acting at the tissue level [13].

Clinical Aspects

The clinical bone manifestations of cortisol excess are determined by the severity and duration of disease, and patient age [2].

In clinical practice, measurement of BMD (bone mass density) at the lumbar spine, hip and femoral neck by dual-energy X-ray absorptiometry (DXA) is the mainstay for diagnosis of osteoporosis and prediction of fracture risk [15]. Skeletal demineralization is graded according to the World Health Organization criteria based on comparisons of the patient's BMD with the average for young adults, after adjusting for race and gender. A T-score ≤–2.5 SD in the hip or spine is defined as osteoporosis, whereas osteopenia is defined as a T-score between –1 and –2.5 SD [15]. Prevalence of osteoporosis at the spine was higher in men as compared with women [16]. However, the densitometric definitions of osteoporosis are applicable only for postmenopausal women and men aged 50 and older, whereas for younger subjects the Z-score (i.e. the number of standard deviations from age-matched controls) ≤2.0 is used to define a BMD 'below the expected range for age' [15]. Since Cushing's syndrome often occurs in men under 50 and in premenopausal women, diagnosis of osteoporosis cannot be easily performed on the basis of BMD alone in this clinical setting. Moreover, BMD appears to be a poor predictor of fracture risk in GIO, differently from what is observed in postmenopausal osteoporosis [17]. In fact, fractures in GIO occur at greater BMDs, consistent with the concept that glucocorticoid excess affects bone quality more than bone quantity, as observed in other endocrine-related secondary forms of osteoporosis [17–20]. This is a clinically relevant finding that has prompted the search for alternative diagnostic tools that are better at reflecting the quality of bone in these patients, such as quantitative ultrasonometry, high-resolution peripheral quantitative computed tomography or measurement of trabecular bone score (TBS) by DXA [21, 22]. Specifically, the assessment of TBS – which is a gray-level texture measurement based on 2D projection images acquired during a DXA lumbar spine scan – was shown to be strongly correlated with bone microarchitecture [22].

In patients with Cushing's syndrome, TBS was reduced and correlated with the number and severity of vertebral fractures, and also with the degree of cortisol excess [23]. In fact, TBS was suggested to be more accurate than BMD in identifying patients at risk for vertebral fractures [23].

Vertebral fractures are the hallmark of GIO [1]. In >50% of the cases, spine fractures occur without specific clinical symptoms and the radiological and morphometric approach has emerged as the method of choice for evaluating the true prevalence and incidence of these fractures in clinical practice [24]. Vertebral fractures are identified, marking the vertebral body with 6 points to describe the vertebral shape and heights. According to the quantitative morphometric approach, vertebral fractures are defined as mild, moderate and severe based on a height ratio decrease of 20–25, 25–40 and >40%, respectively [25]. Quantitative morphometry is usually performed on spinal X-ray images, although the quantitative approach may also be applied to images of the spine acquired by DXA [21]. To have a global measure of vertebral fracture severity, the spine deformity index can be calculated by summing the score of each vertebral fracture assigned on the basis of the grade of fracture (score 1, 2 or 3 for mild, moderate and severe fractures, respectively) [26]. The severity of prevalent vertebral fractures is a strong clinical marker of disease progression, predicts future fractures independently of BMD and has been suggested as indicative of significant architectural deterioration of bone [27]. Vertebral fractures were shown to occur in about 50% of patients with Cushing's syndrome with higher prevalence in males as compared to females [28]. Moreover, the European Registry on Cushing's Syndrome (ERCUSYN) revealed that vertebral fractures were more prevalent in ectopic Cushing's syndrome as compared with pituitary Cushing's disease (44 vs. 25%) [28]. Bone fractures occurred in 62% of patients with osteoporosis and in 42% of patients with osteopenia. Additionally, 25% of patients with normal BMD experienced a bone fracture [28]. However, incident vertebral fractures were shown to develop even in patients with stable BMD during a short-term follow-up [29].

Therapeutic Aspects

Most of the literature data on the treatment of GIO, as well as related therapeutic guidelines, are derived from studies performed in patients exposed to exogenous glucocorticoid excess [30, 31]. However, endogenous GIO has some peculiar aspects that could make it difficult to translate the clinical and therapeutic approach from the exogenous to endogenous GIO [9]. A first peculiar aspect worthy of consideration is the potential recovery of bone health after resolution of hypercortisolism, an opportunity that cannot be commonly achieved in patients with exogenous GIO in whom glucocorticoids are taken for therapeutic purposes. As a matter of fact, several authors have reported normalization of bone turnover and improvement, although not always normalization, in BMD after resolution of hypercortisolism [32]. However, there are also patients with a persistently high fracture risk after the cure of hypercortisolism [33] and other patients (e.g. those with ectopic ACTH secretion and Cushing's disease) in whom the resolution of hypercortisolism may take a long time, implying a multistep therapeutic approach [34], while vertebral fractures tend to occur early during the natural history of disease [1]. In all these clinical conditions, a skeletal-specific approach should be undertaken regardless of the degree of underlying hypercortisolism. The American College of Rheumatology (ACR) and the International Osteoporosis Foundation (IOF) recommend to identify and possibly correct coexistent risk factors contributing to increase the fracture risk in patients exposed to glucocorticoid excess [30, 31]. The correction of hypovitaminosis D and the negative calcium balance associated with hypercortisolism is an intuitive approach to reduce fracture risk in patients with GIO, mainly in those with endogenous hypercortisolism in whom adequate amounts of vitamin D and calcium are likely required to support the rapid mineralization of the newly formed bone matrix occurring after removal of the cause of glucocorticoid excess [9]. Supplementations with calcium and vitamin D are very important and are cost-effective measures that can be applied to everyone with GIO. Corticosteroids induce vitamin D resistance and it has been suggested that a higher value for serum 25-OH-vitamin D (40–60 ng/ml) should be targeted with respect to the general population [35]. To achieve this goal, patients may require up to 2,000 UI of vitamin D_3 daily [35].

Hypercortisolism may induce suppression of the gonadal and GH-IGF-1 axes, which may contribute to the skeletal fragility [1]. Although sex steroids were shown to protect the skeleton from deleterious effects of glucocorticoids excess in an experimental condition [36], there are no data on the antifracture effects of sex steroid replacement therapy in humans with endogenous hypercortisolism. Moreover, estrogen administration may potentially worsen the prothrombotic state of patients with endogenous hypercortisolism [30, 31]. Theoretically, a window of opportunity may exist for GH treatment in patients with GIO [6], although there could be some concerns about the potential drawbacks of such an approach in patients chronically exposed to glucocorticoid excess. In fact, both recombinant GH and glucocorticoid treatment are known to induce insulin resistance in hepatic and peripheral tissues, potentially resulting in worsened glucose tolerance [37, 38].

Besides the correction of coexistent risk factors for fractures, antiosteoporotic drugs may be needed in some patients in whom fracture risk could not be normalized by correction of hypercortisolism [9]. The ACR and IOF recommend to use bisphosphonates as first-line therapy in patients with exogenous GIO [30, 31]. Alendronate and clodronate were tested in patients with endogenous hypercortisolism and demonstrated positive effects on BMD [39, 40], whereas data on fractures in this clinical context are still lacking. Moreover, it is unclear whether bisphosphonates may negatively influence the recovery of bone remodeling after resolution of cortisol excess [9].

Since GIO is mainly characterized by an impairment of bone formation and quality, teriparatide could be considered an interesting therapeutic option for either exogenous or endogenous GIO [41]. In patients with endogenous GIO, teriparatide, oppositely to bisphosphonates, may favor the recovery of bone remodeling after resolution of hypercortisolism. However, clinical experiences with this 'anabolic' treatment are yet to be reported in patients with endogenous hypercortisolism.

Conclusion

All patients with endogenous hypercortisolism should undergo a complete evaluation of bone metabolic status, including both hormonal and radiological studies (i.e. spine X-ray and DXA) to determine the risk of developing a new fracture (mainly vertebral). Prevention with calcium and vitamin D supplements is mandatory, while antiosteoporotic therapy should be considered depending on individual risks assessments. When choosing a pharmacological therapy, it is important to have in mind that resolution of hypercortisolism, which is not always simple, rapid or complete, may improve or normalize BMD and microarchitecture. Bisphosphonates have long been considered the primary antiosteoporotic treatment, although their mechanism of action does not seem to fully support their therapeutic role in GIO. Anabolic therapies seem to target more precisely the pathogenic mechanisms underlying bone fragility in GIO, although clinical experiences in endogenous hypercortisolism has so far been limited.

References

1 Mazziotti G, Angeli A, Bilezikian JP, Canalis E, Giustina A: Glucocorticoid-induced osteoporosis: an update. Trends Endocrinol Metab 2006;7:144–149.
2 Mancini T, Doga M, Mazziotti G, Giustina A: Cushing's syndrome and bone. Pituitary 2005;7:1–4.
3 Vestergaard P, Lindholm J, Jørgensen JO, Hagen C, Hoeck HC, Laurberg P, Rejnmark L, Brixen K, Kristensen LØ, Feldt-Rasmussen U, Mosekilde L: Increased risk of osteoporotic fractures in patients with Cushing's syndrome. Eur J Endocrinol 2002;146:51–56.
4 Trementino L, Appolloni G, Ceccoli L, Marcelli G, Concettoni C, Boscaro M, Arnaldi G: Bone complications in patients with Cushing's syndrome: looking for clinical, biochemical, and genetic determinants. Osteoporos Int 2014;25:913–921.
5 Canalis E, Giustina A, Bilezikian JP: Mechanisms of anabolic therapies for osteoporosis. N Engl J Med 2007;357:905–916.
6 Mazziotti G, Giustina A: Glucocorticoids and the regulation of growth hormone secretion. Nat Rev Endocrinol 2013;9:265–276.
7 Giustina A, Mazziotti G, Canalis E: Growth hormone, insulin-like growth factors, and the skeleton. Endocr Rev 2008;29:535–559.
8 Adler RA, Giustina A: Parathyroid hormone and glucocorticoid-induced osteoporosis; in Bilezikian JP (ed): The Parathyroids, ed 3. Amsterdam, Elsevier, 2014, vol 59, pp 837–841.
9 Scillitani G, Mazziotti G, Di Somma C, Moretti S, Stigliano A, Pivonello R, Giustina A, Colao A: Treatment of skeletal impairment in patients with endogenous hypercortisolism: when and how? Osteoporos Int 2014;25:441–446.
10 Minetto M, Reimondo G, Osella G, Ventura M, Angeli A, Terzolo M: Bone loss is more severe in primary adrenal than in pituitary-dependent Cushing's syndrome. Osteoporos Int 2004;15:855–861.
11 Morelli V, Donadio F, Eller-Vainicher C, Cirello V, Olgiati L, Savoca C, Cairoli E, Salcuni AS, Beck-Peccoz P, Chiodini I: Role of glucocorticoid receptor polymorphism in adrenal incidentalomas. Eur J Clin Invest 2010;40:803–811.

12 Szappanos A, Patócs A, Tőke J, Boyle B, Sereg M, Majnik J, Borgulya G, Varga I, Likó I, Rácz K, Tóth M: BclI polymorphism of the glucocorticoid receptor gene is associated with decreased bone mineral density in patients with endogenous hypercortisolism. Clin Endocrinol 2009;71:636–643.
13 Mazziotti G, Porcelli T, Bianchi A, Cimino V, Patelli I, Mejia C, Fusco A, Giampietro A, De Marinis L, Giustina A: Glucocorticoid replacement therapy and vertebral fractures in hypopituitary adult males with GH deficiency. Eur J Endocrinol 2010;163:15–20.
14 Hwang JY, Lee SH, Kim GS, Koh JM, Go MJ, Kim YJ, Kim HC, Kim TH, Hong JM, Park EK, Lee JY, Kim SY: HSD11B1 polymorphisms predicted bone mineral density and fracture risk in postmenopausal women without a clinically apparent hypercortisolemia. Bone 2009;45:1098–1103.
15 Schousboe JT, Shepherd JA, Bilezikian JP, Baim S: Executive summary of the 2013 International Society for Clinical Densitometry Position Development Conference on bone densitometry. J Clin Densitom 2013;16:455–466.
16 Pecori Giraldi F, Moro M, Cavagnini F; Study Group on the Hypothalamo-Pituitary-Adrenal Axis of the Italian Society of Endocrinology: Gender-related differences in the presentation and course of Cushing's disease. J Clin Endocrinol Metab 2003;88:1554–1558.
17 Mazziotti G, Bilezikian J, Canalis E, Cocchi D, Giustina A: New understanding and treatments for osteoporosis. Endocrine 2012;41:58–69.
18 Bonadonna S, Mazziotti G, Nuzzo M, Bianchi A, Fusco A, De Marinis L, Giustina A: Increased prevalence of radiological spinal deformities in active acromegaly: a cross-sectional study in postmenopausal women. J Bone Miner Res 2005;20:1837–1844.
19 Mazziotti G, Bianchi A, Bonadonna S, Nuzzo M, Cimino V, Fusco A, De Marinis L, Giustina A: Increased prevalence of radiological spinal deformities in adult patients with GH deficiency: influence of GH replacement therapy. J Bone Miner Res 2006;21:520–528.
20 Mancini T, Mazziotti G, Doga M, Carpinteri R, Simetovic N, Vescovi PP, Giustina A: Vertebral fractures in males with type 2 diabetes treated with rosiglitazone. Bone 2009;45:784–748.
21 Griffith JF, Genant HK: New advances in imaging osteoporosis and its complications. Endocrine 2012;42:39–51.
22 Ulivieri FM, Silva BC, Sardanelli F, Hans D, Bilezikian JP, Caudarella R: Utility of the trabecular bone score (TBS) in secondary osteoporosis. Endocrine 2014;47:435–448.
23 Eller-Vainicher C, Morelli V, Ulivieri FM, Palmieri S, Zhukouskaya VV, Cairoli E, Pino R, Naccarato A, Scillitani A, Beck-Peccoz P, Chiodini I: Bone quality, as measured by trabecular bone score in patients with adrenal incidentalomas with and without subclinical hypercortisolism. J Bone Miner Res 2012;10:2223–2230.
24 Angeli A, Guglielmi G, Dovio A, Capelli G, de Feo D, Giannini S, Giorgino R,Moro L, Giustina A: High prevalence of asymptomatic vertebral fractures in post-menopausal women receiving chronic glucocorticoid therapy: a cross-sectional outpatient study. Bone 2006;39:253–259.
25 Genant HK, Jergas M, Palermo L, Nevitt M, Valentin RS, Black D, Cummings SR: Comparison of semiquantitative visual and quantitative morphometric assessment of prevalent and incident vertebral fractures in osteoporosis. The Study of Osteoporotic Fractures Research Group. J Bone Miner Res 1996;11:984–996.
26 Siris ES, Genant HK, Laster AJ, Chen P, Misurski DA, Krege JH: Enhanced prediction of fracture risk combining vertebral fracture status and BMD. Osteoporos Int 2007;18:761–770.
27 Di Somma C, Rubino M, Faggiano A, Vuolo L, Contaldi P, Tafuri N, Andretti M, Savastano S, Colao A: Spinal deformity index in patients with type 2 diabetes. Endocrine 2013;43:651–658.
28 Valassi E, Santos A, Yaneva M, Tóth M, Strasburger CJ, Chanson P, Wass JA, Chabre O, Pfeifer M, Feelders RA, Tsagarakis S, Trainer PJ, Franz H, Zopf K, Zacharieva S, Lamberts SW, Tabarin A, Webb SM: The European Registry on Cushing's syndrome: 2-year experience. Baseline demographic and clinical characteristics. Eur J Endocrinol 2011;165:383–392.
29 Morelli V, Eller-Vainicher C, Salcuni AS, Coletti F, Iorio L, Muscogiuri G, Della Casa S, Arosio M, Ambrosi B, Beck-Pecoz P, Chiodini I: Risk of new vertebral fractures in patients with adrenal incidentaloma with and without subcliclinal hypercortisolim: a multicenter longitudinal study. J Bone Miner Res 2011;26:1816–1821.
30 American College of Rheumatology Ad Hoc Committee on Glucocorticoid-Induced Osteoporosis: Recommendations for the prevention and treatment of glucocorticoid-induced osteoporosis. Arthritis Rheum 2001;44:1496–1503.
31 Lekamwasam S, Adachi JD, Agnusdei D, Bilezikian J, Boonen S, Borgström F, Cooper C, Diez Perez A, Eastell R, Hofbauer LC, Kanis JA, Langdahl BL, Lesnyak O, Lorenc R, McCloskey E, Messina OD, Napoli N, Obermayer-Pietsch B, Ralston SH, Sambrook PN, Silverman S, Sosa M, Stepan J, Suppan G, Wahl DA, Compston JE; Joint IOF-ECTS GIO Guidelines Working Group: A framework for the development of guidelines for the management of glucocorticoid-induced osteoporosis. Osteoporos Int 2012;23:2257–2276.
32 Randazzo ME, Grossrubatscher E, Ciaramella P, Vanzulli A, Loli P: Spontaneous recovery of bone mass after cure of endogenous hypercortisolism. Pituitary 2012;15:193–201.

33 Faggiano A, Pivonello R, Filippella M, Di Somma C, Orio F Jr, Lombard G, Colao A: Spine abnormalities and damage in patients cured from Cushing's disease. Pituitary 2001;4:153–161.
34 Mancini T, Porcelli T, Giustina A: Treatment of Cushing disease: overview and recent findings. Ther Clin Risk Manag 2010;6:505–516.
35 Canalis E, Mazziotti G, Giustina A, Bilezikian JP: Glucocorticoid-induced osteoporosis: pathophysiology and therapy. Osteoporos Int 2007;18:1319–1328.
36 Weinstein RS, Jia D, Powers CC, Stewart SA, Jilka RL, Parfitt AM, Manolagas SC: The skeletal effects of glucocorticoid excess override those of orchidectomy in mice. Endocrinology 2004;145:1980–1987.
37 Bismuth E, Chevenne D, Czernichow P, Simon D: Moderate deterioration in glucose tolerance during high-dose growth hormone therapy in glucocorticoid treated patients with juvenile idiopathic arthritis. Horm Res Paediatr 2010;73:465–472.
38 Mazziotti G, Gazzaruso C, Giustina A: Diabetes in Cushing syndrome: basic and clinical aspects. Trends Endocrinol Metab 2011;22:499–506.
39 Di Somma C, Colao A, Pivonello R, Klain M, Faggiano A, Tripodi FS, Merola B, Salvatore M, Lombardi G: Effectiveness of chronic treatment with alendronate in the osteoporosis of Cushing's disease. Clin Endocrinol 1998;48:655–662.
40 Tauchmanova L, Pivonello R, Di Somma C; Rossi R, De Martino MC, Camera L, Klain M, Salvatore M, Lombardi G, Colao A: Bone demineralization and vertebral fractures in endogenous cortisol excess: role of disease etiology and gonadal status. J Clin Endocrinol Metab 2006;91:1779–1784.
41 Carpinteri R, Porcelli T, Mejia C, Patelli I, Bilezikian JP, Canalis E, Angeli A, Giustina A, Mazziotti G: Glucocorticoid-induced osteoporosis and parathyroid hormone. J Endocrinol Invest 2010;33(7 suppl):16–21.

Prof. Andrea Giustina, MD, PhD
Chair of Endocrinology, University of Brescia
Via Biseo 17
IT–25123 Brescia (Italy)
E-Mail a.giustina@libero.it

Arvat E, Falorni A (eds): Cortisol Excess and Insufficiency.
Front Horm Res. Basel, Karger, 2016, vol 46, pp 74–86 (DOI: 10.1159/000443868)

Cortisol Excess and the Brain

Eugenia Resmini • Alicia Santos • Susan M. Webb

Department of Endocrinology/Medicine, Hospital Sant Pau, Centro de Investigación Biomédica en Red de Enfermedades Raras (CIBER-ER, Unidad 747), IIB-Sant Pau, ISCIII, and Universitat Autònoma de Barcelona (UAB), Barcelona, Spain

Abstract

Until the last decade, little was known about the effects of chronic hypercortisolism on the brain. In the last few years, new data have arisen thanks to advances in imaging techniques; therefore, it is now possible to investigate brain activity in vivo. Memory impairments are present in patients with Cushing's syndrome (CS) and are related to hippocampal damage; functional dysfunctions would precede structural abnormalities as detected by brain imaging. Earlier diagnosis and rapid normalization of hypercortisolism could stop the progression of hippocampal damage and memory impairments. Impairments of executive functions (including decision-making) and other functions such as visuoconstructive skills, language, motor functions and information processing speed are also present in CS patients. There is controversy concerning the reversibility of brain impairment. It seems that longer disease duration and older age are associated with less recovery of brain functioning. Conversely, earlier diagnosis and rapid normalization of hypercortisolism appear to stop progression of brain damage and functional impairments. Moreover, brain tissue functioning and neuroplasticity can be influenced by many factors. Currently available studies appear to be complementary, evaluating the same phenomenon from different points of view, but are often not directly comparable. Finally, CS patients have a high prevalence of psychopathology, such as depression and anxiety which do not completely revert after cure. Thus, psychological or psychiatric evaluation could be recommended in CS patients, so that treatment may be prescribed if required.

The brain can be divided into cortical and subcortical structures (fig. 1). The cortical structure involves the cerebral cortex (the exterior layer on the brain surface) which covers the different (frontal, temporal, parietal and occipital) lobes. Subcortical structures are those situated below the cortex. They include the hippocampus, amygdala, thalamus, hypothalamus, basal ganglia and cerebellum, among others.

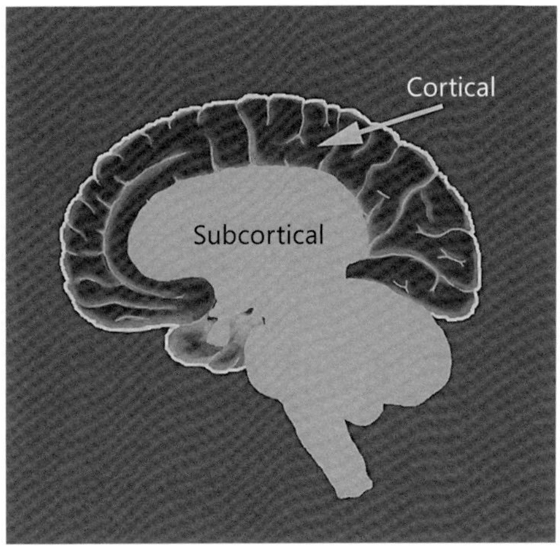

Fig. 1. Cortical and subcortical areas of the brain.

The hypothalamic-pituitary-adrenal axis plays an essential role in stress responses and stress-related psychiatric disorders. Chronic hypercortisolism during stress response leads to a cascade of processes in the brain which determine region-specific alterations in dendrite and spine morphology and reduction of neurogenesis [1]. Circulating corticosteroids reach every organ, coordinating brain and body functions towards coping with stress, recovery and adaptation.

The exact mechanisms involved in brain damage during chronic stress and/or chronic glucocorticoid (GC) exposure are poorly understood. Animal models represent an accessible substrate to study mechanisms and risk factors contributing to stress-related disorders; however, the link between animal models and the human brain is still far from clear.

Cushing's syndrome (CS), an example of chronic endogenous hypercortisolism, is associated with deficits in concentration and memory, as well as a wide range of cognitive impairments; therefore, it is a good human model to evaluate the effects of cortisol excess on the brain.

Structural and Functional Alterations

Hippocampus

The hippocampus, a subcortical brain area critical for learning and memory, is rich in GC receptors and for this reason particularly vulnerable to GC excess [1]. Animal studies have shown that the hippocampus is sensitive to both deficiency and elevation of GC [2, 3]. Administration of exogenous GC or exposure to endogenous hypercortisolism due to chronic social and experimental stress also induces changes in hippocampal pyramidal cell morphology and cell loss, impairing memory performance in animals [4]. Thus, the hippocampus is a structure particularly studied in CS patients.

Loss of volume of the hippocampus has been demonstrated to recover 1 year after surgery, in parallel with improvements in depression, anxiety, obsessive-compulsive and paranoid subscales of the Symptom Checklist 90 (SCL-90) questionnaire, which evaluates psychopathology symptoms [5].

In children with CS, loss of volume of the amygdala, a structure next to the hippocampus, did not improve after control of hypercortisolemia [6], while in adolescents, functional imaging (which reflects brain functional activations, not structure) showed greater activation in the left amygdala (related to emotional memory) and right anterior hippocampus (usually associated with verbal and visual memory, during an emotional task) [7].

A recent study has demonstrated that verbal and visual memory performance are worse in CS patients than in controls, but only the patients with severe memory impairments also have reduced hippocampal volumes (HV) [8]. In this study, brain atrophy and reduction in total and cortical gray matter volumes have also been observed in CS patients compared with controls; however, subcortical gray matter reduction has only been seen in patients with severe memory impairment, parallel to reduced HV. This would suggest that GC exposure initially determines cortical gray matter atrophy, persistent after control of hypercortisolism; only after longer exposure to GC would it also determine hippocampal reduction, especially in older subjects. Moreover, the negative effect of GC excess on memory and HV does not seem to be totally reversible after biochemical cure since there were no differences between active and cured CS, or between HV or memory performance [8].

A shorter exposure to hypercortisolism by an earlier diagnosis and successful treatment of CS would probably avert the progression of memory dysfunction and the reduction of HV, which is an important take-home message for clinicians in the daily management of these patients.

In contrast, another study described a significant increase in right and left HV in patients with Cushing's disease after transsphenoidal surgery [9]. It involved a small number of subjects who were younger than in other studies; since the resolution of MRI was lower and disease duration not indicated, comparison of the different studies is difficult.

All these available data suggest that longer disease duration and older age impact negatively on the possibility to recover brain function. Moreover, brain tissue functioning and neuroplasticity can be influenced by many factors; the currently available studies appear to be complementary because they study the same phenomenon from different points of view, but are often not directly comparable. The volume measures may be underestimating the change in neural structures [10]; indeed, it is reasonable to assume that initial functional abnormalities would precede structural abnormalities after GC overexposure since memory is generally impaired in all CS patients. Consequently, there is a need to detect brain functional abnormalities, with a non-invasive technique. ^{1}H-MR-spectroscopy is a sensitive, non-invasive imaging technique. It provides information on biochemical composition of brain tissue in vivo by measuring metabolites containing protons, allowing functional evaluation of the brain. It is routinely preceded by MRI, which is used to select a volume of interest, where proton spectra of brain metabolites will be acquired. Thus, ^{1}H-MR-spectroscopy may detect and identify subtle functional alterations in the brain, despite an apparently normal structure, by assessing concentrations of neuronal components. It can also indirectly deliver information on glial and neuronal integrity, potential cell loss and metabolic alterations in the brain, and has been used to study hippocampal metabolites in CS patients [11].

Using ^{1}H-MR-spectroscopy, persistently abnormal metabolites have been found in the head of both hippocampi of CS patients, despite endocrine cure of hypercortisolism [11]. Low levels of N-acetyl-aspartate indicate neuronal dysfunction and/or loss, while high levels of glutamate + glutamine suggest concomitant glial proliferation as a repair mechanism. These altered brain metabolites could be considered early markers of GC neurotoxicity, would precede hippocampal volume reduction and could be involved in the memory impairments evidenced in these patients [11]. These alterations could explain worse memory performance in CS patients with normal HV. Thus, an earlier diagnosis and a rapid normalization of hypercortisolism would avoid the progression of hippocampal damage and memory impairments.

Longitudinal studies to further clarify these preliminary observations would allow evaluating whether these metabolite impairments are also present in other areas of the brain of CS patients and even in patients using high doses of GC drugs.

Frontal Cortex

GC receptors are also abundant in the frontal cortex [12], an area able to inhibit and regulate hypothalamic-pituitary-adrenal responses to acute stress [13]. The frontal cortex is involved in executive functions, such as decision-making, and in emotional stress responses [14].

Hypercortisolemia secondary to stress has been related to loss of prefrontal cortex control over subcortical areas, and promotes more risk-taking behaviour [15]. In fact, Coates and Herbert [16] observed that increased cortisol levels may shift risk preferences and even affect the ability to engage in rational choices. Moreover, higher salivary cortisol levels after induced stress and exogenous administration of GC have been shown to be negatively related to decision-making in healthy subjects [17].

Neuroimaging allows accurate quantification of cortical thickness and specific MRI postprocessing software can assess gray matter alterations and correlate its structures with cognitive function. In particular, analysis of cortical thickness has been shown to be more accurate in depicting gray matter loss than other more established tools like voxel-based morphometry [18]. Frontal gray matter volume loss has been associated with impairments in decision-making in chronic alcohol consumption, which determines high circulating cortisol levels [19].

The decision-making process has been evaluated in CS patients, using the Iowa Gambling Task (IGT) and exploring its relationship with cortical thickness measured by 3-tesla MRI [20]. CS patients failed to learn advantageous strategies during the IGT and their behaviour was driven by short-term reward and long-term punishment. This suggested that CS patients had learning problems because they did not use previous experience during the test as a feedback factor to regulate their choices. Moreover, these cognitive alterations were accompanied by decreased cortical thickness, mainly in specific frontal areas (the left superior frontal cortex, left precentral cortex, left insular cortex, left and right rostral anterior cingulate cortex, and right caudal middle frontal cortex).

The hippocampus may interact with the frontal cortex to sustain emotional regulation and to maintain contextual information needed to represent and monitor motivationally relevant goals. The relationship between lower performance in verbal memory (a function related to the hippocampus) and impaired decision-making (a function related to the frontal cortex) showed in this study supports this idea.

Interestingly, no differences have been evidenced between patients cured of CS and those with active hypercortisolism, suggesting an incomplete recovery of the gray matter of the brain after endocrine remission of hypercortisolism [20]. These neuropsychological and morphological frontal alterations described after cortisol normalization provide further support to the concept that chronic hypercortisolism promotes brain changes which are not completely reversible after endocrine remission. Awareness of these persistent alterations would justify a specific neuropsychological assessment of patients exposed to high cortisol levels.

Cerebellum

Animal studies have demonstrated a high density of GC receptors in the cerebellum [21], a structure classically related to motor control, coordination and balance. Nevertheless, it is also involved in emotional control and many cognitive functions, including executive functions, memory (visual, declarative, procedural and verbal working), visuospatial skills, information processing speed, fluency, language and emotional processing [22].

Cerebellar atrophy has been found in patients suffering from depression and post-traumatic stress disorder, two situations where hypercortisolism is supposed to be involved. Additionally, cerebellar reduction has also been found in patients with rheumatoid arthritis who require GC treatment. Cerebellar volume has also been studied in both active and remitted CS patients [22]. Active CS patients had a smaller cerebellar cortex than controls, but not patients in remission. Interestingly, cerebellar volumes were negatively correlated to circulating triglyceride levels and age, so patients with higher triglycerides and older age at diagnosis had the smallest cerebellar cortex [22]. These data suggest that high triglycerides, together with cortisol exposure, could have an aging-like effect, inducing a volumetric reduction of the cerebellum. Aging is known to lead to a volumetric reduction of several parts of the brain, including the cerebellum. On the other hand, aging is usually related to reduced neurogenesis; therefore, suffering from CS at an older age could also be a risk for smaller cerebellar volume. Additionally, right cerebellar cortex volume positively correlated to quality of life, measured with the Cushing QoL questionnaire. This finding, not reported before, may be explained by the involvement of the cerebellum in the modulation of emotional responses. Finally, the left cerebellar cortex volume was correlated to visual memory, indicating that patients with a smaller cerebellar cortex volume would also have poorer visual memory.

The fact that patients in remission did not have smaller cerebellar cortex volumes is encouraging, suggesting that cerebellar reduction during GC excess may be reversible, at least in part. In fact, another study in CS patients in remission found an increase of the left posterior lobe of the cerebellum in comparison to healthy controls [23]. According to the authors, after chronic exposure to hypercortisolism, a neuronal reorganization may occur in the brain, leading to dendritic hypertrophy in some structures and to atrophy in others. Longitudinal studies will be necessary in the future to confirm these hypotheses.

Other Brain Areas

Few data are available on the effect of chronic GC exposure to other brain regions; however, long-term exposure to hypercortisolism damages neuronal cells [3, 4, 24]. Hypercortisolism in CS has been associated with loss of global cerebral volume, although a loss of brain cells has not been clearly demonstrated [25]. Increased widths of the 3rd ventricle or the bicaudate diameter were also described as partially reversible after control of hypercortisolism [26]. CS patients had smaller gray matter volumes in the anterior cingulate cortex compared with controls [23].

The pathogenesis of brain volume loss induced by chronic GC excess is probably multifactorial [26], but the mechanisms involved are not fully understood. They may include effects of GC on several growth factors and receptors including brain-derived neurotrophic factor, nerve growth factor, basal fibroblast growth factor and vascular mechanisms. Most studies of the effects of GC on the brain have been conducted essentially in hippocampal cells in culture and it is unknown whether the same mechanisms apply to neurons in other brain regions.

Widespread changes of white matter integrity in the brain, related to the severity of depression, have also been described in CS patients in remission, suggesting persistent structural effects of hypercortisolism [27]. The potential reversibility of the premature loss of brain volume in CS after correction of hypercortisolism seems to depend on age and disease duration, as previously reported. Indeed, signs of cerebral atrophy should be evaluated in patients suffering from CS, and all of the brain regions should be evaluated.

Cognitive and Psychological Alterations

Memory

Memory is the most studied cognitive function in hypercortisolism, and impairments in both verbal and visual memory have been described. In the 1980s, Whelan et al. [28] already noticed that two thirds of their CS patients had some sort of cognitive deficit. In particular, 37% of the patients had alterations in visual memory, showing a poor performance on the Benton Visual Retention Test, and 31% of the patients had alterations in verbal memory, showing a poor performance in Memory for Unrelated Sentences from the Michigan Neuropsychological Test Battery.

Several studies later confirmed deficient memory in hypercortisolemic patients. For verbal memory, in 2000 Forget et al. [29] found impairments measured with the California Verbal Learning Test and León-Carrión et al. [30] also found a poorer performance in verbal memory than controls in a sample of 15 active CS patients. There is some controversy regarding logical memory, as two studies found poor performance in CS patients [31, 32] while another did not [29]. On the other hand, poor performance on learning and delayed recall on paired associates from the Wechsler Memory Scale (WMS) has also been found [32]. Regarding visual memory, several studies have found poorer performance in CS patients in comparison to controls (measured with the Visual Memory Test from the WMS) [29, 31, 33], and only one study did not find any impairment [32]. Santos et al. [22] also found that patients with active CS had a worse performance than controls in visual memory measured with the Rey-Osterrieth complex figure (ROCF).

The reversibility of these problems is still matter of debate. There is data suggesting an improvement in memory after hypercortisolism control in verbal memory in a small sample of 7 patients [34], and in logic memory, both learning and retrieval improved after surgery in a small sample of 8 patients [31]. Another study also found improvements in learning (52% of the patients in logical memory learning, 61% of the patients in paired associates learning and 53% on the Selective Reminding Test) [35]. A longitudinal study found an improvement in the Selective Reminding Test list-learning task, with younger patients having quicker improvement than older patients (at 3–5 vs. at 13–18 months) [36]. By contrast, another longitudinal study did not find any visual or verbal memory improvement in 13 CS patients 1 year after surgery [37].

Nevertheless, it seems that some degree of memory impairment may still be present after endocrine cure [38]. Resmini et al. [8] found verbal and visual memory impairments in a sample of 33 patients (22 cured) measured with the ROCF and the Rey Auditory Verbal Learning Task. Furthermore, Tiemensma et al. [38] studied a large cohort of 74 patients in remission and found poorer associative learning in the WMS than with controls (but not in comparison to non-functioning pituitary adenomas). In addition, they found a worse memory quotient in the WMS and poorer performance in the visual memory test ROCF (immediate and delayed recall) in comparison to both controls and non-functioning adenomas.

Executive Functions and Attention

Several studies in CS have found some sort of attention or executive dysfunction, even if there is some controversy on the exact neuropsychological tests which are impaired. Executive functions involve multiple capacities that help to regulate behaviour and skills, such as the ability to focus attention and select relevant information, planning, abstract thinking, inhibition, rule acquisition, or flexibility.

Regarding working memory (measured with the digit span backwards test), data are controversial as one study found poorer performance than controls [31] while two did not [22, 29]. The same occurs for Trail Making Test B scores, a test which evaluates both working memory and task-switching ability, as some studies have found impairment [29, 33] while another did not [31]. Nevertheless, these impairments are not seen in patients in remission [38, 39].

Similar results are found for verbal fluency. One study found poorer performance in comparison to controls in letter and category fluency [29], although others did not [22, 31]. However, improvement was found after treatment in a longitudinal study [36], and interestingly there was an age effect (only younger patients improved). Unfortunately, this may not mean complete recovery of fluency skills, as even patients in remission who demonstrate normal fluency show poorer figure fluency in comparison to non-functioning pituitary adenomas [38].

Regarding inhibition, one study found poorer performance in active patients than controls in the colour naming with interference of the Stroop Test [29], while another did not [30]. However, this impairment was not found in patients in remission [38], although planning measured with the Tower of Hanoi test does not seem to be impaired in CS [30]. Crespo et al. [20], using the IGT, did observe that CS patients had decision-making problems.

A pattern of high number of intrusions or repetitions in neuropsychological tests is usually an indicator of executive dysfunction. This was found in two studies with active CS patients using Luria's Memory Words Revised [30] and the California Verbal Learning Test [33]; in a study with patients in remission, a higher number of repetitions in the Figure Fluency Test was found [38].

Some studies have reported attention impairments in CS. These patients had a similar performance to that of controls aged 15 years older in several attention tasks, while they performed worse than controls matched for age (Visual Target Detection, Trail Making Test A and Stroop) [33]. Nevertheless, selective attention, measured with the Bells Test or with an adapted letter cancellation task, does not seem to be impaired in active CS patients [29, 30], and attention span, measured with the digit span forward test, was impaired in active CS patients in one study [29] but not in another [31]. Information in longitudinal studies regarding improvement after cure is also controversial [31, 36, 37]. Nevertheless, studies of patients in remission indicate that they are still impaired [39] and tend to have poorer concentration than controls measured with the WMS [38]. For sustained attention, similar performance was found in patients in remission in comparison to controls using the Attention Network Test [39].

Other Cognitive Functions

Most studies involving CS have found some sort of impairment in other cognitive functions, although not all agree on the exact functions that are impaired. A summary of the findings on the different studies involving cognitive function in CS can be found in table 1.

Table 1. Summary of findings on the different studies involving CS: cognitive impairment or improvement in different neuropsychological functions

Cognitive function	Impairment or poorer performance than controls found?		Improvement after cure?	
	yes	no	yes	no
Memory				
Verbal	8[a], 28–31, 38[b]		31, 34–36	37
Visual	8[a], 22, 28, 29, 31, 33, 38[b]	32		37
Executive functions and attention				
Working memory	29, 31, 33	22, 38[b]		
Verbal fluency	29	22, 31, 38[b]	36	
Inhibition	29	30, 38[b]		
Planning		30		
Decision-making	20[a]			
Attention				
Selective	29, 33, 38[b]	30, 31	31	36, 37
Sustained		39[b]		
Other functions				
Visuoconstructive skills	29, 31–33, 37	22, 30	37, 40	
Language	29, 31, 32	22, 33	35	
Motor functions	22[b], 28, 29	31, 32, 38[b], 39[b]		
Information processing speed	29, 31, 38[b], 39[b], 40	32		

Numbers refer to studies in the reference list. [a] Involved a sample that included together both patients with active CS and patients in remission. [b] Involved only patients in remission.

Several studies have found poorer performance than in controls in tests evaluating visuoconstructive skills, such as object assembly, block design or visual reproduction [29, 31, 32, 33, 37], but one did not [22]. It is important to mention that the version of these tests differed between studies. Even if a longitudinal study found a slight increase in block design and object assembly scores 1 year after cure, this also occurred in controls, suggesting that this improvement may be independent of hypercortisolism [40]. In fact, these improvements in both tests were not found in another longitudinal study which re-evaluated 13 CS patients, in which improvements in another visuospatial task (Hooper Visual Organization) were found [37]. For other tests involving visuospatial skills, namely Judgement Line Orientation, Corsi's Tests or the Street Completion Test, no impairment was found in CS patients [29, 30].

Regarding language, results are also controversial, as some of the studies found poorer performance than controls measured with vocabulary and comprehension [29, 31, 32], while other studies did not [22, 33]. Another suggested that 25% of the patients improved on the vocabulary test after remission [35].

Regarding arithmetic performance, Whelan et al. [28] found impairment in 41% of his patients. One study also found poorer performance in active patients than controls [32], while two did not [29, 33]. Interestingly, another study found an improvement in 50% of the patients after cure [35].

Results regarding motor functions are also controversial. In the 1980s, Whelan et al. [28] found that 40% of the patients had impairment in a fine motor task (Purdue Pegboard), while differences were not found in another study [32]. For the Grooved Pegboard, another fine motor task, a recent study showed that only patients in remission had a tendency to poor performance [22]. Nevertheless, the small sample of patients with active CS enrolled in these studies may have precluded finding impairments. For Trail Making Test A, a task which requires gross motor skills, some studies found poorer performance in active CS patients than controls [29], while others did not [22, 31], although performance in patients in remission seemed to be normal [38, 39].

Most studies have found impairment on the Symbol Digit Substitution Test, a test that involves several neuropsychological components (including information processing speed, attention capacity, working memory and motor speed) [29, 31, 40], while only one did not [32]. In fact, impairment was still present in CS patients in remission [38, 39].

In conclusion, apart from memory, there is still a need to understand the impact of prior exposure to chronic hypercortisolism on cognition and the involved mechanisms. However, many studies in CS patients in remission have still found impairment after cure in different cognitive functions [41]. The heterogeneity of results suggests that different mechanisms may be involved in cognitive alterations, which are perhaps mediated by chronic exposure to hypercortisolism. Moreover, cardiovascular risk has been also recently associated with impairments in cognitive function [42]. Investigations involving larger samples of patients with active CS would be of great interest to analyse the impact of possible confounding factors. On the other hand, longitudinal studies including a high number of patients and followed over longer periods would be helpful to clarify exactly which aspects can improve after control of hypercortisolism.

Psychopathology and Personality

CS has been related to significant psychopathology [43]. Most studies agree that hypercortisolism may lead to increased anxiety and depression, which is still present even after biological cure [22, 39, 44]. Depression is usually the most prevalent characteristic, and has been associated with female sex, older age, higher baseline urinary cortisol, more severe clinical condition and absence of detectable pituitary adenoma [45].

There are few data describing an improvement in depressed mood, anxiety or somatic symptoms after cortisol normalization [37]. Dorn et al. [43] found that the presence of psychopathology decreased after cure. Using the SCL-90, improvements were found after treatment in the subscales of somatization, depression, anxiety, obsessive-compulsion and paranoid ideation in one study [5].

Regarding personality, Sonino et al. [46] did not find specific differences between patients in remission and controls in any personality dimensions measured with the Tridimensional Personality Questionnaire. Nevertheless, a larger subsequent study found an increased prevalence of maladaptive personality traits in patients in remission. They showed worse performance than non-functioning pituitary adenomas in 11 of 18 personality scales [47]. When patients were compared to healthy controls they had worse performance on 10 subscales, although when depression and anxiety were included as covariates only affective lability and anxiousness remained significant [44].

In conclusion, CS patients seem to have a high prevalence of psychopathology, which very often involves depression and anxiety, and does not completely revert after endocrine cure. Psychological or psychiatric evaluation may be recommended in CS patients, and treatment prescribed if required.

References

1 Joëls M, Karst H, Krugers HJ, Lucassen PJ: Chronic stress: implications for neuronal morphology, function and neurogenesis. Front Neuroendocrinol 2007;28:72–96.

2 Sapolsky RM, Stein-Behrens BA, Armanini MP: Long-term adrenalectomy causes loss of dentate gyrus and pyramidal neurons in the adult hippocampus. Exp Neurol 1990;114:246–249.

3 Watanabe Y, Gould E, McEwen BS: Stress induces atrophy of apical dendrites of hippocampus CA3 pyramidal neurons. Brain Res 1992;588:341–345.

4 Sapolsky RM, Uno H, Rebert CS, Finch CE: Hippocampal damage associated with prolonged glucocorticoid exposure in primates. J Neurosci 1990;10:2897–2902.

5 Starkman MN, Giordani B, Gebarski SS, Schteingart DE: Improvement in mood and ideation associated with increase in right caudate volume. J Affect Disord 2007;101:139–147.

6 Merke DP, Giedd JN, Keil MF, Mehlinger SL, Wiggs EA, Holzer S, Rawson E, Vaituzis AC, Stratakis CA, Chrousos GP: Children experience cognitive decline despite reversal of brain atrophy one year after resolution of Cushing's syndrome. J Clin Endocrinol Metab 2005;90:2531–2536.

7 Maheu FS, Mazzone L, Merke DP, Keil MF, Stratakis CA, Pine DS, Ernst M: Altered amygdala and hippocampus function in adolescents with hypercortisolemia: a functional magnetic resonance imaging study of Cushing syndrome. Dev Psychopathol 2008;20:1177–1189.

8 Resmini E, Santos A, Gómez-Anson B, Vives Y, Pires P, Crespo I, Portella MJ, de Juan-Delago M, Barahona MJ, Webb SM: Verbal and visual memory performance and hippocampal volumes, measured by 3-Tesla magnetic resonance imaging, in patients with Cushing's syndrome. J Clin Endocrinol Metab 2012;97:663–671.

9 Toffanin T, Nifosì F, Follador H, Passamani A, Zonta F, Ferri G, Scanarini M, Amistà P, Pigato G, Scaroni C, Mantero F, Carollo C, Perini GI: Volumetric MRI analysis of hippocampal subregions in Cushing's disease: a model for glucocorticoids neural modulation. Eur Psychiatry 2011;26:64–67.

10 Patil CG, Lad SP, Katznelson L, Laws ER Jr: Brain atrophy and cognitive deficits in Cushing's disease. Neurosurg Focus 2007;23:E11.

11 Resmini E, Santos A, Gómez-Anson B, López-Mourelo O, Pires P, Vives-Gilabert Y, Crespo I, Portella MJ, de Juan-Delago M, Webb SM: Hippocampal dysfunction in cured Cushing's syndrome patients, detected by ^{1}H-MR-spectroscopy. Clin Endocrinol (Oxf) 2013;79:700–707.

12 Sánchez MM, Young LJ, Plotsky PM, Insel TR: Distribution of glucocorticoid receptors in the rhesus brain: relative absence of glucocorticoid receptors in the hippocampal formation. J Neurosci 2000;20:4657–4668.

13 Radley JJ, Rocher AB, Miller M, Janssen WG, Liston C, Hof PR, McEwen BS, Morrison JH: Repeated stress induces dendritic spine loss in the rat medial prefrontal cortex. Cereb Cortex 2006;16:313–320.

14 Miller EK, Freedman DJ, Wallis JD: The prefrontal cortex: categories, concepts and cognition. Phil Trans R Soc Lond B Biol Sci 2002;357:1123–1136.

15 De Kloet R, Joëls M, Holsboer F: Stress and the brain, from adaptation to disease. Nat Rev Neurosci 2005;6:463–475.

16 Coates JM, Herbert J: Endogenous steroids and financial risk taking on a London trading floor. Proc Natl Acad Sci USA 2008;105:6167–6172.
17 Santos-Ruiz A, García-Rios MC, Fernández-Sánchez JC, Pérez-Garcia M, Muñoz-Garcia MA, Peralta-Ramirez MI: Can decision-making skills affect responses to psychological stress in healthy women? Psychoneuroendocrinology 2012;37:1912–1921.
18 Pereira JB, Ibarretxe-Bilbao N, Marti MJ, Compta Y, Junqué C, Bargallo N, Tolosa E: Assessment of cortical degeneration in patients with Parkinson's disease by voxel-based morphometry, cortical folding, and cortical thickness. Hum Brain Mapp 2012;33:2521–2534.
19 Le Berre AP, Rauchs G, La Joie R, Mézenge F, Boudehent C, Vabret F, Segobin S, Viader F, Allain P, Eustache F, Pitel AL, Beaunieux H: Impaired decision-making and brain shrinkage in alcoholism. Eur Psychiatry 2014;29:125–133.
20 Crespo I, Granell E, Santos A, Valassi E, Vives-Gilabert Y, De Juan-Delago M, Webb SM, Gómez-Ansón B, Resmini E: Impaired decision-making and selective cortical frontal thinning in Cushing's syndrome. Clin Endocrinol (Oxf) 2014 Dec;81:826–833.
21 Sánchez MM, Young LJ, Plotsky PM, Insel TR: Distribution of corticosteroid receptors in the rhesus brain: relative absence of glucocorticoid receptors in the hippocampal formation. J Neurosci 2000;20:4657–4668.
22 Santos A, Resmini E, Crespo I, Pires P, Vives-Gilabert Y, Granell E, Valassi E, Gómez-Ansón B, Martínez-Momblán MA, Mataró M, Webb SM: Small cerebellar cortex volume in patients with active Cushing's syndrome. Eur J Endocrinol 2014;171:461–469.
23 Andela CD, van der Werff SJ, Pannekoek JN, van den Berg SM, Meijer OC, van Buchem MA, Rombousts SA, van der Mast RC, Romijn JA, Tiemensma J, Biermasz NR, van der Wee NJ, Pereira AM: Smaller grey matter volumes in the anterior cingulate cortex and greater cerebellar volumes in patients with long-term remission of Cushing's disease: a case-control study. Eur J Endocrinol 2013;169:811–819.
24 Swaab DF, Bao AM, Lucassen PJ: The stress system in the human brain in depression and neurodegeneration. Ageing Res Rev 2005;4:141–194.
25 Bourdeau I, Bard C, Forget H, Boulanger Y, Cohen H, Lacroix A: Cognitive function and cerebral assessment in patients who have Cushing's Syndrome. Endocrinol Metab Clin North Am 2005;34:357–369.
26 Bourdeau I, Bard C, Noel B, Leclerc I, Cordeau MP, Belair M, Lesage J, Lafontaine L, Lacroix A: Loss of brain volume in endogenous Cushing's syndrome and its reversibility after correction of hypercortisolism. J Clin Endocrinol Metab 2002;87:1949–1954.
27 Van der Werff SJ, Andela CD, Nienke Pannekoek J, Meijer OC, van Buchem MA, Rombouts SA, van der Mast RC, Biermasz NR, Pereira AM, van der Wee NJ: Widespread reductions of white matter integrity in patients with long-term remission of Cushing's disease. Neuroimage Clin 2014;4:659–667.
28 Whelan TB, Schteingart DE, Starkman MN, Smith A: Neuropsychological deficits in Cushing's syndrome. J Nerv Ment Dis 1980;168:753–757.
29 Forget H, Lacroix A, Somma M, Cohen H: Cognitive decline in patients with Cushing's syndrome. J Intl Neuropsychol Soc 2000;6:20–29.
30 León-Carrión J, Atutxa AM, Mangas MA, Soto-Moreno A, Pumar A, Leon-Justel A, Martín-Rodriguez JF, Venegas E, Domínguez-Morales MR, Leal-Cerro A: A clinical profile of memory impairment in humans due to endogenous glucocorticoid excess. Clin Endocrinol (Oxf) 2009;70:192–200.
31 Mauri M, Sinforiani E, Bono G, Vignati F, Berselli ME, Attanasio R, Nappi G: Memory impairment in Cushing's disease. Acta Neurol Scand 1993;87:52–55.
32 Starkman MN, Giordani B, Berent S, Schork MA, Schteingart DE: Elevated cortisol levels in Cushing's disease are associated with cognitive decrements. Psychosom Med 2001;63:985–993.
33 Michaud K, Forget H, Cohen H: Chronic glucocorticoid hypersecretion in Cushing's syndrome exacerbates cognitive aging. Brain Cogn 2009;71:1–8.
34 Martignoni E, Costa A, Sinforiani E, Liuzzi A, Chiodini P, Mauri M, Bono G, Nappi G: The brain as a target for adrenocortical steroids: cognitive implications. Psychoneuroendocrinology 1992;17:343–354.
35 Starkman MN, Giordani B, Gebarski SS, Schteingart DE: Improvement in learning associated with increase in hippocampal formation volume. Biol Psychiatry 2003;53:233–238.
36 Hook JN, Giordani B, Schteingart DE, Guire K, Giles J, Ryan K, Gebarski SS, Langenecker SA, Starkman MN: Patterns of cognitive change over time and relationship to age following successful treatment of Cushing's disease. J Int Neuropsychol Soc 2007;13:21–29.
37 Forget H, Lacroix A, Cohen H: Persistent cognitive impairment following surgical treatment of Cushing's syndrome. Psychoneuroendocrinology 2002;27:367–383.
38 Tiemensma J,Koksoorn NE, Biermasz NR, Keijser BJ, Wassenaar MJ, Middelkoop HA, Pereira AM, Romijn JA: Subtle cognitive impairments in patients with long-term cure of Cushing's disease. J Clin Endocrinol Metab 2010;95:2699–2714.
39 Ragnarsson O, Berglund P, Eder DN, Johannsson G: Long-term cognitive impairments and attentional deficits in patients with Cushing's disease and cortisol-producing adrenal adenoma in remission. J Clin Endocrinol Metab 2012;97:1640–1648.

40 Dorn LD, Cerrone P: Cognitive function in patients with Cushing syndrome: a longitudinal perspective. Clin Nurs Res 2000;9:420–440.
41 Andela CD, van Haalen FM, Ragnarsson O, Papakokkinou E, Johannsson G, Santos A, Webb SM, Biermasz NR, van der Wee NJ, Pereira AM: MECHANISMS IN ENDOCRINOLOGY: Cushing's syndrome causes irreversible effects on the human brain: a systematic review of structural and functional magnetic resonance imaging studies. Eur J Endocrinol 2015;173:R1–R14.
42 Santos A, Resmini E, Gómez-Ansón B, Crespo I, Granell E, Valassi E, Pires P, Vives-Gilabert Y, Martínez-Momblán MA, de Juan M, Mataró M, Webb SM: Cardiovascular risk and white matter lesions after endocrine control of Cushing's syndrome. Eur J Endocrinol 2015;173:765–775.
43 Dorn LD, Burgess ES, Friedman TC, Dubbert B, Gold PW, Chrousos GP: The longitudinal course of psychopathology in Cushing's syndrome after correction of hypercortisolism. J Clin Endocrinol Metab 1997;82:912–919.
44 Tiemensma J, Biermasz NR, Middelkoop HA, van der Masr RC, Romijn JA, Pereira AM: Increased prevalence of psychopathology and maladaptative personality traits after long-term cure of Cushing's disease. J Clin Endocrinol Metab 2010;95:129–141.
45 Sonino N, Fava GA, Raffi AR, Boscaro M, Fallo F: Clinical correlates of major depression in Cushing's disease. Psychopathology 1998;31:302–306.
46 Sonino N, Bonnini S, Fallo F, Boscaro M, Fava GA: Personality characteristics and quality of life in patients treated for Cushing's syndrome. Clin Endocrinol (Oxf) 2006;64:314–318.
47 Sonino N, Ruini C, Navarrini C, Ottolini F, Sirri L, Paoletta A, Fallo F, Boscaro M, Fava GA: Psychosocial impairment in patients treated for pituitary disease: a controlled study. Clin Endocrinol (Oxf) 2007;67:719–726.

Eugenia Resmini, MD, PhD
Department of Endocrinology, Hospital de Sant Pau
C.S. Antoni Maria Claret 167
ES–08025 Barcelona (Spain)
E-Mail eresmini@santpau.cat

Arvat E, Falorni A (eds): Cortisol Excess and Insufficiency.
Front Horm Res. Basel, Karger, 2016, vol 46, pp 87–105 (DOI: 10.1159/000443869)

Update on Hypercortisolism Therapy

Giorgio Arnaldi • Laura Trementino

Clinic of Endocrinology and Metabolic Diseases, Ospedali Riuniti di Ancona University Hospital, Ancona, Italy

Abstract

Treating Cushing's syndrome is very challenging and should be tailored to the patient. Surgery is considered the gold standard treatment for both pituitary adrenocorticotropic hormone (ACTH)-secreting adenomas, ectopic ACTH-secreting tumors and adrenal tumors, as the chance to be successful is high, especially for adrenal tumors, when performed in specialized centers by expert surgeons. Pituitary radiotherapy represents a second-line treatment in patients not cured with surgery, or when medical treatment is not suitable/efficacious, although the rate of cure is largely variable and achieved only in the long term, and is associated with the risk of developing secondary hypopituitarism. Several drugs, acting at the pituitary, adrenal or peripheral tissue level, are available. Medical treatment is indicated as second-line therapy for patients unsuccessfully treated with pituitary surgery, or in those awaiting radiotherapy to become effective, or prior to adrenalectomy, and as the first-line approach to prepare patients for surgery, especially those with severe comorbidities, or in those not suitable/refusing surgery. The success rate of medical therapy is variable, depending on the cause and severity of hypercortisolism, and is often associated with important side effects.

In the majority of patients, endogenous chronic cortisol excess or Cushing's syndrome (CS) is due to an adrenocorticotropic hormone (ACTH)-secreting pituitary adenoma or Cushing's disease (CD). Other possible causes are ectopic ACTH-secreting tumors, and benign and malignant glucocorticoid (GC)-producing adrenocortical tumors [1–3]. Hypercortisolism, regardless of the cause, is characterized by a complex phenotype that includes obesity, muscle weakness, hypertension, diabetes mellitus, dyslipidemia, hypercoagulability, osteoporosis and bone fractures, menstrual disorders, cognitive impairment, and depression [4, 5]. It is also associated with increased mortality, mainly due to cardiovascular disorders, venous thrombotic disease or infectious diseases. Indeed, recent data show that, with effective therapy, survival is not different from the general population, whereas persistent/recurrent disease is associated with poor outcome (2.8- to 16-fold greater than the general population risk) [6, 7]. For these reasons, it is important to normalize cortisol secretion as rapidly as possible.

Surgery

Surgery is the gold standard treatment for hypercortisolism (i.e. adrenalectomy for adrenal tumor(s) or adrenal hyperplasia, selective transsphenoidal pituitary adenomectomy for ACTH-secreting pituitary adenomas). The surgeon's experience is a major determinant for the outcome of pituitary surgery, which remains very challenging (65–90% remission rates in patients with microadenomas and approximately 46% for macroadenomas) [8]. Whether preoperative MRI identification of the tumor improves the surgical outcome remains debatable.

The endoscopic transsphenoidal approach improves the panoramic visualization through the wide angle of view and powerful light devices. For this reason, this technique has progressively replaced microscopic transsphenoidal surgery in many specialized centers [9, 10]. Surgical outcomes appear similar between the microscopic and endoscopic techniques, especially in microadenomas, although a direct comparison is not possible [11]. Recently, the endoscopic approach has shown excellent results in the treatment of pediatric patients with CD [12].

The complication rates of pituitary surgery are relatively low in expert centers. In a survey of 18 retrospective series involving more than 3,000 patients (all with at least 40 patients with a follow-up of ≥6 months), the prevalence of anterior pituitary damage was <20% in most series (range 2–41) and 3–9% for permanent diabetes insipidus, with the risk of hypopituitarism related to the extension of the hypophysectomy. Other less common surgical complications include cerebrospinal fluid leak (0–8%), meningitis (0–3%), neurological deficits (0–2%), hematomas (<1%), thromboembolic events (0–4%), and wound or nasoseptal complications (0–4%) [13].

Unfortunately, postsurgical recurrence of CD is higher than in other pituitary tumors: 5–10% at 5 years and 10–20% at 10 years, with young age being a significant risk factor for relapse. The median interval of recurrence ranges from 2.3 to 7.2 years after pituitary surgery, although the risk of relapse persists over 10 years [8]. In other words, undetectable postoperative cortisol values predict a more positive outcome but do not eliminate the possibility of recurrence, even during long-term follow-up.

The management of patients with persistent or recurrent CD after surgery is controversial. Treatment options include secondary pituitary surgery, pituitary radiotherapy (RT) and bilateral adrenalectomy, although no treatment has proven to be fully satisfactory. The size and shape of the residual tumor can be used to establish which patients are candidates for repeated surgery, although there is an overall lower rate of success than the initial operation and a significantly higher risk of hypopituitarism [8]. A multidisciplinary approach is required to identify and select the combination of treatments for each patient [14].

In skilled hands adrenal tumors can be successfully treated by unilateral laparoscopic adrenalectomy, which is curative in most cases of adrenal CS. Resection of an ectopic ACTH-producing tumor is curative in the absence of metastatic disease.

Pituitary Radiotherapy

Pituitary RT is a second-line treatment for persistent hypercortisolism when surgery fails. Interestingly, the first patient with hypercortisolism treated with pituitary RT was reported by Harvey Cushing himself. In conventional RT treatments, a total dose of 35–55 Gray (Gy) is administered in daily fractions of 1.8–2 Gy over 4–5 weeks. Stereotactic irradiation can be given as a single-fraction dose using a multiheaded cobalt unit (Gamma Knife), a linear accelerator (LINAC) or a proton beam. In addition, there are reports of some success by CyberKnife RT for CD in small numbers of patients. Generally, a single dose of 20 Gy is biologically equivalent to a fractionated dose of 50–110 Gy [15, 16].

RT is efficacious in controlling hypercortisolemia in approximately 50–60% of patients within 2–5 years, and success rates increase over time (up to 89% has been reported). However, the results are very different between series, depending on the doses administered, time of follow-up, criteria used to define disease control and patient selection. It is noteworthy that tumor volume was better controlled than cortisol levels, ranging from 83 to 100% [17–19]. Similarly to what happens in patients treated with surgery, recurrences may occur even several years after RT, so long-term monitoring is required [8].

Despite the initial enthusiasm, the outcomes of stereotactic radiosurgery have been shown to be similar to fractionated RT. In particular, there is no clear evidence that radiosurgery reduces the time needed to achieve disease control or the risk of hypopituitarism (50–70% of the cases), which represent the most important disadvantages associated with RT, thus requiring regular monitoring of pituitary function and special attention to suggestive symptoms. Other radiation risks include neuropathy of the optic (1–2%) and other cranial (2–4%) nerves, and secondary neoplasia within the radiation field (mostly meningiomas). Data are not sufficient to establish the effects of RT on cerebrovascular and neurocognitive function [20, 21].

Awaiting the beneficial effect of RT, patients should be treated with medical therapy to reduce hypercortisolism. Medical treatment should then be withdrawn at 6- to 12-month intervals to evaluate RT efficacy.

Bilateral Adrenalectomy

Bilateral adrenalectomy, preferably performed by laparoscopic approach, provides immediate cure in patients with CD treated unsuccessfully by surgery and/or RT. Additional indications are ectopic ACTH tumors when the source remains occult or cannot be removed, and bilateral primary adrenal hypercortisolism (primary pigmented nodular adrenocortical disease and ACTH-independent macronodular adrenocortical hyperplasia) [22].

Unexpectedly, up to 10% of patients experience recurrence years after bilateral adrenalectomy, due to adrenal remnants or accessory glands. A recent review including 1,320 patients showed a surgical morbidity of 18% and a median mortality of 3%. In particular, in CD patients the surgical mortality was <1%. Adrenal crises occurred in 9.3 cases/100 patients/year. Overall mortality was 17% during a 41-month (range: 14–294) follow-up, with 46% of the cases registered within the first year after surgery, suggesting the importance of a careful management of morbidities [23]. Apart from surgical risk, major issues related to bilateral adrenalectomy are the need for lifelong monitoring of GC- and mineralocorticoid-replacement therapy and the risk of Nelson's syndrome (29–47% at 10 years) [24].

The management of Nelson's syndrome or corticotroph tumor progression is still debated. It has been pointed out that the risk and time of progression are variable, and not accelerated by pregnancy; it can be detected early by repeated plasma ACTH assays and pituitary MRI follow-up, and, when it occurs, early stages are manageable [14]. A visible remnant and increased plasma ACTH levels are considered risk factors [25]. Routine pituitary RT after adrenalectomy has been suggested, but not routinely performed [14].

Medical Treatment

The rationale for medical treatment varies considerably, ranging from a temporary and palliative measure, to a resource in the management of difficult cases. Indeed, medical therapy represents a second-line treatment in patients unsuccessfully treated with pituitary surgery, or in those waiting for RT to become effective, prior to adrenalectomy. Moreover, it can be used as a first-line approach to prepare patients for surgery, especially those with severe comorbidities like diabetes, hypertension and marked coagulation abnormalities. Finally, it is an option for all patients who are not suitable for surgery, have few chances of surgical cure or refuse surgery [8].

Targets of medical treatment can be at the pituitary, adrenal or peripheral tissue level. Drugs include inhibitors of ACTH secretion, steroidogenesis inhibitors and GC receptor antagonists [8, 26]. The main features of the various medical treatments are summarized in table 1.

Table 1. Main features of currently available drugs for the treatment of CS

Drug	Administration	Daily dosage	Efficacy (UFC 24 h normalized)	Adverse effects	Notes
Pituitary-directed drugs					
Cabergoline	Orally weekly (fractionated)	1–7 mg	30–40%	Dizziness and nausea Cardiac valvulopathy?	Relatively small studies; escape; low cost; off-label use
Pasireotide	Subcutaneously twice a day	450–1,200 μg	26% (67% in clinical practice)	Hyperglycemia, diarrhea, nausea, cholelithiasis, hypocortisolism	The only drug approved after RCT; diabetes mellitus risk; better efficacy in mild hypercortisolism; rapid onset of action
Adrenal-directed drugs					
Ketoconazole	Orally twice/ thrice a day	400–1,200 mg	45–49%	Hepatotoxicity, gastrointestinal disturbances, hypocortisolism, male hypogonadism and gynecomastia	Rare severe; hepatotoxicity → need for close monitoring of liver function; important drug interactions; acidic gastric environment is necessary for optimal absorption; rapid onset of action; off-label use in many countries
Metyrapone	Orally thrice a day	750–5,000 mg	43%	Hirsutism, acne, hypokalemia, hypertension, nausea, hypocortisolism	Increase of androgens may limit the long-term use in women; increase of mineralocorticoid precursors may cause hypokalemia, edema and hypertension; a reliable cortisol assay without cross-reactivity with precursors is needed; used during pregnancy, although efficacy and safety not fully established; rapid onset of action; off-label use in many countries
Mitotane	Orally twice/thrice a day	500–6,000 mg	72–80%	Gastrointestinal and neurologic disturbances, hypercholesterolemia, hypothyroidism, male hypogonadism, hypocortisolism	Poor tolerability; need for mitotanemia monitoring; increase of CBG with limitation in measurement of serum cortisol; slow onset of action; approved for adrenal cancer
Etomidate	Intravenously (bolus followed by infusion)	0.03 mg/kg/h		Sedation, myoclonus, hypotension, hypocortisolism	Requires monitoring for ICU; rapid onset of action; off-label use
GC-receptor blockade					
Mifepristone	Orally once a day	300–600 mg	60% diabetics (clinical improvement due to lack of biomarker)	Hypokalemia, hypertension, hypocortisolism, fatigue, nausea, endometrial thickening	Need for clinical evaluation to assess efficacy; lack of biochemical markers to monitor response and avoid adrenal insufficiency; suspected hypocortisolism should be treated with dexamethasone at high doses; hypokalemia should be treated with mineralocorticoid antagonists; important drug interactions; contraindicated in women planning pregnancy; approved by FDA for treatment of hyperglycemia in patients with CS

CBG = Corticosteroid-binding globulin; ICU = intensive care unit; RCT = randomized controlled trial.

Pituitary-Directed Drugs

Cabergoline

Two different mechanisms of action underlie the potential efficacy of dopaminergic drugs in the treatment of CD: the neuromodulation of ACTH and a direct action on ACTH-secreting pituitary tumors [27–29].

Type 2 dopamine (D_2) receptor is present in murine corticotroph tumor cells (AtT-20), in normal human pituitary glands and in more than 75% of human corticotroph pituitary adenomas [28, 29]. Although corticotroph adenomas can express both D_2 isoforms, D_2-long is the predominant isoform. The role of these isoforms in the regulation of ACTH secretion remains to be determined. In a small series of human corticotroph pituitary tumors, a significant in vitro inhibition of ACTH secretion was found in all D_2-positive tumors, but not in D_2-negative cases by either bromocriptine or cabergoline [28, 29].

In clinical practice, bromocriptine can significantly reduce cortisol secretion although normalization is observed in <20% of the patients and the efficacy is generally transitory [26, 27].

A study reported a significant reduction of cortisol levels in 6 out of 10 patients, but a normalization in only 4 of them after 3 months of cabergoline treatment. All cabergoline-responsive cases were associated with D_2 expression in primary cultured tumor cells, whereas all but one of the nonresponders did not express D_2 receptors [30].

The long-term efficacy and safety of cabergoline was confirmed in an open-label prospective study performed in 20 patients with persistent CD after surgery. At the 24-month follow-up, with a median cabergoline dose of 3.5 mg/week (1–7 mg/week), 40% of patients had improved from a clinical point of view and cortisol secretion was controlled [30]. The presence of mild hyperprolactinemia was associated with an initial, but not chronic, response to cabergoline. The prevalence of overweight/obesity decreased from 87.5% at baseline to 62.5%, and hypertension nearly normalized in the majority of patients. After 24 months of treatment, glucose and insulin levels, as well as HOMA-IR, significantly decreased; the prevalence of diabetes mellitus and impaired glucose tolerance decreased from 25 and 37.5% at baseline to 10 and 20%, respectively. It is important to remember that cabergoline may have a direct effect on hypertension and glucose metabolism, independently from cortisol effect. In addition, cabergoline induced tumor shrinkage in 20% of the patients with visible adenomas. Two patients reported hypotension associated with severe asthenia, and 2 others did not tolerate the treatment; no significant cardiac valve dysfunction (except for a slight worsening of tricuspid regurgitation in 1 case) or adrenal insufficiency was observed [31].

A retrospective study performed in 30 patients confirmed that short-term treatment with cabergoline improves cortisol secretion in 50% of the cases, and could normalize urinary cortisol excretion in 36% of cases. Long-term follow-up (mean: 37 months) demonstrated sustained treatment effectiveness in 30% of the subjects with persistent or recurrent disease. No correlation between basal prolactin levels and response to cabergoline therapy was observed [32]. Vilar et al. [33] reported a complete response in 25% of the 12 patients treated with cabergoline (maximal dose: 3 mg/week over 6 months) only, whereas a reduction of cortisol values ranging from 15 to nearly 50% was observed in the remaining ones. Finally, a normalization of urinary cortisol was obtained in 2 of 6 patients (33%) treated with cabergoline at doses ranging from 0.5 to 3 mg/week for 6 months [34].

An escape phenomenon was observed in up to 30% of the patients, although the pathogenic mechanism remains to be clarified. Cabergoline has also been suggested in combination with other medications in patients with CD. Larger trials are needed to establish the role and the modalities of combination therapies [30, 34].

In conclusion, cabergoline appears potentially efficacious in patients with CD, although at the moment it remains a pituitary-directed off-label treatment. As a tentative practical guideline for CD treatment, cabergoline might be reserved for patients with mild hypercortisolism. The mean doses (2–3.5 mg/week) administered in the various studies were higher than those typically suggested to treat hyperprolactinemia. The starting dose is usually 1 mg twice a week, and the dosage may be increased up to 7 mg/week, depending on cortisol response. Serum prolactin levels did not predict long-term cortisol response. Echocardiographic monitoring should be performed in patients who require long-term treatment, especially at high doses.

Pasireotide

ACTH-secreting pituitary adenomas express somatostatin receptors, mainly somatostatin-receptor subtype 5 (sst5) [8], whose activation inhibits ACTH secretion, providing a therapeutic target for patients with CD [35].

Pasireotide is a multireceptor ligand somatostatin analogue that binds to four of the five sst, with the highest affinity for sst5 [36]. In vitro, it inhibits basal and corticotropin-releasing hormone-stimulated ACTH release from human ACTH-secreting pituitary tumors and AtT-20 murine corticotroph tumor cells. In AtT-20 cells, pretreatment administration of dexamethasone did not affect the sensitivity of the cells to the inhibitory effect of pasireotide, suggesting that sst5 is relatively resistant to negative control induced by GCs [35].

Pasireotide is the first medical therapy specifically designed and developed as a pituitary-targeted treatment for patients with CD. In a phase II open-label, single-arm, multicenter study, 39 patients with de novo, persistent or recurrent CD were treated with 600 μg of pasireotide subcutaneously twice daily [37]. After 15 days, the mean urinary free cortisol (UFC) level decreased significantly by 45%. Normalization of UFC was found in 17% of the patients, while levels were reduced in 76% of the patients. Serum cortisol levels and plasma ACTH levels were also reduced. Steady-state plasma concentrations of pasireotide were achieved within 5 days of treatment, and serum levels were higher in responders than in nonresponders.

The phase III trial was a randomized, double-blind, multicenter study that included 162 patients with de novo, persistent or recurrent CD ineligible for surgery [38].

Patients were randomized to receive pasireotide 600 μg (n = 82) or 900 μg (n = 80) subcutaneously twice daily for 12 months.

After 3 months of treatment, patients with a mean UFC level not exceeding 2 × ULN or the baseline level were kept on their randomly assigned dose; all others received an additional 300 μg twice daily. Fifteen percent (12/82) of the patients in the 600-μg and 26% (21/80) of the patients in the 900-μg twice-daily dose group achieved UFC levels less than or equal to ULN (primary end point of the study) after 6 months of treatment.

Of the 103 patients with UFC values available at baseline and at month 6, a reduction was observed in 88% of the cases, being significant – either normalization or ≥50% reduction from baseline – in 49%. The reduction in mean UFC levels was rapid and sustained. At month 12, UFC levels normalized in 13% of patients in the 600-μg group and in 25% of those in the 900-μg group. The lower normalization rate observed in the 600-μg twice-daily group was considered to be due to the higher percentage of patients with severe hypercortisolism included in that group.

A reduction of serum and salivary cortisol and plasma ACTH, as well as an improvement of signs and symptoms of CD, were also observed. On the basis of the phase III study results, pasireotide was approved in Europe and the US for the treatment of adults with CD for whom surgery has failed or is not an option.

In a subsequent publication of this large trial, Pivonello et al. [39] analyzed changes in clinical signs and symptoms secondary to treatment with pasireotide, and found significant reductions in blood pressure, body weight, waist circumference and LDL cholesterol, as well as in facial rubor and supraclavicular and dorsal fat pads. Pasireotide treatment was also associated with a significant improvement in scores obtained from questionnaires investigating quality of life [31].

Interestingly, the clinical benefit achieved during treatment with pasireotide was independent from UFC normalization, as it occurred also in patients with reduced, but not normalized, UFC levels [37–39].

The long-term benefit associated with pasireotide treatment was confirmed by the results of the 2-year extended phase II and III studies [40, 41], as well as by a series of case reports from single-center experiences describing treatment efficacy after 5 years of treatment [42, 43].

The phase III study also reported a reduction in tumor volume at month 12 of 9 and 44% in the 600- and 900-μg twice-daily dose group, respectively. These data were confirmed by two subsequent studies [44, 45].

Significant tumor shrinkage was observed in a patient with an ACTH-secreting pituitary macroadenoma during 24 months of pasireotide treatment, with changes in tumor volume detectable at month 6 [44, 45]. Simeoli et al. [45] reported the radiological disappearance of an ACTH-secreting pituitary microadenoma in 1 case.

The safety profile of pasireotide appears similar to other somatostatin analogues with respect to gastrointestinal symptoms and gallstones, while the frequency of hyperglycemia is higher.

The phase III study reported a 73% prevalence of hyperglycemia, with 6% of patients discontinuing treatment due to it [38]. Irrespective of dosage, glucose and glycosylated hemoglobin (HbA1c) levels increased soon after pasireotide initiation: from 5.8% at baseline to 7.2 and 7.4% in the 600- and 900-μg groups, respectively, at month 6, with preexisting diabetes or impaired glucose tolerance being major risk factors [38]. Therefore, a careful monitoring of glucose levels during pasireotide treatment is mandatory. Studies in healthy volunteers have shown that hyperglycemia associated with pasireotide treatment results from a decrease in incretin and insulin secretion, with no change in insulin sensitivity [46]. Based on these data, the preferential use of DPP-4 inhibitors as well as GLP-1 analogues has been recommended for the management of hyperglycemia during pasireotide in CD. Pivonello et al. [39] reported that glucose control during pasireotide treatment was independent from UFC response, while single case reports suggest the possible normalization of glycemic levels, as well as a significant improvement of preexisting diabetes mellitus, after continuative treatment with pasireotide and control of underlying disease [42, 43]. Hypocortisolism-related adverse events were reported in 13 patients (8%) [38]. The safety profile of pasireotide at the 24-month follow-up was similar to that reported at the 12-month follow-up, with no new safety issues identified during the extension period [40, 41].

Interestingly, the results of the phase III trial also suggested that poorly responsive patients may be identified within the first few months of treatment, and pasireotide is apparently more effective in normalizing UFC in patients with lower baseline cortisol levels [38]. On the contrary, subsequent small studies suggested that UFC normalization may be delayed, especially in patients with severe hypercortisolism [43, 47]. In addition, in clinical practice the efficacy of pasireotide seems to be greater than that reported in clinical trials, with an UFC normalization rate of >60% [47].

A substudy of the phase II trial conducted at one of the original study centers supports the usefulness of late-night salivary cortisol as a simple and noninvasive biomarker to monitor the early response to treatment [48]. The potential role of late-night salivary cortisol in predicting long-term response to treatment is also supported by a more recent publication [47]. In particular, a late-night salivary cortisol percentage fall >27%, as well as a normalization of this parameter, during a 600-μg acute pasireotide suppression test was associated with a probability of 100% of achieving a favorable response to treatment in the medium/long term. Further studies must be carried out to confirm these preliminary results.

Finally, pasireotide may be effective as preoperative treatment in critically ill CD patients in whom a surgical approach is considered hazardous and needs to be delayed [49], as well as in the medical management of Nelson's syndrome [50].

Other Pituitary-Directed Drugs

Based on clinical and experimental evidence, which suggests neurohumoral influences of antiserotonergic drugs on ACTH-secreting pituitary adenomas, some authors have suggested their use in the treatment of CD [51, 52]. However, these drugs are generally ineffective and are not routinely recommended [8]. A possible indication for their use may be for patients with a mild form of hypercortisolism.

In a small series of patients with CD, nuclear receptor ligands have also been used. Nuclear hormone receptor peroxisome proliferator-activated receptor-γ is highly expressed in human corticotroph tumor cells [53]. However, open and nonrandomized clinical trials with peroxisome proliferator-activated receptor-γ agonists do not replicate the effects of rosiglitazone in experimental CD [54–58]. Although effective in some patients, especially in those with diabetes mellitus, the use of these drugs does not appear to be of clear clinical utility.

In a murine tumoral corticotroph cell line and experimental CS, retinoic acid, a ligand of the Nur orphan receptor subfamily, was able to inhibit cell proliferation, ACTH secretion and proopiomelanocortin synthesis. In addition, direct inhibition of corticosterone secretion and cell proliferation was also observed in adrenal cells [59]. A prospective proof-of-concept study showed that the oral administration of 10–80 mg/day of retinoic acid was able to reduce UFC in 5 of the 7 patients treated, with complete normalization achieved in 3 of them [60]. Further clinical trials are necessary to evaluate efficacy and safety of retinoids in CD.

Recently, gefitinib, an epidermal growth factor receptor tyrosine kinase inhibitor, has been shown to attenuate ACTH secretion, inhibit cell proliferation and induce apoptosis in mouse corticotroph epidermal growth factor receptor transfectants [61].

Adrenal-Directed Drugs

Differently from pituitary-directed drugs, adrenal steroid synthesis inhibitors are effective in the majority of the cases of hypercortisolism, independently from their origin [8, 62]. The most commonly used drugs are ketoconazole, metyrapone, mitotane and etomidate. LCI699, a potent inhibitor of 11β-hydroxylase and 18-hydroxylase (aldosterone synthase), and the nonracemic KTZ (2S,4R KTZ) are two promising compounds currently under investigation. All these drugs competitively inhibit adrenal enzyme activity and decrease cortisol secretion, but do not treat the underlying tumor or restore normal hypothalamic-pituitary-adrenal axis secretory dynamics.

Ketoconazole

Introduced in the late 1970s as an antifungal agent, the imidazole derivative ketoconazole was noted to cause gynecomastia and reduce plasma testosterone and serum cortisol levels. In the following years, ketoconazole was shown to interfere with cytochrome P450 enzymes in several organs (i.e. adrenal glands, testes, ovaries, liver, kidneys) [62]. First used in 1983 to treat CS, it is currently the most frequently used hypocortisolemic agent.

Ketoconazole is a potent inhibitor of adrenal steroidogenesis through the inhibition of cytochrome P450 enzymes, including the cholesterol side-chain cleavage complex, 17,20-lyase, 11-hydroxylase and 17-hydroxylase. Its action is rapid, dose-dependent and fully reversible (which is not always the case with mitotane) [62]. Prolonged administration in patients with CD is neither associated with a compensatory rise, nor with a decrease of ACTH levels. This phenomenon, however, does not seem to involve a specific effect on ACTH secretion, but rather some sort of adjustment in the sensitivity of the hypothalamic-pituitary-adrenal axis.

The efficacy of ketoconazole treatment is difficult to establish as the rate of control of hypercortisolism ranges between 14 and 100%, depending on the criteria used to define normalization, patient characteristics, previous treatment, medication type and doses, and length of follow-up. As most of the reports include both patients naïve for treatment and previously treated with surgery and/or RT, results are difficult to interpret. The reduction/normalization of cortisol production is paralleled by the regression and/or rapid improvement of clinical symptoms, like diabetes mellitus, hypokalemia, hypertension, hirsutism and depression [63, 64]. However, escape from pharmacological control has been reported in some cases [63, 64].

In a retrospective analysis, Castinetti et al. [65] found normalization of urinary cortisol in 45% of patients (mean follow-up: 23 months; range: 6–72). Control of the disease was observed during the first month in 8 patients, and after 3 months in 9 patients. The controlled patients also presented clinical regression of signs of hypercortisolism, including lowering of blood pressure and loss of weight (mean: 1–2 kg at 3 months, and 5 kg at the 1-year follow-up). Blood pressure was normal in all controlled patients at 3–6 months after initiation of ketoconazole. In diabetic patients, metabolic control was also improved. Ketoconazole was stopped in the first week of treatment in 5 patients (13%) because of clinical or biological intolerance. The treatment was safe and adrenal insufficiency was not observed. Interestingly, during treatment, the tumor became visible on pituitary MRI in 5 patients, allowing these patients to undergo pituitary surgery 12–30 months later.

Similar results were observed in a retrospective study by Valassi et al. [66] in patients treated with steroidogenesis inhibitors prior to surgery between 1983 and 2010: normalization of UFC and clinical control was achieved in 9 out of 17 patients treated with ketoconazole only [66]. More recently, Castinetti et al. [64] published the results of the French Retrospective Study on Ketoconazole Outcome (FReSKO) including retrospective data of 200 patients followed in 14 French centers. Forty patients received ketoconazole before surgery, 32 as primary treatment and 128 after unsuccessful surgery or following RT. At the last follow-up (mean: 14.4 months), 49.2% of the patients had normalized UFC levels and 25.6% had a decrease ≥50%, while 25.4% had unchanged levels. In addition, at the last follow-up, clinical signs were improved in 55.2%, hypertension in 40%, hypokalemia in 38.4% and diabetes in 59% of affected patients. The proportion of males was higher in the uncontrolled than in the controlled group. However, most males (59%) had at least a 50% decrease of UFC (including 39% with normal UFC at the last visit).

Because of its different selectivity (effective blockade of cholesterol side-chain cleavage and 17 hydroxylase/C17–20 lyase activities), ketoconazole has antiandrogenic properties which can have favorable effects on female hirsutism, but may be disturbing for male patients as it may cause hypogonadism and gynecomastia [64]. Treatment is usually started at a dose of 200 mg twice daily, with higher doses (up to 1,200 mg/day) required to bring UFC to normal limits. The treatment is generally well tolerated. Alteration of liver function is the most common side effect, with severe liver failure in rare cases. Due to potential fatal hepatotoxicity, in 2013/2014 the Food and Drug Administration (FDA) and the European Medicines Agency (EMA) restricted its use as an antifungal agent. Thus, monitoring liver function is necessary during treatment. Reversible elevation of transaminases occurs in approximately 5–10% of the patients. Other adverse reactions include skin and gastrointestinal disorders, and, very rarely, adrenal insufficiency.

As a widespread inhibitor of CYP enzymes, ketoconazole may simultaneously affect several physiologic functions including vitamin D metabolism and cholesterol synthesis; for this reason, differently from mitotane, ketoconazole decreases cholesterol levels. Discontinuation is recommended when transaminases increase by more than 3 times ULN. Taken together, available data – although not generated by large randomized clinical trials – place ketoconazole among the well-known and use-established therapeutic tools to treat hypercortisolism [8, 62]. Interestingly, ketoconazole is a racemic mixture of two cis-enantiomers: 2S,4R and 2R,4S. Stereoisomers have different pharmacological properties. 2S,4R ketoconazole has higher antisteroidogenetic activity and its efficacy in CS is currently under investigation in a phase III trial.

Metyrapone

Metyrapone primarily acts on the 11β/18-hydroxylase enzyme. It is administered orally and absorbed quickly with a rapid onset of action, but a short half-life (2 h), thus requiring multiple doses (up to 6) per day. Generally, peak concentration is reached 1 h after administration, but there is interindividual variability. The main metabolite is metyrapol (reduced form), which is as potent as metyrapone to inhibit CYP11B1, but takes about twice as long as metyrapone to be eliminated from the plasma. The treatment with metyrapone is effective in all types of CS, with biochemical control and clinical improvement observed in 50–75% of the patients; as there are no major adverse effects, it can be used as a long-term treatment if needed [8, 62, 67]. The drug was approved by the EMA in April 2014 and, although not specifically approved for use during pregnancy, it has been occasionally administered to pregnant women with no apparent adverse events. It can be used alone or in combination with other drugs or pituitary RT. Although metyrapone effectively decreases cortisol levels, a substantial number of patients may require combination treatment to achieve eucortisolemia [66, 68].

Metyrapone is administered orally, usually beginning with a daily dose of 0.5–1 g (in 2–4 fractioned doses) and increased every few days to a maximal dose of 6 g/day. It is important to remember that a reliable cortisol assay (LC-MS/MS) without cross-reactivity with precursors is needed to monitor patients during treatment.

In patients with pituitary and ectopic ACTH-secreting tumors, metyrapone, while reducing cortisol, increases ACTH secretion with an overstimulation of adrenal androgen and mineralocorticoid precursor (e.g. desoxycorticosterone) production. However, adverse effects due to increased androgens (acne, hirsutism) and mineralocorticoid precursor (hypokalemia, edema), as a consequence of 11β/18-hydroxylase inhibition, are infrequent and can be reversed by adding aminoglutethimide, which has a predominant effect on the cholesterol side-chain cleavage complex [69]. Finally, it is important to remember that adrenal insufficiency has also been observed.

Osilodrostat

Osilodrostat (LCI699) is an orally active inhibitor of aldosterone synthase (CYP11B2). Originally developed to treat resistant hypertension, cardiac failure and renal disease, when administered at higher doses it also inhibits 11β-hydroxylase (CYP11B1). It is rapidly absorbed with a peak blood concentration at 1 h after oral administration, and a half-life of 4–5 h.

It is currently the most potent inhibitor of 11β-hydroxylase. Although LCI699 and metyrapone have a similar mechanism of action, LCI699 has a 3-fold higher affinity for its targeted steroidogenic enzyme, and it has a more than 2-fold longer half-life. An open-label, proof-of-concept, single-arm study has been conducted to assess the safety and tolerability of LCI699 in CD [70]. After 10 weeks of treatment, UFC levels normalized or were reduced >50% in all 12 patients. Cortisol decrease led to a compensatory increase in ACTH levels (3- to 4-fold), as well as in cortisol and aldosterone precursors (11-deoxycortisol and 11-deoxycorticosterone) and androgen levels. Both systolic and diastolic pressure improved. LCI699 was generally well tolerated, although an overall weight increase (average: 2.4 kg) was observed, together with edema (1 patient) and hypokalemia (4 patients). Based on these promising results, evaluation of LCI699 is currently being evaluated more extensively in patients with CD.

Mitotane

In 1949 Nelson noticed that dogs treated with the insecticide dichlorodiphenyldichloroethane (DDD) developed adrenal cortical atrophy. This observation led to the development of adrenolytic agent DDD mitotane (o.p'DDD), an isomer of the insecticide. Patients with CD have been treated with mitotane since 1961, although only few retrospective studies have been performed. Recently, in a series of 76 patients, Baudry et al. [71] showed that mitotane treatment induced a remission in 72% of the patients after a median of 7 months. However, 71% of the patients who did not receive alternative therapy relapsed after 5–68 months (median: 13.2).

Various mechanisms of action have been suggested, including adrenocorticolytic effects, modifications of steroid metabolism and direct inhibition of steroidogenesis (cholesterol side-chain cleavage and 11β/18-hydroxylase activities). Extensive metabolism is required for the drug to be active, and it takes weeks to reduce cortisol secretion. Mitotane is a lipid-soluble compound and its pharmacokinetics is characterized by a prevalent accumulation in adipose tissue and prolonged half-life (18–159 days) [71]. It is licensed for the symptomatic treatment of advanced or inoperable adrenocortical carcinoma (functional or not), but it has also been used off-label for the management of CS.

The dose and mitotane plasma levels required to control hypercortisolism are lower than those needed to achieve antineoplastic activity, with medians around 2.7 g of mitotane per day and 8.5 mg/l, respectively [71, 72]. Daily doses (2–4 g, fractioned in 2–3 doses) should be titrated to maintain UFC in the normal range, avoiding excessive suppression of adrenal function. Careful monitoring of mitotane plasma concentrations may be helpful in long-term treatment. Since selectivity is not high, extra-adrenal effects are likely. GC replacement is needed and patients should be monitored for adrenal insufficiency and toxic effects. Replacement therapy doses are higher than usual because mitotane increases the metabolism of exogenous GCs and blood levels of hormone-binding proteins. Urinary and salivary cortisol measurement should be performed to monitor its effect. At the doses used to treat CD, mitotane has less adrenolytic effects on the zona glomerulosa, thus mineralocorticoid replacement may not be required. Mitotane strongly activates CYP3A4 and increases hydrocortisone clearance [72]. The most common side effects associated with treatment are gastrointestinal (i.e. dyspepsia, anorexia, nausea and diarrhea) and neurological (i.e. fatigue, somnolence, confusion and dizziness). Hypercholesterolemia is also common and may require treatment with statins. Gynecomastia has also been observed.

Etomidate

Etomidate is a short-acting intravenous anesthetic agent. This compound is an imidazole derivative and suppresses adrenal steroid synthesis (both cortisol and aldosterone) by inhibiting cholesterol side-chain cleavage and 11β-hydroxylase. It also appears to depress the function of the central nervous system by interfering with the GABA system [8, 73].

The suppressive effects of etomidate on steroidogenesis are immediate and may persist for several days (up to 14) after discontinuation of the drug. Intravenously, etomidate (in an alcohol-based vehicle in Europe and in an aqueous solution of propylene glycol in the US) can be used safely for a prolonged period as an adrenostatic agent in patients with severe hypercortisolism when oral therapy is not possible, and in those who are not an immediate surgical candidate [73]. It should be infused with continuous monitoring of hemodynamics and periodic assessment of adrenal function.

GC Receptor Blockers (Mifepristone)

Mifepristone (RU486) was the first potent GC antagonist available for clinical use. It also binds competitively to androgen and progestin receptors. To date, only a few patients with CS have been treated [8].

Recently, Fleseriu et al. [74] published the largest prospective multicenter, open-label trial of mifepristone in CS (SESIMEC). This study, including 50 subjects (43 with

CD) treated with 300–1,200 mg/day of mifepristone, demonstrated that this drug is effective in treating clinical and metabolic features related to hypercortisolism. In particular, 60% of the 29 patients with glucose intolerance or diabetes were defined as 'responders'. There was continued improvement in glucose tolerance measured at weeks 6, 10, 16 and 24. Of the 12 patients treated with insulin at baseline, 7 reduced their daily dose by 50%. There was also a significant reduction in mean HbA1c over the course of treatment. Hypertension improved in 40% of cases, and at least one other clinical parameter (i.e. weight, depression, cognition or quality of life) improved in 87% of cases. Three cases of severe hypokalemia were reported; other adverse events included symptoms of cortisol insufficiency (i.e. fatigue, nausea, vomiting, arthralgia and headache) and related to the drug antiprogestin effect (i.e. endometrial thickening). ACTH levels increased more than 2-fold in 31/43 patients with CD during a follow-up of 11.3 months; 3 macroadenomas increased in size, while 2 regressed [75]. A drawback of this drug, with its long half-life, is the lack of biochemical markers to monitor response and avoid adrenal insufficiency. Suspected adrenal insufficiency should be treated with dexamethasone at high doses. Mifepristone is approved in the United States for control of hypercortisolism-induce hyperglycemia in patients with CS who failed surgery or who are not surgical candidates.

Combination Therapy

The use of different combinations of drugs may increase the effectiveness while decreasing side effects. Treatment should be tailored to each patient, as no universally valid treatment strategy exists. The different drugs should be selected according to their properties, the particular situation of each patient and, potentially in the near future, the pattern of receptor expression of corticotroph tumors.

The presence of both sst and dopamine receptors in human corticotroph adenomas, together with the inhibition of ACTH secretion due to their activation may suggest a potential combined therapeutic approach in selected patients with CD. If the functional heterodimerization of these receptors occurs in vivo as it has already been well demonstrated in vitro, the combination of cabergoline and pasireotide and/or other sst5-targeted analogues and/or dopastatin (a chimeric dopamine-somatostatin analogue) could be an exciting concept, increasing medical treatment options in these patients. This potential clinical strategy has not been evaluated yet, and future trials are awaited with interest.

Finally, the combined use of pituitary-directed and adrenal-directed drugs is worthy of further investigations in the attempt to improve therapeutic success rates. Additive effects of ketoconazole and octreotide have been observed in the management of patients with CS, including CD.

References

1 Arnaldi G, Angeli A, Atkinson AB, Bertagna X, Cavagnini F, Chrousos GP, Fava GA, Findling JW, Gaillard RC, Grossman AB, Kola B, Lacroix A, Mancini T, Mantero F, Newell-Price J, Nieman LK, Sonino N, Vance ML, Giustina A, Boscaro M: Diagnosis and complications of Cushing's syndrome: a consensus statement. J Clin Endocrinol Metab 2003;8:5593–5602.

2 Nieman LK, Biller BM, Findling JW, Newell-Price J, Savage MO, Stewart PM, Montori VM: The diagnosis of Cushing's syndrome: an Endocrine Society Clinical Practice Guideline. J Clin Endocrinol Metab 2008;93:1526–1540.

3 Lacroix A, Feelders RA, Stratakis CA, Nieman LK: Cushing's syndrome. Lancet 2015;386:913–927.

4 Arnaldi G, Mancini T, Tirabassi G, Trementino L, Boscaro M: Advances in the epidemiology, pathogenesis, and management of Cushing's syndrome complications. J Endocrinol Invest 2012;35:434–448.

5 Mancini T, Kola B, Mantero F, Boscaro M, Arnaldi G: High cardiovascular risk in patients with Cushing's syndrome according to 1999 WHO/ISH guidelines. Clin Endocrinol (Oxf) 2004;61:768–777.

6 Clayton RN, Raskauskiene D, Reulen RC, Jones PW: Mortality and morbidity in Cushing's disease over 50 years in Stoke-on-Trent, UK: audit and meta-analysis of literature. J Clin Endocrinol Metab 2011;96:632–642.

7 van Haalen FM, Broersen LH, Jorgensen JO, Pereira AM, Dekkers OM: Management of endocrine disease: mortality remains increased in Cushing's disease despite biochemical remission: a systematic review and meta-analysis. Eur J Endocrinol 2015;172:R143–R149.

8 Biller BM, Grossman AB, Stewart PM, Melmed S, Bertagna X, Bertherat J, Buchfelder M, Colao A, Hermus AR, Hofland LJ, Klibanski A, Lacroix A, Lindsay JR, Newell-Price J, Nieman LK, Petersenn S, Sonino N, Stalla GK, Swearingen B, Vance ML, Wass JA, Boscaro M: Treatment of adrenocorticotropin-dependent Cushing's syndrome: a consensus statement. J Clin Endocrinol Metab 2008;93:2454–2462.

9 Laws ER Jr, Barkhoudarian G: The transition from microscopic to endoscopic transsphenoidal surgery: the experience at Brigham and Women's Hospital. World Neurosurg 2014;82(6 Suppl):S152–S154.

10 Cappabianca P, Cavallo LM, Solari D, Esposito F: Endoscopic endonasal transsphenoidal approach to pituitary adenomas. J Neurosurg 2015;122:473–474.

11 Wagenmakers MA, Boogaarts HD, Roerink SH, Timmers HJ, Stikkelbroeck NM, Smit JW, van Lindert EJ, Netea-Maier RT, Grotenhuis JA, Hermus AR: Endoscopic transsphenoidal pituitary surgery: a good and safe primary treatment option for Cushing's disease, even in case of macroadenomas or invasive adenomas. Eur J Endocrinol 2013;169:329–337.

12 Storr HL, Drake WM, Evanson J, Matson M, Berney DM, Grossman AB, Akker SA, Monson JP, Alusi G, Savage MO, Sabin I: Endonasal endoscopic transsphenoidal pituitary surgery: early experience and outcome in paediatric Cushing's disease. Clin Endocrinol (Oxf) 2014;80:270–276.

13 Kelly DF: Transsphenoidal surgery for Cushing's disease: a review of success rates, remission predictors, management of failed surgery, and Nelson's syndrome. Neurosurg Focus 2007;23:E5.

14 Bertagna X, Guignat L: Approach to the Cushing's disease patient with persistent/recurrent hypercortisolism after pituitary surgery. J Clin Endocrinol Metab 2013;98:1307–1318.

15 Ding D, Starke RM, Sheehan JP: Treatment paradigms for pituitary adenomas: defining the roles of radiosurgery and radiation therapy. J Neurooncol 2014;117:445–457.

16 Jagannathan J, Yen CP, Pouratian N, Laws ER, Sheehan JP: Stereotactic radiosurgery for pituitary adenomas: a comprehensive review of indications, techniques and long-term results using the Gamma Knife. J Neurooncol 2009;92:345–356.

17 Loeffler JS, Shih HA: Radiation therapy in the management of pituitary adenomas. J Clin Endocrinol Metab 2011;96:1992–2003.

18 Budyal S, Lila AR, Jalali R, Gupta T, Kasliwal R, Jagtap VS, Bandgar T, Menon P, Shah NS: Encouraging efficacy of modern conformal fractionated radiotherapy in patients with uncured Cushing's disease. Pituitary 2014;17:60–67.

19 Marek J, Ježková J, Hána V, Kršek M, Liščák R, Vladyka V, Pecen L: Gamma Knife radiosurgery for Cushing's disease and Nelson's syndrome. Pituitary 2015;18:376–384.

20 Lecumberri B, Estrada J, García-Uría J, Millán I, Pallardo LF, Caballero L, Lucas T: Neurocognitive long-term impact of two-field conventional radiotherapy in adult patients with operated pituitary adenomas. Pituitary 2015;18:782–795.

21 Losa M, Picozzi P, Redaelli MG, Laurenzi A, Mortini P: Pituitary radiotherapy for Cushing's disease. Neuroendocrinology 2010;92(suppl 1):107–110.

22 Reincke M, Ritzel K, Osswald A, Berr CM, Stalla GK, Hallfeldt K, Reisch N, Schopohl J, Beuschlein F: A critical re-appraisal of bilateral adrenalectomy for ACTH-dependent Cushing's syndrome. Eur J Endocrinol 2015;173:M23–M32.

23 Ritzel K, Beuschlein F, Mickisch A, Osswald A, Schneider HJ, Schopohl J, Reincke M: Clinical review: outcome of bilateral adrenalectomy in Cushing's syndrome: a systematic review. J Clin Endocrinol Metab 2013;98:3939–3948.

24 Osswald A, Plomer E, Dimopoulou C, Milian M, Blaser R, Ritzel K, Mickisch A, Knerr F, Stanojevic M, Hallfeldt K, Schopohl J, Kuhn KA, Stalla G, Beuschlein F, Reincke M: Favorable long-term outcomes of bilateral adrenalectomy in Cushing's disease. Eur J Endocrinol 2014;171:209–215.
25 Assie G, Bahurel H, Coste J, Silvera S, Kujas M, Dugue MA, Karray F, Dousset B, Bertherat J, Legmann P, Bertagna X: Corticotroph tumor progression after adrenalectomy in Cushing's Disease: a reappraisal of Nelson's syndrome. J Clin Endocrinol Metab 2007;92:172–179.
26 Pivonello R, De Leo M, Cozzolino A, Colao A: The treatment of Cushing's disease. Endocr Rev 2015;36: 385–486.
27 Arnaldi G, Cardinaletti M, Boscaro M: Advances in medical treatment of Cushing's disease. Expert Rev Endocrinol Metab 2007;2:735–743.
28 Pivonello R, Ferone D, Lombardi G, Colao A, Lamberts SW, Hofland LJ: Novel insights in dopamine receptor physiology. Eur J Endocrinol 2007;156 (suppl 1):S13–S21.
29 Pivonello R, Ferone D, de Herder WW: Dopamine receptor expression and function in corticotroph pituitary tumors. J Clin Endocrinol Metab 2004;89: 2452–2462.
30 Pivonello R, De Martino MC, Cappabianca P, De Leo M, Faggiano A, Lombardi G, Hofland LJ, Lamberts SW, Colao A: The medical treatment of Cushing's disease: effectiveness of chronic treatment with the dopamine agonist cabergoline in patients unsuccessfully treated by surgery. J Clin Endocrinol Metab 2009;94:223–230.
31 Webb SM, Ware JE, Forsythe A, Yang M, Badia X, Nelson LM, Signorovitch JE, McLeod L, Maldonado M, Zgliczynski W, de Block C, Portocarrero-Ortiz L, Gadelha M: Treatment effectiveness of pasireotide on health-related quality of life in patients with Cushing's disease. Eur J Endocrinol 2014;171:89–98.
32 Godbout A, Manavela M, Danilowicz K, Beauregard H, Bruno OD, Lacroix A: Cabergoline monotherapy in the long-term treatment of Cushing's disease. Eur J Endocrinol 2010;163:709–716.
33 Vilar L, Naves LA, Azevedo MF, Arruda MJ, Arahata CM, Moura ESL, Agra R, Pontes L, Montenegro L, Albuquerque JL, Canadas V: Effectiveness of cabergoline in monotherapy and combined with ketoconazole in the management of Cushing's disease. Pituitary 2010;13:123–129.
34 Barbot M, Albiger N, Ceccato F, Zilio M, Frigo AC, Denaro L, Mantero F, Scaroni C: Combination therapy for Cushing's disease: effectiveness of two schedules of treatment: should we start with cabergoline or ketoconazole? Pituitary 2014;17:109–117.
35 Hofland LJ, van der Hoek J, Feelders R, van Aken MO, van Koetsveld PM, Waaijers M, Sprij-Mooij D, Bruns C, Weckbecker G, de Herder WW, Beckers A, Lamberts SW: The multi-ligand somatostatin analogue SOM230 inhibits ACTH secretion by cultured human corticotroph adenomas via somatostatin receptor type 5. Eur J Endocrinol 2005;152:645–654.
36 Bruns C, Lewis I, Briner U, Meno- Tetang G, Weckbecker G: SOM230: a novel somatostatin peptidomimetic with broad somatotropin release inhibiting factor (SRIF) receptor binding and a unique antisecretory profile. Eur J Endocrinol 2002;146:707–716.
37 Boscaro M, Ludlam WH, Atkinson B, Glusman JE, Petersenn S, Reincke M, Snyder P, Tabarin A, Biller BM, Findling J, Melmed S, Darby CH, Hu K, Wang Y, Freda PU, Grossman AB, Frohman LA, Bertherat J: Treatment of pituitary-dependent Cushing's disease with the multireceptor ligand somatostatin analog pasireotide (SOM230): a multicenter, phase II trial. J Clin Endocrinol Metab 2009;94:115–122.
38 Colao A, Petersenn S, Newell-Price J, Findling JW, Gu F, Maldonado M, Schoenherr U, Mills D, Salgado LR, Biller BM; Pasireotide B2305 Study Group: A 12-month phase 3 study of pasireotide in Cushing's disease. N Engl J Med 2012;366:914–924.
39 Pivonello R, Petersenn S, Newell-Price J, Findling JW, Gu F, Maldonado M, Trovato A, Hughes G, Salgado LR, Lacroix A, Schopohl J, Biller BM; Pasireotide B2305 Study Group: Pasireotide treatment significantly improves clinical signs and symptoms in patients with Cushing's disease: results from a phase III study. Clin Endocrinol (Oxf) 2014;81:408–417.
40 Boscaro M, Bertherat J, Findling J, Fleseriu M, Atkinson AB, Petersenn S, Schopohl J, Snyder P, Hughes G, Trovato A, Hu K, Maldonado M, Biller BM: Extended treatment of Cushing's disease with pasireotide: results from a 2-year, phase II study. Pituitary 2014;17:320–326.
41 Schopohl J, Gu F, Rubens R, Van Gaal L, Bertherat J, Ligueros-Saylan M, Trovato A, Hughes G, Salgado LR, Boscaro M, Pivonello R: Pasireotide can induce sustained decreases in urinary cortisol and provide clinical benefit in patients with Cushing's disease: results from an open-ended, open-label extension trial. Pituitary 2015;18:604–612.
42 MacKenzie-Feder J, Bourdeau I, Vallette S, Beauregard H, Ste-Marie LG, Lacroix A: Pasireotide monotherapy in Cushing's disease: a single-centre experience with 5-year extension of phase III trial. Pituitary 2014;17:519–529.
43 Trementino L, Cardinaletti M, Concettoni C, Marcelli G, Boscaro M, Arnaldi G: Up-to 5-year efficacy of pasireotide in a patient with Cushing's disease and pre-existing diabetes: literature review and clinical practice considerations. Pituitary 2015;18:359–365.
44 Shimon I, Rot L, Inbar E: Pituitary-directed medical therapy with pasireotide for a corticotroph macroadenoma: pituitary volume reduction and literature review. Pituitary 2012;15:608–613.

45 Simeoli C, Auriemma RS, Tortora F, De Leo M, Iacuaniello D, Cozzolino A, De Martino MC, Pivonello C, Mainolfi CG, Rossi R, Cirillo S, Colao A, Pivonello R: The treatment with pasireotide in Cushing's disease: effects of long-term treatment on tumor mass in the experience of a single center. Endocrine 2015;50:725–740.
46 Henry RR, Ciaraldi TP, Armstrong D, Burke P, Ligueros-Saylan M, Mudaliar S: Hyperglycemia associated with pasireotide: results from a mechanistic study in healthy volunteers. J Clin Endocrinol Metab 2013;98:3446–3453.
47 Trementino L, Zilio M, Marcelli G, Michetti G, Barbot M, Ceccato F, Boscaro M,Scaroni C, Arnaldi G: The role of an acute pasireotide suppression test in predicting response to treatment in patients with Cushing's disease: findings from a pilot study. Endocrine 2015;50:154–161.
48 Trementino L, Cardinaletti M, Concettoni C, Marcelli G, Polenta B, Spinello M, Boscaro M, Arnaldi G: Salivary cortisol is a useful tool to assess the early response to pasireotide in patients with Cushing's disease. Pituitary 2015;18:60–67.
49 Cannavo S, Messina E, Albani A, Ferrau F, Barresi V, Priola S, Esposito F, Angileri F: Clinical management of critically ill patients with Cushing's disease due to ACTH-secreting pituitary macroadenomas: effectiveness of presurgical treatment with pasireotide. Endocrine 2015, Epub ahead of print.
50 Katznelson L: Sustained improvements in plasma ACTH and clinical status in a patient with Nelson's syndrome treated with pasireotide LAR, a multireceptor somatostatin analog. J Clin Endocrinol Metab 2013;98:1803–1807.
51 Krieger DT, Amorosa L, Linick F: Cyproheptadine-induced remission of Cushing's disease. N Engl J Med 1975;293:893–896.
52 Sonino N, Fava GA, Fallo F, Franceschetto A, Belluardo P, Boscaro M: Effect of the serotonin antagonists ritanserin and ketanserin in Cushing's disease. Pituitary 2000;3:55–59.
53 Heaney AP, Fernando M, Yong WH, Melmed S: Functional PPAR-gamma receptor is a novel therapeutic target for ACTH-secreting pituitary adenomas. Nat Med 2002;8:1281–1287.
54 Ambrosi B, Dall'Asta C, Cannavo S, Libe R, Vigo T, Epaminonda P, Chiodini I, Ferrero S, Trimarchi F, Arosio M, Beck-Peccoz P: Effects of chronic administration of PPAR-gamma ligand rosiglitazone in Cushing's disease. Eur J Endocrinol 2004;151:173–178.
55 Pecori Giraldi F, Scaroni C, Arvat E, Martin M, Giordano R, Albiger N, Leao AA, Picu A, Mantero F, Cavagnini F: Effect of protracted treatment with rosiglitazone, a PPAR-gamma agonist, in patients with Cushing's disease. Clin Endocrinol 2006;64: 219–224.
56 Cannavo S, Arosio M, Almoto B, Dall'Asta C, Ambrosi B: Effectiveness of long-term rosiglitazone administration in patients with Cushing's disease. Clin Endocrinol (Oxf) 2005;63:118–119.
57 Suri D, Weiss RE: Effect of pioglitazone on adrenocorticotropic hormone and cortisol secretion in Cushing's disease. J Clin Endocrinol Metab 2005;90: 1340–1346.
58 Morcos M, Fohr B, Tafel J, Pfisterer F, Hamann A, Humpert P, Bode H, Schwenger V, Zeier M, Becker C, Kasperk C, Schilling T, Hammes HP, Bierhaus A, Nawroth PP: Long-term treatment of central Cushing's syndrome with rosiglitazone. Exp Clin Endocrinol Diabetes 2007;115:292–297.
59 Pàez-Pereda M KD, Hopfner U, Theodoropuolou M, Pagotto U, Uhl E, Losa M, Stalla J, Grubler Y, Missale C, Arzt E, Stalla GK: Retinoic acid prevents experimental Cushing's syndrome. J Clin Invest 2001;108:1123–1131.
60 Pecori Giraldi F, Ambrogio AG, Andrioli M, Sanguin F, Karamouzis I, Corsello SM, Scaroni C, Arvat E, Pontecorvi A, Cavagnini F: Potential role for retinoic acid in patients with Cushing's disease. J Clin Endocrinol Metab 2012;97:3577–3583.
61 Fukuoka H, Cooper O, Ben-Shlomo A, Mamelak A, Ren SG, Bruyette D, Melmed S: EGFR as a therapeutic target for human, canine, and mouse ACTH-secreting pituitary adenomas. J Clin Invest 2011;121: 4712–4721.
62 Daniel E, Newell-Price JD: Therapy of endocrine disease: steroidogenesis enzyme inhibitors in Cushing's syndrome. Eur J Endocrinol 2015;172:R263–R280.
63 Sonino N, Boscaro M, Paoletta A, Mantero F, Ziliotto D: Ketoconazole treatment in Cushing's syndrome: experience in 34 patients. Clin Endocrinol (Oxf) 1991;35:347–352.
64 Castinetti F, Guignat L, Giraud P, Muller M, Kamenicky P, Drui D, Caron P, Luca F, Donadille B, Vantyghem MC, Bihan H, Delemer B, Raverot G, Motte E, Philippon M, Morange I, Conte-Devolx B, Quinquis L, Martinie M, Vezzosi D, Le Bras M, Baudry C, Christin-Maitre S, Goichot B, Chanson P, Young J, Chabre O, Tabarin A, Bertherat J, Brue T: Ketoconazole in Cushing's disease: is it worth a try? J Clin Endocrinol Metab 2014;99:1623–1630.
65 Castinetti F, Morange I, Jaquet P, Conte-Devolx B, Brue T: Ketoconazole revisited: a preoperative or postoperative treatment in Cushing's disease. Eur J Endocrinol 2008;158:91–99.
66 Valassi E, Crespo I, Gich I, Rodriguez J, Webb SM: A reappraisal of the medical therapy with steroidogenesis inhibitors in Cushing's syndrome. Clin Endocrinol (Oxf) 2012;7:735–742.

67 Daniel E, Aylwin S, Mustafa O, Ball S, Munir A, Boelaert K, Chortis V, Cuthbertson DJ, Daousi C, Rajeev SP, Davis J, Cheer K, Drake W, Gunganah K, Grossman A, Gurnell M, Powlson AS, Karavitaki N, Huguet I, Kearney T, Mohit K, Meeran K, Hill N, Rees A, Lansdown AJ, Trainer PJ, Minder AE, Newell-Price J: Effectiveness of metyrapone in 195 patients with Cushing's syndrome. J Clin Endocrinol Metab 2015;100:4146–4154.
68 Kamenický P, Droumaguet C, Salenave S, Blanchard A, Jublanc C, Gautier JF, Brailly-Tabard S, Leboulleux S, Schlumberger M, Baudin E, Chanson P, Young J: Mitotane, metyrapone, and ketoconazole combination therapy as an alternative to rescue adrenalectomy for severe ACTH-dependent Cushing's syndrome. J Clin Endocrinol Metab 2011;96:2796–2804.
69 Sonino N, Boscaro M, Ambroso G, Merola G, Mantero F: Prolonged treatment of Cushing's disease with metyrapone and aminoglutethimide. IRCS Med Sci 1986;14:485–486.
70 Bertagna X, Pivonello R, Fleseriu M, Zhang Y, Robinson P, Taylor A, Watson CE, Maldonado M, Hamrahian AH, Boscaro M, Biller BM: LCI699, a potent 11β-hydroxylase inhibitor, normalizes urinary cortisol in patients with Cushing's disease: results from a multicenter, proof-of-concept study. J Clin Endocrinol Metab 2014;99:1375–1383.
71 Baudry C, Coste J, Bou Khalil R, Silvera S, Guignat L, Guibourdenche J, Abbas H, Legmann P, Bertagna X, Bertherat J: Efficiency and tolerance of mitotane in Cushing's disease in 76 patients from a single center. Eur J Endocrinol 2012;167:473–481.
72 Chortis V, Taylor AE, Schneider P, Tomlinson JW, Hughes BA, O'Neil DM, Libe R, Allolio B, Bertagna X, Bertherat J, Beuschlein F, Fassnacht M, Karavitaki N, Mannelli M, Mantero F, Opocher G, Porfiri E, Quinkler M, Sherlock M, Terzolo M, Nightingale P, Shackleton CHL, Stewart PM, Hahner S, Arlt W: Mitotane therapy in adrenocortical cancer induces CYP3A4 and inhibits 5α-reductase, explaining the need for personalized glucocorticoid and androgen replacement. J Clin Endocrinol Metab 2013;98:161–171.
73 Preda VA, Sen J, Karavitaki N, Grossman AB: Etomidate in the management of hypercortisolaemia in Cushing's syndrome: a review. Eur J Endocrinol 2012;167:137–143.
74 Fleseriu M, Biller BMK, Findling JW, Molitch ME, Schteingart DE, Gross C: Mifepristone, a glucocorticoid receptor antagonist, produces clinical and metabolic benefits in patients with Cushing's syndrome. J Clin Endocrinol Metab 2012;97:2039–2049.
75 Fleseriu M, Findling JW, Koch CA, Schlaffer SM, Buchfelder M, Gross C: Changes in plasma ACTH levels and corticotroph tumor size in patients with Cushing's disease during long-term treatment with the glucocorticoid receptor antagonist mifepristone. J Clin Endocrinol Metab 2014;99:3718–3727.

Professor Giorgio Arnaldi, MD, PhD
Clinic of Endocrinology and Metabolic Diseases
Ospedali Riuniti di Ancona University Hospital
IT–60100 Ancona (Italy)
E-Mail gioarnaldi@gmail.com

Arvat E, Falorni A (eds): Cortisol Excess and Insufficiency.
Front Horm Res. Basel, Karger, 2016, vol 46, pp 106–114 (DOI: 10.1159/000443870)

Is Adrenal Insufficiency a Rare Disease?

Per Dahlqvist[a] · Magnus Isaksson[b] · Sophie Bensing[c]

[a]Department of Public Health and Clinical Medicine, Umeå University, Umeå, [b]Department of Medical Sciences, Uppsala University, Uppsala, and [c]Department of Molecular Medicine and Surgery, Karolinska Institutet, Stockholm, Sweden

Abstract

Adrenal insufficiency (AI) is a potentially life-threatening condition and it is of utmost importance to identify and adequately manage affected individuals. Diagnosis is often delayed, probably partly because diseases of the adrenal or pituitary region that cause primary AI (PAI) or central AI are relatively rare conditions. However, iatrogenic AI, i.e. the physiological downregulation of the hypothalamic-pituitary-adrenal axis and adrenal atrophy caused by glucocorticoid treatment for different inflammatory conditions is likely to be considerably more common. The type of glucocorticoid, dose and duration of treatment are factors to consider when trying to predict the risk of developing symptoms of AI. However, the considerable individual variation in the sensitivity for developing iatrogenic AI impedes prediction. In industrialized countries, autoimmune adrenalitis accounts for the majority of cases of PAI. Among children, genetic conditions – in particular congenital adrenal hyperplasia – need to be considered. Important risk groups for central AI are patients with tumours in the hypothalamic-pituitary region, moderate-to-severe traumatic head injury and patients who receive cranial radiotherapy or cytotoxic T-lymphocyte antigen 4 blockade treatment. Structured endocrine follow-up is essential in these groups. Health workers need to be attentive to these potentially fatal conditions and at-risk populations should be carefully informed about symptoms and signs of AI.

Patients suffering from adrenal insufficiency (AI) have a deficient production or action of glucocorticoids. Primary AI (PAI) is present if the adrenal cortex itself is affected. Central AI results from pituitary or hypothalamic disease that hampers the release of adrenocorticotropic hormone (ACTH) from the pituitary and/or corticotropin-releasing hormone from the hypothalamus with subsequent loss of stimulation of adrenal cortisol synthesis. Exogenous glucocorticoids exert negative feedback on the hypothalamic-pituitary-adrenal axis by inhibiting the release of corticotropin-releasing hormone and ACTH, which can cause iatrogenic AI. Irrespective of the cause, AI is a potentially life-threatening condition and to identify and adequately manage affected individuals is of utmost importance. This chapter gives an overview of the epidemiology of the different forms of AI, emphasizing some patient groups that are important not to overlook.

Primary Adrenal Insufficiency

AI was first described by Thomas Addison, a physician working at Guy's Hospital in London. In a monograph published in 1855, he described the typical symptoms and clinical findings of 11 patients suffering from PAI. Back in Addison's day and well into the 20th century, tuberculosis was the predominant cause of PAI. Nowadays, PAI from infectious disorders has dramatically declined in industrialized countries (<10%) and instead autoimmune adrenalitis accounts for the majority of cases (>80%) [1, 2]. Other causes include genetic (e.g. X-linked adrenoleukodystrophy, adrenal hypolasia congenita, triple A syndrome, familiar glucocorticoid deficiency, Smith-Lemli-Opitz syndrome and Kearns-Sayre syndrome), haemorrhagic, metastatic and infiltrative disorders and drugs, but these are all rare in adult patients. It is important to note that infections, like tuberculosis and HIV, still account for a substantial and probably underestimated number of PAI cases in developing countries either from direct destruction, opportunistic infections or medication (e.g. rifampicin, protease inhibitors and ketoconazole). The symptoms of PAI are often unspecific, making it difficult to recognize and correctly diagnose a patient. Considerable delay in the diagnosis, often months and sometimes years, has recently been reported [3]. Many patients are severely ill at diagnosis and fatalities among undiagnosed cases are described in historic as well as contemporary reports [4]. Thus, the awareness of PAI is still insufficient, which stresses the need for better training of medical staff.

Autoimmune PAI

Autoimmune PAI has a female preponderance and commonly presents in young and middle-aged adults [2, 5]. The disease may appear clinically isolated (<40%), but more often is seen together with other autoimmune diseases as part of an autoimmune polyendocrine syndrome (APS) [1]. APS1 is a rare monogenic autosomal recessive disease with chronic mucocutaneous candidiasis, hypoparathyroidism and PAI as major components [6]. The prevalence of APS1 is estimated at 1:80,000 worldwide, but more common in Iranian Jews (1:9,000), Sardinians (1:14,000) and Finns (1:25,000) [6]. APS2 is a considerably more common disorder, often featuring PAI in combination with type 1 diabetes and/or autoimmune thyroid disease. If PAI is considered in a patient, a concomitant autoimmune disease certainly increases clinical suspicion. In 1992, the enzyme steroid 21-hydroxylase was identified as the major autoantigen in autoimmune PAI [7]. Autoantibodies against 21-hydroxylase are present in the majority (>90%) of patients with autoimmune PAI, but not in patients with non-autoimmune forms (0%) [2, 8]. Thus, 21-hydroxylase autoantibody analysis should be the test of first choice in the mandatory evaluation of the aetiological diagnosis of PAI [9].

Congenital Adrenal Hyperplasia
In children, autoimmune PAI is relatively uncommon while genetic causes dominate [10]. Congenital adrenal hyperplasia (CAH), an autosomal recessive disorder affecting 1/10,000–1/20,000 newborns [11, 12], is the most common genetic cause of PAI. More than 90% of CAH results from 21-hydroxylase deficiency caused by mutations in the *CYP21A2* gene (OMIM 613815). Different mutations result in no or some residual enzyme activity, causing variable degrees of cortisol and mineralocorticoid deficiency together with concurrent adrenal androgen excess. If not promptly diagnosed and treated, severe forms of CAH may result in fatal adrenal crisis already in early infancy. Many countries have introduced neonatal screening programs for CAH, and some have proven to be very effective in detecting severe cases and thereby reducing mortality [12]. In nations without screening CAH, cases are demonstrably missed and contribute to neonatal deaths [13].

Epidemiology of PAI
PAI is considered a rare disease, but the prevalence has gradually increased in contemporary developed economies. Robust European registry data have recently estimated the prevalence rate of autoimmune PAI to be 87–144 cases per million [1, 5, 14, 15]. The European incidence has been estimated to be 4–6 cases per million per year and is proposed to be rising [5, 14]. Why the incidence of autoimmune PAI seems to be increasing in Europe in the last decades is poorly understood, but improved clinical awareness and diagnostic tools are probably chiefly responsible. A general increase of autoimmune diseases other than autoimmune PAI has been observed, including type 1 diabetes mellitus and coeliac disease, indicating that environmental factors may also contribute. Limited epidemiological data exist from the rest of the world, but generally report lower prevalence – the lowest being 5 cases per million from Japan [16]. The global variations in the incidence and prevalence of PAI could relate to genetic variation, environmental factors, access to adequate diagnostics tools and difficulties identifying all cases in a population since nationwide patient registry data of good quality are not frequently available.

Central Adrenal Insufficiency

Central AI is more common than PAI [17]. Two Spanish population-based studies found prevalence rates of ACTH deficiency to be 23–28/100,000 [18, 19]. The most frequent cause is a pituitary adenoma, causing hypopituitarism by mass effect of the tumour itself or by treatment with surgery and/or radiotherapy [18]. However, other tumours in the hypothalamic-pituitary region, such as craniopharyngiomas, meningiomas, and intrasellar and suprasellar metastases can also cause central AI. Other causes include cranial radiotherapy, traumatic brain injury (TBI), lymphocytic hypophysitis, Sheehan's syndrome, and infections or infiltrative disease of the pituitary [17]. Central AI is usually found together with other pituitary hormone deficiencies, except for a few rare genetic causes and some cases of lymphocytic hypophysitis. Importantly, the increased mortality in patients with pituitary insufficiency is largely attributable to the ACTH deficiency (mainly due to increased mortality in infections) [17, 20].

Pituitary Tumours
Recent studies report a prevalence of clinically relevant pituitary adenomas of 76–94/100,000 [21, 22] and an incidence of 4/100,000 per year [23]. In the Swedish Pituitary Registry, 18% of 4,263 patients with pituitary adenomas (1991–2013) had ACTH deficiency at diagnosis. ACTH deficiency was more common in patients with non-functioning pituitary adenomas and much less frequent in patients with microadenomas (<1 cm). ACTH deficiency was increased to 27% in 3,253 patients at follow-up 1 year after diagnosis (unpubl. data). Based on this, the prevalence of ACTH deficiency due to pituitary adenoma can be estimated to be around 23/100,000 inhabitants and the incidence close to 1/100,000 per year. To this should be added patients with other, rarer tumours like craniopharyngiomas, where ACTH deficiency may be more prevalent. Consequently, assessment of adrenal function is essential in all patients with tumours in the hypothalamic-pituitary region at diagnosis and after surgery and radiation.

Traumatic Brain Injury and Subarachnoid Haemorrhage
TBI is a major cause of death and disability among young adults. An estimated 775,000 patients are hospitalized in Europe every year due to TBI. The pituitary is vulnerable to head trauma due to its anatomical location, fragile structure and vascular supply. Hypothalamic and pituitary damage caused by TBI has been recognized for almost a century, but was until recently considered rare [24]. The chronic sequelae after TBI (i.e. fatigue, memory impairment and emotional lability) have close resemblance with symptoms of hypopituitarism and may therefore be difficult to recognize in TBI patients. During the last decade, several studies have shown permanent post-traumatic hypopituitarism in 25–68% of patients after TBI [24]. The risk of post-traumatic hypopituitarism appears to be higher after more severe TBI [25]. However, the reported prevalence of permanent post-traumatic hypopituitarism varies considerably, which may be due to differences in trauma severity, time after TBI and diagnostic criteria for hypopituitarism, i.e. the reported prevalence of central AI after TBI varies from 0 to 60% assessed by basal serum cortisol or ACTH stimulation or insulin-tolerance tests [26]. Later studies with strict definitions of pituitary hormone deficiencies show con-

siderably lower prevalence of permanent ACTH insufficiency after TBI, i.e. 1–13% [24, 25, 27]. A similar high prevalence of pituitary insufficiency, including ACTH deficiency, has been reported after aneurysmal subarachnoid haemorrhage. Taken together, this suggests that pituitary insufficiency, including central AI, may be an often overlooked, treatable complication, which may hamper rehabilitation and impair long-term outcome after TBI and subarachnoid haemorrhage. Consequently, patients with at least moderate or severe TBI should complete laboratory screening for pituitary insufficiency.

Radiotherapy

Remarkable improvements in childhood cancer treatment over the last decades have increased 5-year survival to almost 80% [28]. Side effects of treatments such as cranial irradiation for intracerebral tumours and total body irradiation for haematological malignancies are often associated with endocrine disorders, including pituitary insufficiency [28]. Growth hormone deficiency is the most common pituitary hormone deficiency, whereas ACTH deficiency is less common. However, the 4-year cumulative incidence of ACTH deficiency was 38% in a study on children treated for central nervous system embryonal tumours, including high doses of radiation to the hypothalamic-pituitary area (median: 44 Gray) [29]. The onset of pituitary insufficiency may occur years after cancer treatment and symptoms may be elusive and progress slowly. More recently acknowledged is that pituitary insufficiency also occurs frequently after cranial radiotherapy for non-pituitary tumours in adult patients. In a meta-analysis including 608 adult patients treated for nasopharyngeal cancer and 205 for intracerebral tumours, ACTH deficiency was present in 22% of the patients (and pituitary insufficiency of any axis in 66%) [30]. Thus, systematic long-term endocrine follow-up is necessary in order to not overlook hormone deficiencies, including a potentially life-threatening AI, in an increasing number of childhood cancer survivors and adults after radiotherapy to the head.

Cytotoxic T-Lymphocyte Antigen 4 Blockade

Ipilimumab is a monoclonal antibody against cytotoxic T-lymphocyte antigen 4 (CTLA-4), used for the treatment of advanced malignant melanoma since 2011. The CTLA-4 receptor, present on T lymphocytes, works as a negative regulator of T-cell activation. Ipilimumab blocks CTLA-4, causing activation of cytotoxic lymphocytes, which results in an immune-mediated antitumour response. The treatment-induced immunostimulation often also results in immune-related side effects, including autoimmune dermatitis with rashes, colitis, hepatitis and hypophysitis. The incidence of hypophysitis secondary to ipilimumab has been reported in clinical trials to range from 0 to 17%, and a recent study even reported it to be as high as 25% with use of high doses [31]. ACTH deficiency frequently occurs among patients with CTLA-4-associated hypophysitis. Therefore, monitoring of pituitary function, especially the hypothalamic-pituitary-adrenal axis is essential in patients treated with CTLA-4 antibodies.

Iatrogenic Adrenal Insufficiency

Epidemiology of Iatrogenic AI

Since their introduction in 1949, glucocorticoids have revolutionized the treatment of inflammatory and immunologically mediated diseases. The use of therapeutic glucocorticoids has gradually increased, and 1% of the population in the United Kingdom was on long-term treatment in 2000 [32]. In 2007, 200,000 patients in Sweden (approx. 2.2% of the population) were treated for 3 weeks or more with oral glucocorticoids [33]. Treatment with exogenous glucocorticoids is consequently widespread. There are reports on adrenal suppression by therapeutic glucocorticoids for all administration routes used. The most well-known connection is with the use of oral glucocorticoids, but there is also evidence of adrenal suppression after treatment with inhaled, topical, rectal, ocular and intra-articular use of glucocorticoids [34].

Iatrogenic AI is considered the most common cause of AI, but the actual prevalence is not firmly established because of difficulties in comparing the different studies conducted to date. The duration of treatment, dose, type of glucocorticoid, diagnostic test, cortisol assay and patient group studied varies considerably. A recent review argues that as many as 46–100% of patients might have iatrogenic AI at withdrawal of glucocorticoid therapy, up to 50% after a week and a few percent after months [35]. Symptoms of hypocortisolism, i.e. iatrogenic AI, are unspecific (weight loss, nausea, fatigue, etc.) and can be difficult to separate from symptoms of the underlying disease for which glucocorticoid treatment was initiated. Furthermore, the correlation between symptoms and biochemical unresponsiveness to exogenous ACTH is poorly studied. This makes clinical decisions on how to treat iatrogenic AI difficult, and to this day there are no prospective studies on the safest way to withdraw glucocorticoid treatment. However, it is crucial to identify and adequately care for patients that cannot mobilize the amount of cortisol needed in stressful conditions during and/or following treatment with glucocorticoids. Contemporary reports of adrenal crisis and fatal cases due to iatrogenic AI still exist, confirming that our awareness and preventive measures of this problem are insufficient. The guidelines for administering stress doses of exogenous glucocorticoids are based on studies of PAI, making clinical decisions about iatrogenic AI a challenge.

Prediction of Iatrogenic AI

The type of glucocorticoid, duration of treatment, and total and highest dose are factors to consider when trying to predict the risk of developing symptoms of AI and in assessing the risk for an adrenal crisis in case of stress during treatment or following cessation of therapy. There is, however, considerable variation between individuals who are susceptible to developing iatrogenic AI, and this evidently impedes prediction. Therapeutic glucocorticoids with a long biological half-life and strong glucocorticoid receptor activation have a greater negative influence on the hypothalamic-pituitary-adrenal axis [36]. Doses less than 5 mg/day of prednisone or equivalent are not thought to induce adrenal suppression, but for higher doses there is a much less clear relationship between the dose used and the development of AI [37]. Short-term treatment (<3 weeks) is generally considered safe even though high-dose, short-term treatment gives transient adrenal suppression, which could be clinically relevant under some circumstances [38]. Long-term treatment can suppress the adrenals for months to years after withdrawal of the glucocorticoid [36].

Conclusions

PAI and central AI are rare but potentially life-threatening conditions, often with long diagnostic delay. The prevalence of iatrogenic AI is probably more common and also potentially fatal. To decrease diagnostic delay and minimize the risk of acute adrenal crisis, it is crucial that health workers are attentive to these conditions and know how to diagnose and adequately care for affected individuals. Also, populations at risk should be carefully informed about symptoms and signs of AI.

Acknowledgements

We thank the Swedish Pituitary Registry for data regarding secondary AI. This work was supported by the Swedish Society for Medical Research (to S.B.).

References

1 Erichsen MM, Lovas K, Skinningsrud B, Wolff AB, Undlien DE, Svartberg J, Fougner KJ, Berg TJ, Bollerslev J, Mella B, Carlson JA, Erlich H, Husebye ES: Clinical, immunological, and genetic features of autoimmune primary adrenal insufficiency: observations from a Norwegian registry. J Clin Endocrinol Metab 2009;94:4882–4890.

2 Betterle C, Scarpa R, Garelli S, Morlin L, Lazzarotto F, Presotto F, Coco G, Masiero S, Parolo A, Albergoni MP, Favero R, Barollo S, Salva M, Basso D, Chen S, Rees Smith B, Furmaniak J, Mantero F: Addison's disease: a survey on 633 patients in Padova. Eur J Endocrinol 2013;169:773–784.

3 Bleicken B, Hahner S, Ventz M, Quinkler M: Delayed diagnosis of adrenal insufficiency is common: a cross-sectional study in 216 patients. Am J Med Sci 2010;339:525–531.

4 Erichsen MM, Lovas K, Fougner KJ, Svartberg J, Hauge ER, Bollerslev J, Berg JP, Mella B, Husebye ES: Normal overall mortality rate in Addison's disease, but young patients are at risk of premature death. Eur J Endocrinol 2009;160:233–237.

5 Bjornsdottir S, Sundstrom A, Ludvigsson JF, Blomqvist P, Kampe O, Bensing S: Drug prescription patterns in patients with Addison's disease: a Swedish population-based cohort study. J Clin Endocrinol Metab 2013;98:2009–2018.

6 Husebye ES, Perheentupa J, Rautemaa R, Kampe O: Clinical manifestations and management of patients with autoimmune polyendocrine syndrome type I. J Intern Med 2009;265:514–529.

7 Winqvist O, Karlsson FA, Kampe O: 21-hydroxylase, a major autoantigen in idiopathic Addison's disease. Lancet 1992;339:1559–1562.

8 Falorni A, Nikoshkov A, Laureti S, Grenbäck E, Hulting AL, Casucci G, Santeusanio F, Brunetti P, Luthman H, Lernmark Å: High diagnostic accuracy for idiopathic Addison's disease with a sensitive radiobinding assay for autoantibodies against recombinant human 21-hydroxylase. J Clin Endocrinol Metab 1995;80:2752–2755.

9 Husebye ES, Allolio B, Arlt W, Badenhoop K, Bensing S, Betterle C, Falorni A, Gan EH, Hulting AL, Kasperlik-Zaluska A, Kämpe O, Løvås K, Meyer G, Pearce SH: Consensus statement on the diagnosis, treatment and follow-up of patients with primary adrenal insufficiency. J Intern Med 2014;275:104–115.

10 Hsieh S, Weir PC: Presentation of primary adrenal insufficiency in childhood. J Clin Endocrinol Metab 2011;96:E925–E928.

11 White PC: Neonatal screening for congenital adrenal hyperplasia. Nat Rev Endocrinol 2009;5:490–498.

12 Gidlof S, Falhammar H, Thilen A, von Dobeln U, Ritzen M, Wedell A, Nordenstrom A: One hundred years of congenital adrenal hyperplasia in Sweden: a retrospective, population-based cohort study. Lancet Diabetes Endocrinol 2013;1:35–42.

13 Grosse SD, Van Vliet G: How many deaths can be prevented by newborn screening for congenital adrenal hyperplasia? Horm Res 2007;67:284–291.

14 Meyer G, Neumann K, Badenhoop K, Linder R: Increasing prevalence of Addison's disease in German females: health insurance data 2008–2012. Eur J Endocrinol 2014;170:367–373.

15 Laureti S, Vecchi L, Santeusanio F, Falorni A: Is the prevalence of Addison's disease underestimated? J Clin Endocrinol Metab 1999;84:1762.

16 Takayanagi R, Miura K, Nakagawa H, Nawata H: Epidemiologic study of adrenal gland disorders in Japan. Biomed Parmacother 2000;54(suppl 1):164s–168s.

17 Crowley RK, Argese N, Tomlinson JW, Stewart PM: Central hypoadrenalism. J Clin Endocrinol Metab 2014;99:4027–4036.

18 Regal M, Paramo C, Sierra SM, Garcia-Mayor RV: Prevalence and incidence of hypopituitarism in an adult Caucasian population in northwestern Spain. Clin Endocrinol (Oxf) 2001;55:735–740.

19 Fernandez-Rodriguez E, Lopez-Raton M, Andujar P, Martinez-Silva IM, Cadarso-Suarez C, Casanueva FF, Bernabeu I: Epidemiology, mortality rate and survival in a homogeneous population of hypopituitary patients. Clin Endocrinol (Oxf) 2013;78:278–284.

20 Burman P, Mattsson AF, Johannsson G, Hoybye C, Holmer H, Dahlqvist P, Berinder K, Engstrom BE, Ekman B, Erfurth EM, Svensson J, Wahlberg J, Karlsson FA: Deaths among adult patients with hypopituitarism: hypocortisolism during acute stress, and de novo malignant brain tumors contribute to an increased mortality. J Clin Endocrinol Metab 2013;98:1466–1475.

21 Fernandez A, Karavitaki N, Wass JA: Prevalence of pituitary adenomas: a community-based, cross-sectional study in Banbury (Oxfordshire, UK). Clin Endocrinol (Oxf) 2010;72:377–382.

22 Daly AF, Rixhon M, Adam C, Dempegioti A, Tichomirowa MA, Beckers A: High prevalence of pituitary adenomas: a cross-sectional study in the province of Liege, Belgium. J Clin Endocrinol Metab 2006;91:4769–4775.

23 Tjornstrand A, Gunnarsson K, Evert M, Holmberg E, Ragnarsson O, Rosen T, Filipsson Nystrom H: The incidence rate of pituitary adenomas in western Sweden for the period 2001–2011. Eur J Endocrinol 2014;171:519–526.

24 Agha A, Thompson CJ: Anterior pituitary dysfunction following traumatic brain injury (TBI). Clin Endocrinol (Oxf) 2006;64:481–488.

25 Klose M, Juul A, Struck J, Morgenthaler NG, Kosteljanetz M, Feldt-Rasmussen U: Acute and long-term pituitary insufficiency in traumatic brain injury: a prospective single-centre study. Clin Endocrinol (Oxf) 2007;67:598–606.

26 Kokshoorn NE, Wassenaar MJ, Biermasz NR, Roelfsema F, Smit JW, Romijn JA, Pereira AM: Hypopituitarism following traumatic brain injury: prevalence is affected by the use of different dynamic tests and different normal values. Eur J Endocrinol 2010;162:11–18.

27 Tanriverdi F, Schneider HJ, Aimaretti G, Masel BE, Casanueva FF, Kelestimur F: Pituitary dysfunction after traumatic brain injury: a clinical and pathophysiological approach. Endocr Rev 2015;36:305–342.

28 Chemaitilly W, Sklar CA: Endocrine complications in long-term survivors of childhood cancers. Endocr Relat Cancer 2010;17:R141–R159.

29 Laughton SJ, Merchant TE, Sklar CA, Kun LE, Fouladi M, Broniscer A, Morris EB, Sanders RP, Krasin MJ, Shelso J, Xiong Z, Wallace D, Gajjar A: Endocrine outcomes for children with embryonal brain tumors after risk-adapted craniospinal and conformal primary-site irradiation and high-dose chemotherapy with stem-cell rescue on the SJMB-96 trial. J Clin Oncol 2008;26:1112–1118.

30 Appelman-Dijkstra NM, Kokshoorn NE, Dekkers OM, Neelis KJ, Biermasz NR, Romijn JA, Smit JW, Pereira AM: Pituitary dysfunction in adult patients after cranial radiotherapy: systematic review and meta-analysis. J Clin Endocrinol Metab 2011;96:2330–2340.

31 Albarel F, Gaudy C, Castinetti F, Carre T, Morange I, Conte-Devolx B, Grob JJ, Brue T: Long-term follow-up of ipilimumab-induced hypophysitis, a common adverse event of the anti-CTLA-4 antibody in melanoma. Eur J Endocrinol 2015;172:195–204.

32 Van Staa TP, Abenhaim L, Cooper C, Zhang B, Leufkens HG: The use of a large pharmacoepidemiological database to study exposure to oral corticosteroids and risk of fractures: validation of study population and results. Pharmacoepidemiol Drug Saf 2000;9:359–366.

33 Calissendorff J, Blomqvist H: Secondary cortisol insufficiency – an undiagnosed condition (in Swedish). Lakartidningen 2007;104:2965–2968.

34 Broersen LH, Pereira AM, Jorgensen JO, Dekkers OM: Adrenal insufficiency in corticosteroids use: systematic review and meta-analysis. J Clin Endocrinol Metab 2015;100:2171–2180.

35 Dinsen S, Baslund B, Klose M, Rasmussen AK, Friis-Hansen L, Hilsted L, Feldt-Rasmussen U: Why glucocorticoid withdrawal may sometimes be as dangerous as the treatment itself. Eur J Int Med 2013;24: 714–720.

36 Kronenberg H, Williams RH: Williams Textbook of Endocrinology, ed 11. Philadelphia, Saunders/Elsevier, 2008.

37 LaRochelle GE Jr, LaRochelle AG, Ratner RE, Borenstein DG: Recovery of the hypothalamic-pituitary-adrenal (HPA) axis in patients with rheumatic diseases receiving low-dose prednisone. Am J Med 1993;95:258–264.

38 Henzen C, Suter A, Lerch E, Urbinelli R, Schorno XH, Briner VA: Suppression and recovery of adrenal response after short-term, high-dose glucocorticoid treatment. Lancet 2000;355:542–545.

Sophie Bensing, MD, PhD
Department of Molecular Medicine and Surgery, Karolinska Institutet
Karolinska University Hospital-Solna D2:04
SE–171 76 Stockholm (Sweden)
E-Mail sophie.bensing@ki.se

Arvat E, Falorni A (eds): Cortisol Excess and Insufficiency.
Front Horm Res. Basel, Karger, 2016, vol 46, pp 115–132 (DOI: 10.1159/000443871)

From Genetic Predisposition to Molecular Mechanisms of Autoimmune Primary Adrenal Insufficiency

Alberto Falorni[a] • Annalisa Brozzetti[a] • Roberto Perniola[b]

[a]Section of Internal Medicine and Endocrine and Metabolic Sciences, Department of Medicine, University of Perugia, Perugia, and [b]Department of Pediatrics – Neonatal Intensive Care, V. Fazzi Regional Hospital, Lecce, Italy

Abstract

Autoimmune Addison's disease (AAD) is a complex disease that results from the interaction of a predisposing genetic background with still unknown environmental factors. Pathogenic variants in the autoimmune regulator *(AIRE)* gene are responsible for autoimmune polyendocrine syndrome type 1, of which AAD is a major disease component. Among the genetic factors for isolated AAD and autoimmune polyendocrine syndrome type 2, a key role is played by HLA class II genes: *HLA-DRB1*0301-DQA1*0501-DQB1*0201* and *DRB1*04-DQA1*0301-DQB1*0302* are positively, and *DRB1*0403* is negatively, associated with genetic risk for AAD. The MHC class I chain-related gene A *(MICA)* allele 5.1 is strongly and positively associated with AAD. Other gene polymorphisms contribute to the genetic risk for AAD, including *CIITA* (MHC class II transactivator), the master regulator of MHC class II expression, cytotoxic T-lymphocyte antigen-4 *(CTLA-4)*, *PTPN22*, *STAT4*, *PD-L1*, *NALP1*, *FCRL3*, *GPR174*, *GATA3*, *NFATC1*, *CYP27B1* and the vitamin D receptor.

In Western countries and Japan, an autoimmune process is responsible for the destruction of the adrenocortical cells and clinical manifestations of primary adrenocortical insufficiency (PAI) in around 80–90% of cases [1]. Autoimmune PAI is also known as autoimmune Addison's disease (AAD), after the name of the physician who in 1855 described the disease and attributed it to a pathology of the adrenal glands. In AAD, autoimmune adrenalitis determines a destructive process of all three layers of the adrenal cortex, with subsequent concomitant deficiency of glucocorticoids, mineralocorticoids and adrenal androgens.

Table 1. Risk of AAD in different populations

Population	Overall risk	References
General adult population	1/7,000–1/7,500	1, 11, 12
First-degree relatives of AAD patients	1/300–1/400	1, 6–8
Patients with thyroid autoimmune diseases or T1DM	1/300–1/400	1, 6–8
Patients with POI or primary hypoparathyroidism	1/10–1/20	1, 13

The autoimmune process responsible for AAD is characterized by the appearance of circulating adrenal cortex autoantibodies (ACA), detected by indirect immunofluorescence on cryostatic tissue sections. The major adrenocortical autoantigen is the cytochrome-P450 (CYP) enzyme steroid 21-hydroxylase (21-OH): the related autoantibodies (21-OH-Ab) are present in approximately 70–80% of patients with AAD and in 85–90% of patients with autoimmune polyendocrine syndrome type 1 (APS1). Although autoantibodies to adrenocortical targets do not seem to be pathogenic, detection of 21-OH-Ab by radioimmunological or radiobinding assays is currently the gold standard marker for identifying AAD in patients with clinical signs of PAI [2, 3]. 21-OH-Ab have a high diagnostic sensitivity and specificity for AAD [4] and have been included in a comprehensive flowchart of immunological, biochemical and imaging data for accurate etiological classification of PAI cases [5].

The appearance of 21-OH-Ab in the serum of patients with other autoimmune diseases but no clinical signs of PAI configures a preclinical AAD [6–8]. It is estimated that around 1–1.5% of patients with autoimmune thyroid diseases (ATD), 1–1.5% of patients with type-1 diabetes mellitus (T1DM) and 4–5% of women with premature primary ovarian insufficiency (POI) are positive for 21-OH-Ab. In these cases, an ACTH stimulation test identifies the patients undergoing an irreversible process of organ damage that ultimately leads to overt AAD: statistically, more than 50% of the subjects with a normal response to the test will exhibit spontaneous remission of preclinical AAD, while an impaired response predicts AAD onset within a few years in 80–95% of cases [6–8].

The concomitant presence of two or more autoimmune endocrine diseases configures the autoimmune polyendocrine syndromes, which are classified according to the disease components [1]. Biochemical or clinical signs of another autoimmune disease are present in more than 60% of AAD patients, and AAD is a major component of both APS1 and autoimmune polyendocrine syndrome type 2 (APS2). APS1 is a rare, inherited disease caused by pathogenic variants in the autoimmune regulator (*AIRE*) gene [9]. Although no association was initially established between APS1 and genes other than *AIRE*, subsequent studies have shown that some disease components, AAD included, recognize specific HLA class II alleles as determinants [10]. APS2 occurs in adult subjects and is characterized by the association of AAD with

ATD, T1DM or both [1]. APS2 and isolated AAD share a common predisposition with other autoimmune endocrine diseases, with a major contribution of HLA genes.

Lastly, population studies suggest a familial and individual susceptibility to AAD (table 1): disease risk is 1/7,500 in the general population [11, 12], but rises to 1/400 in first-degree relatives of AAD patients and in patients with ATD or T1DM. In women with autoimmune POI, the risk for (preclinical or clinical) AAD is 1/10–1/20 [13].

AIRE and Autoimmune Addison's Disease

As indicated, APS1 is a monogenic disease with autosomal recessive inheritance, caused by pathogenic variants in the *AIRE* gene, which is located on chromosome 21 and encodes for the homonymous protein, AIRE [9]. The syndrome is also known by the acronym APECED (autoimmune polyendocrinopathy-candidiasis-ectodermal dystrophy) to better depict the main types of clinical manifestations [14]. Major components of APS1 are chronic mucocutaneous candidiasis, hypoparathyroidism and AAD. Clinical diagnosis requires the coexistence of two major components; only one major component is sufficient if a first-degree relative of the patient was already diagnosed with APS1 [14]. AAD occurs in about three quarters of APS1 patients, with no gender preponderance. Onset of AAD-related symptoms is usually observed at the beginning of the second decade of life. Various other endocrine and non-endocrine diseases, which include autoimmune POI in the female sex, atrophic gastritis with pernicious anaemia, ATD, T1DM, malabsorption and autoimmune hepatitis, may be observed. Dystrophies of the ectodermal tissues, such as alopecia, vitiligo, interstitial keratitis, nail dystrophy and calcifications of the tympanic membrane, complete the clinical picture [14]. Typically, sera from APS1 patients test positive for many autoantibody specificities, including those to two further adreno-cortical/gonadal autoantigens, namely CYP enzymes 17α-hydroxylase and side-chain cleavage [15]. More recent studies have shown that almost all APS1 patients exhibit positivity for autoantibodies to type-1 interferons (IFN), mainly IFNα_2 and IFNω [16]. Because of their sensitivity and early appearance, it has been suggested that assay of such autoantibodies should be used in a diagnostic flowchart to identify atypical forms of APS1 [16]. In addition, autoantibodies to interleukins (IL) produced by T-helper-17 cells, such as IL-17A, IL-17F and IL-22, have been documented in APS1 patients [17].

AIRE acts as a regulator, especially activator, of gene transcription. The biophysical and biochemical properties of AIRE are connected with the domains that compose the amino-acid chain [18]. At the N-terminal end of the molecule, the homogeneously staining region or caspase-recruitment domain is responsible for the intracellular compartmentalization of AIRE, mediates its homomerization and is presumably implied in proapoptotic activity. The middle SAND domain contains several amino-acid basic groups, which could be engaged in electrostatic interaction with the phosphate groups of DNA. Interestingly, an AIRE variant lying in the SAND domain, p.Gly228Trp, has been associated with autosomal dominant inheritance of APS1, featured by unusually high prevalence of ATD [19]. Similar evidence has been observed in mice bearing the corresponding amino-acid substitution [20]. Lastly, AIRE comprises, at the C-terminal end, two plant-homeodomain (PHD) fingers, named PHD1 and PHD2, which represent cysteine-rich sequences and enclose a Cys4HisCys3 motif coordinating two zinc ions. Similarly to PHD belonging to other transcription factors, AIRE PHD1 would be able to 'read' the post-translational modifications of the histones, in particular the degree of methylation of the amino acids placed in the tail of histone H3: this interaction is critical in conditioning, either permissively or repressively, the downstream events. On the other hand, PHD2, which is unable to bind to the histones, would confer to AIRE the actual property of promoting the gene transcription.

Some pathogenic AIRE variants are prevalent in certain geographical areas. Typically, p.Arg257* is found in Finnish and Northern European APS1 patients [9], while p.Leu323Serfs* is common in British patients [21], and p.Arg139* is typical of Sardinian patients [22]. In any case, AIRE variants do not provide for a genotype-phenotype correlation, and the set of disease components and severity of the clinical picture are rather influenced, as indicated, by other genetic traits, mainly HLA class II alleles [10].

The murine *Aire* gene, similarly to the human homolog, reaches a significant expression only in a subset of medullary thymic epithelial cells and, albeit to a lesser degree, in thymic dendritic cells [23, 24]. Importantly, medullary thymic epithelial cells are a privileged site of promiscuous gene expression, a phenomenon characterized by transcription of genes encoding for autoantigens ordinarily restricted to specific extrathymic tissues. Thymic self-representation is finalized to the presentation of the autoantigens to the maturing thymocytes: the negative selection and consequent apoptosis of the thymocytes bearing T-cell receptors with critical affinity/avidity for the interacting epitopes represents the main mechanism of central tolerance and avoids the release of autoreactive mature T cells in the periphery. A body of evidence indicates that Aire drives the transcription of the genes encoding for tissue-specific autoantigens in medullary thymic epithelial cells, and that Aire deficiency compromises the above program of self-tolerance [25, 26].

Murine models of disease highlight that species-specific variables affect the clinical picture emerging from Aire deficiency: although *Aire*-deficient (*Aire*$^{-/-}$) mice exhibit lymphocyte infiltration of various organs accompanied by appearance of several autoantibody specificities, the resulting phenotype does not match with that of human APS1 [27, 28]. Moreover, the use of highly inbred murine lines demonstrates how genetic background determines (at the intraspecies level) the susceptibility to the onset of single disease components, and ultimately dictates the severity of the phenotype [29, 30].

With regard to the involvement of the adrenal cortex in *Aire*$^{-/-}$ mice, it should be underlined that, although in some cases adrenal glands were undetectable at dissection, neither lymphocyte infiltration of the adrenocortical tissue nor clinical signs resembling those of human PAI have been reported [27, 28]. Again, autoantibodies to CYP enzymes are unusual in *Aire*$^{-/-}$ mice [31]. In what is an even more enigmatic issue, dependency from Aire of the genes encoding the above molecules is uncertain in itself [32], so it seems correct to conclude that the link between adrenocortical autoimmunity and human AIRE/murine Aire needs to be clarified.

MHC Class I and Class II Polymorphisms and Autoimmune Addison's Disease

A long series of studies have confirmed that the major histocompatibility complex plays a major role in genetic susceptibility for AAD [33–42] (table 2).

Initial studies demonstrated an association between the risk of AAD (as well as of other endocrine autoimmune diseases) and HLA-B8. These studies were limited in some cases by the lack of accurate immunological testing and the inclusion of patients with 'clinically idiopathic Addison's disease', not necessarily of autoimmune origin. Subsequent studies showed that no significant association exists between B8 and APS II, thus opening a controversial debate on the actual role of B8 in genetic predisposition for polyglandular autoimmunity.

The demonstration that T1DM is primarily associated with the polymorphism of class II genes and that the association with HLA-B polymorphism was secondary to linkage disequilibrium with DR and DQ genes paved the way for subsequent studies of the genetic association of class II genes with other endocrine autoimmune diseases, including AAD. In 1986, Maclaren and Riley [33] provided the first demonstration of the association of HLA-DR3 and -DR4 with AAD. Interestingly, the same alleles were found similarly associated with T1DM, and the association persisted even in the subgroup of 37 AAD patients without T1DM [33].

Further studies confirmed the conclusions of the Maclaren and Riley's report. More specifically, a study published in 1991 [34] showed that DR3 was associated with the disease with a relative risk of 3.2, while the association with DR4 was subdivided according to the DQ specificity: DQw8 (subsequently denominated *DQB1*0302*) was associated with AAD only in DR4+ individuals with T1DM, while DQw7 (*DQB1*0301*) conferred genetic risk for AAD in patients without T1DM.

The differential association of *DQB1*0301* and **0302* with T1DM and AAD is presumably at the basis of discordant results generated by studies published during the 1990s. Badenhoop et al. [36] studied 53 patients with Addison's disease, 171 patients with T1DM, 271 with Graves' disease, 65 with Hashimoto's thyroiditis and 271 healthy controls, and demonstrated a common genetic association of the studied diseases with *HLA-DQB1*0501-DQB1*0201* (the DQ haplotype in linkage disequilibrium with *DRB1*0301*). In the same study, *DQA1*0301-DQB1*0302* (the haplotype

Table 2. Genes found associated with the risk for non-APS1 AAD

Gene	Chromosome	References
HLA-DRB1	6p21.3	33–42
HLA-DQA1	6p21.3	33–42
HLA-DQB1	6p21.3	33–42
MICA	6p21.33	39, 50, 51
MICB	6p21.3	39
CIITA	16p13	53, 54
CTLA4	2q33	55–59
PTPN22	1p13.3-p13.1	63–65
VDR	12q13.11	60
CYP27B1	12q14.1	61
STAT4	2q32.2-q32.3	62
GATA3	10p15	62
NFKB1	4q24	62
IL23A	12q13.3	62
CD274/PD-L1	9p24	66
NLRP1	17p13.2	67
FCRL3	1q21-q22	68
GPR174	Xq21.1	69
NFATC1	18q23	70

CIITA = Class II, major histocompatibility complex, transactivator; *CTLA4* = cytotoxic T-lymphocyte-associated protein 4; *CYP27B1* = cytochrome P450, family 27, subfamily B, polypeptide 1; *FCRL3* = Fc receptor-like 3; *GATA3* = GATA-binding protein 3; *GPR174* = G protein-coupled receptor 174; *HLA* = human leukocyte antigen; *IL23A* = interleukin 23, α-subunit p19; *MICA* = MHC class I polypeptide-related sequence A; *MICB* = MHC class I polypeptide-related sequence B; *NFATC1* = nuclear factor of activated T cells, cytoplasmic, calcineurin-dependent 1; *NFKB1* = nuclear factor of kappa light polypeptide gene enhancer in B cells 1; *NLRP1*: NLR family, pyrin domain containing 1; *PD-L1* = programmed death ligand 1; *STAT4* = signal transducer and activator of transcription 4.

in linkage disequilibrium with *DRB1*04*) was significantly associated only with T1DM, but not with AAD. In a subsequent Italian study [39], a strong significant association was observed only with *DRB1*0301-DQA1*0501-DQB1*0201* (DR3-DQ2; OR = 4.77, 95% CI: 1.78–12.8), but not with *DRB1*04-DQA1*0301-DQB1*0302* (DR4-DQ8). The results of these latter two studies are at variance with those of a US study published in 1999 [38] that showed a strong association with both DQ2 and DQ8, and a preferential expression of the subtype *DRB1*0404* in AAD. The controversy regarding the association between *DRB1*04-DQA1*0301-DQB1*0302* (DR4-DQ8) and AAD was apparently resolved by two European studies published in 2002 [40] and 2005 [42].

In the Norwegian study by Myhre et al. [40], a strong and statistically significant association was detected for *DRB1*04-DQA1*0301-DQB1*0302* (DR4-DQ8; OR = 2.5, 96%: 1.6–3.8). The same study confirmed the findings of the previous US report [38], regarding the association with *DRB1*04* subtypes, as **0404*, but not **0401*, was preferentially found in patients with AAD, contrarily to what was observed in T1DM. Among the other HLA haplotypes, *DRB1*01-DQA1*01-DQB1*0501* and *DRB1*13-DQA1*0103-DQB1*0603* were negatively and significantly associated with the risk for AAD (OR = 0.1 and 0.2, respectively) [40].

The Italian study [42] confirmed that both *DQA1*0501-DQB1*0201* and *DQA1*0301-DQB1*0302* are strongly and significantly associated with AAD (with an OR higher than 6 and higher than 5, respectively). These associations were confirmed in both APS II patients (n = 78) and patients with isolated AAD (n = 88), thus confirming the conclusions of the Norwegian study and demonstrating that both haplotypes confer genetic susceptibility for AAD, also in Italy. The large number of AAD and healthy control subjects enrolled in that study [42] enabled the demonstration that the subtype *DRB1*0403* was absent in 56 DRB1*04-positive AAD patients, as well as in 113 DRB1*04-positive T1DM patients. However, *DRB1*0403* was the most frequent subtype among healthy control subjects from central Italy (representing 27% of 127 DRB1*04-positive individuals). Thus, that study [42] provided the first demonstration of the strong genetic protection conferred by *DRB1*0403* for AAD, similarly to what was observed in T1DM.

The molecular mechanisms of HLA class II genetic predisposition are not yet fully understood. A hypothesis is that the peptide-binding pocket of the predisposing DR and DQ variants would favour the lodging of autoantigen-derived peptides and their presentation to CD4+ T cells. However, this hypothesis does not explain why a long series of autoimmune diseases shares the same HLA predisposition, as for instance *DRB1*0301-DQA1*0501-DQB1*0201* in T1DM, AAD, Hashimoto's thyroiditis, Graves' disease, coeliac disease or systemic lupus erythematosus, and no evident similarities in amino-acid sequence or biologic function are shared by the relevant autoantigens. In addition, the predisposing alleles may vary in different ethnic groups also in relation to different linkage disequilibrium. An alternative hypothesis is that the predisposing HLA molecules would have a modest ability of binding peptides from autoantigens, thus reducing the efficacy of clonal deletion of autoreactive T cells in the thymus, still enabling peripheral activation of autoreactive CD4+ cells.

Occurrence of ACA and/or 21-OH-Ab in patients with other endocrine autoimmune diseases identifies the so-called preclinical Addison's disease. The overall risk to develop clinical AAD is as high as 30–40% in autoantibody-positive individuals [6–8]. Initial studies tested the effect of HLA DR polymorphism on the clinical progression towards AAD in adrenal autoantibody-positive individuals [7]. In a study of 43 ACA-positive individuals from northern Italy, subdivided into two groups, subjects progressing towards clinical or subclinical AAD at follow-up (n = 22) and subjects maintaining normal adrenal function (n = 21), DR3 was the only allele found positively associated with progression of the disease, even though the strength of this marker was lower than that of other major factors, such as high ACA levels, impaired response to the ACTH stimulation test or presence of two or more concomitant autoimmune diseases [7]. In a larger, more recent study of 100 ACA-positive individuals from northern Italy, Coco et al. [8] observed that the presence of DR3 and/or DR4 was not associated with risk of progression towards clinical AAD at multivariate analysis. Thus, the HLA class II status appears to modulate the risk for the development of an adrenal autoimmune process, but progression to clinical disease is influenced by other variables.

Baker et al. [43] have shown that the class I allele HLA-B15 is protective for the development of clinical AAD in subjects positive for 21-OH-Ab, thus further stressing the importance of negatively associated/protective alleles in the risk for the disease.

Other HLA Genes

Around 8% of the human genome consists of retrovirus-like elements, corresponding to 50–1,000 proviral copies of different full-length human endogenous retrovirus elements per haploid human genome with up to 25,000 copies of solitary long terminal repeats (LTR) distributed on most human chromosomes [44].

The DQ-LTR13 retrovirus-like element is located close to the *DQB1* gene (1.3 Kb upstream), outside the deletion in the 5′ flanking region of the *DQB1* gene. It was reported that the presence of DQ-LTR13 would be significantly increased in T1DM and AAD patients [45], and it has been hypothesized that DQ-LTR13 might play a role in pathogenesis of human autoimmunity [46]. DQ-LTR13 would function as an upstream regulatory element increasing the activity of the *DQB1*0302* promoter and decreasing that of the *DQB1*0201* promoter [46]. The decreased activity of the *DQB1*0201* promoter in the presence of DQ-LTR13 is in line with the strong association of *DRB1*03-DQA1*0501-DQB1*0201*-LTR13– with endocrine autoimmune diseases observed in some studies [45]. It has been speculated [46] that the different effect of DQ-LTR13 on high-risk DQB1 alleles might be related to a different interaction with an allelic polymorphism described in the 5′-flanking region of the DQB1 gene and characterized by a TG dinucleotide which is present on the *DQB1*0302* allele, but absent in the *DQB1*0201* allele. According to this hypothesis, *DQB1*0201* would be associated with AAD and other endocrine autoimmune diseases independently of the presence of DQ-LTR13, while *DQB1*0302* would increase genetic risk only when in combination with the DQ-LTR13 retrovirus-like element.

A subsequent Italian study [42] confirmed that the DQ-LTR13 retrovirus-like element is significantly increased both in T1DM and in AAD patients as compared to healthy control subjects (OR = 2.20 and 1.95, respectively), but showed for the first time that the DQ-LTR13 element is virtually absent among subjects carrying the *DRB1*0403* allele. Multivariate logistic regression analysis demonstrated that *DQB1*0201* and *DQB1*0302* resulted positively and *DRB1*0403* negatively and independently associated with both T1DM and AAD, while the association with DQ-LTR13 disappeared for both diseases [42], thus showing that the association of DQ-LTR13 with human endocrine autoimmune diseases is secondary to a positive linkage disequilibrium with *DQB1*0302* and a negative linkage disequilibrium with *DRB1*0403*.

A distinct family of MHC genes is located within the class III region and has been denominated MHC class I chain-related genes (MIC) [47]. The MIC family consists of 5 pseudogenes, *MICC, MICD, MICE, MICF* and *MICG,* and 2 functional genes, *MICA* and *MICB* [47]. MICA molecules are not expressed constitutively, and they are under the control of heat shock promoter elements, viral infections, bacterial infections or oxidative stress. MICA was first identified to be expressed in the cells of intestinal epithelium where it is recognized by γδ T cells. It has been suggested that the stress-induced expression of MICA and MICB may serve as an immune surveillance mechanism for the detection of damaged, infected or transformed epithelial cells.

MICA have no role in antigen presentation, but function as signals of cellular distress, and trigger a range of effector mechanisms, including cellular cytotoxicity, cytokine secretion and cellular proliferation. MICA expression has been suggested also in a population of stellate cells located in the subcapsular thymic cortex, which suggests a possible role of MICA and its activating receptor NKG2D in the selection or maturation of the T-cell repertoire. Engagement of NKG2D by MICA activates cytolytic responses from γδ T cells and NK cells against transfectants and epithelial tumours expressing MICA.

Analysis of the *MICA* gene revealed a trinucleotide repeat (GCT) microsatellite polymorphism within the transmembrane region. So far, 5 major alleles of exon 5 of the MICA gene, which consist of 4, 5, 6 and 9 repetitions of GCT, or 5 repetitions of GCT with an additional nucleotide insertion (GGCT), have been identified. These alleles have been accordingly named A4, A5, A6, A9 and A5.1, and the sizes are, respectively, 179, 182, 185, 194 and 183 bp [48, 49]. *MICA* 10, 7 and 8 have also been reported.

The *MICA* gene polymorphism was found to be associated with genetic risk for AAD [39]. More specifically, *MICA5.1* was positively associated with the disease with an OR of 6.52 [39]. The association of *MICA5.1* with Addison's disease was not dependent on the concomitant presence of other autoimmune diseases, as 8/10 (80%) subjects with isolated Addison's were also carrying this allele [39]. Conversely, *MICA6* was negatively associated with ADD (OR = 0.13, corrected p = 0.002) [39].

A subsequent independent study from the US confirmed the association of *MICA5.1* with ADD [50]. A study performed in 21-OH-Ab-positive individuals showed that at the 2-year follow-up, individuals homozygous for *MICA5.1* had a significantly higher progression toward clinical AAD than subjects not homozygous for *MICA5.1* (40% progression vs. 0%) [51], which suggests that homozygosity for *MICA5.1* may increase progression to clinically overt adrenal insufficiency among 21-OH-Ab-positive subjects.

The strong linkage disequilibrium existing within the *DRB1*03-DQA1*0501-DQB1*0201-MICA5.1-HLA-B*-extended haplotype has so far limited the possibility to demonstrate unequivocally that the *MICA* gene polymorphism is independently associated with the risk for human autoimmune diseases. Further studies on large populations are needed to address this specific question.

Class II Transactivator and Autoimmune Addison's Disease

HLA class II expression on antigen-presenting cells is under the control of the class II transactivator (CIITA), the master regulator for *HLA-D* gene expression. CIITA controls both the constitutive and the IFNγ-inducible expression of HLA molecules. CIITA exhibits a cell-specific, cytokine-inducible and differentiation-specific expression, and is expressed in the same cells expressing class II molecules, namely B cells, monocytes, dendritic cells and activated T cells [52].

Hypothetically, modulation of the expression of HLA class II determinants in antigen-presenting cells may represent a critical factor in the activation and maintenance of an organ-specific autoimmune process. CIITA/MHC2TA is encoded by a gene that has been mapped to chromosome 16p13. *CIITA/MHC2TA* is characterized by the presence of several single nucleotide polymorphisms (SNPs) in both the promoter type III (responsible for constitutive CIITA expression in B cells) and the coding sequence.

The association of the polymorphism of *CIITA/MHC2TA* with AAD was initially shown in an Italian study on 128 AAD patients and 406 healthy control subjects [53] (table 2). In that study [53], the frequency of allele –168G of *CIITA/MHC2TA* was significantly increased among affected patients (39% alleles), as compared to 29% in controls ($p = 0.003$). The OR of the association was 1.72 (95% CI: 1.06–2.78). Interestingly, the association of *CIITA/MHC2TA* gene polymorphism with the risk for AAD continued to be statistically significant also at the multivariate logistic regression analysis, which included class II haplotypes in the analysis [53]. A subsequent study, from another European population, confirmed that the polymorphism of *CIITA/MHC2TA* is associated with genetic risk for AAD [54].

The molecular mechanisms of *CIITA/MHC2TA* genetic predisposition for AAD are currently unknown. It could be speculated that *CIITA/MHC2TA* polymorphism may influence the expression of MHC molecules which, in turn, may be related to the risk for the development of autoimmune and inflammatory diseases.

CTLA4 and Autoimmune Addison's Disease

The activation of T cells requires both a signal provided by antigen-TCR engagement and a co-stimulatory signal mainly provided by the interaction of CD28 with its ligand B7.1/B7.2 on antigen-presenting cells. The cytotoxic T-lymphocyte antigen-4 (CTLA-4) is another co-stimulatory molecule that binds to B7.1/B7.2, but provides a negative signal to T-cell activation via transduction of an intracellular signal and modulation of tryptophan catabolism in B7-expressing dendritic cells. The inhibitory effect of CTLA-4 on T-cell activation has motivated a long series of investigations aimed at testing the association of *CTLA4* gene polymorphism with human autoimmune diseases. Thus, *CTLA4* polymorphism has been found to be associated with Graves' disease, Hashimoto's thyroiditis, T1DM, primary biliary cirrhosis, multiple sclerosis, coeliac disease and rheumatoid arthritis.

The first study of the association of *CTLA4* exon 1 polymorphism (49A/G) with AAD was performed in a German population by Donner et al. [55] (table 2). In that study, although no statistically significant association was found, patients with Addison's disease carrying *DQA1*0501* were significantly more *CTLA-4 Ala17* (G allele) positive than controls with the same *DQA1* allele. Subsequently, a statistically significant association of the *CTLA4* microsatellite polymorphism [variant lengths of a dinucleotide (AT)n repeat] within exon 3 was shown in English patients, but not in Norwegian, Finnish or Estonian patients [56]. The increased frequency of the *CTLA4* G allele in AAD was shown 2 years later in a larger study that enrolled 90 patients, of which 49 had isolated AAD and 41 had APS2 [57]. The association appeared stronger in patients with APS2 (OR = 1.73, 95% CI: 1.05–2.84) than in patients with isolated AAD (OR = 1.56, 95% CI: 0.98–2.49). In an Italian study of AAD patients [58], the *CTLA4* G allele was found in 40% of AAD patient alleles, as compared to 27% healthy control alleles, the difference was statistically significant ($p < 0.0001$) at an estimated OR of 2.66 (95% CI: 1.83–3.86). A meta-analysis of the available studies confirmed the positive genetic association between *CTLA4* gene polymorphism and AAD [58]. Recently, the EURADRENAL consortium analysed 16 SNPs in the extended *CTLA* gene locus encompassing *CD28, CTLA4* and *ICOS* in 382 Norwegian and 309 UK AAD patients, and found a significant disease association with 4 SNPs (including the *rs231755* SNP analysed in the previous Italian study) in the Norwegian, but not in the UK, population [59]. Again, a meta-analysis of available data confirmed the positive association of *rs231755* SNP with AAD in the European population. Haplotype analysis revealed that also the *CTLA4* haplotype *PROMOTER_1661(A)-rs231726 (T)-rs1896286 (T)* was significantly associated with AAD, while the *CD28* and *ICOS* polymorphisms did not contribute independently [59].

A polymorphism that alters CTLA4 function would be predicted to influence regulation of T-cell responses, possibly favouring autoreactivity and the development of autoimmune conditions. The G allele of *rs231775* confers higher T-cell proliferation than the A allele, which may be associated with increased risk for the development of autoimmune processes. Furthermore, this SNP is located on the peptide leader sequence of CTLA-4 and may also interfere with mRNA stability.

Other Genes and Autoimmune Addison's Disease

In a German study, a significant association was found between the polymorphism of the vitamin D receptor (VDR) and AAD [60] (table 2). The study analysed the *Fok*I, *Bsm*I, *Apa*I and *Taq*I polymorphisms of the *VDR* gene. Both the 'ff' and the 'tt' genotypes were found significantly more frequently among AAD patients than among healthy control subjects (OR = 2.75 and 2.42, respectively). Because of the documented effect of vitamin D on immune regulation, the association between the VDR polymorphism and endocrine autoimmune diseases is of interest, but further studies are needed to confirm the association and to elucidate the mechanisms by which distinct receptor variants might confer disease susceptibility. A significant association was also found between AAD and the polymorphism of the *CYP27B1* gene [61]. CYP27B1 (25-hydroxyvitamin D_3-1α-hydroxylase) is a mitochondrial P450 enzyme, which catalyses the conversion of 25-hydroxyvitamin D_3 to $1{,}25(OH)_2D_3$, the most active natural vitamin D metabolite. In a study of 124 AAD patients and 320 German healthy control subjects [61], the –1260CC genotype was significantly more frequent among patients than controls (table 2). A similar positive association was found also with Hashimoto's thyroiditis, Graves' disease and T1DM [61]. The positive association with the *CYP27B1* gene polymorphism (recently confirmed by a large European multicentre study of the EURADRENAL consortium [62]) complements the findings with the VDR polymorphisms, thus suggesting that the regulation of 25-hydroxyvitamin D_3-1α-hydroxylase might affect the local abundance of calcitriol and influence the regulation of antigen-presenting, dendritic and regulatory T cells.

An initial study [63] reported a weak association between the *PTPN22* gene polymorphism, which encodes for lymphoid tyrosine phosphatase (LYP), and AAD (table 2). In that study, however, the association did not reach statistical significance when the *PTPN22* genotypes were taken into consideration, while a weak, but significant, increase of the T-allele frequency was observed among Addison patients, as compared to healthy control subjects. A subsequent German study [64] did not find a significant association between the same polymorphism (more recently denominated *PTPN22* 1858C/T) and the risk for AAD. However, very recently, the hypothesis that this gene polymorphism may contribute to the genetic risk for AAD has found support from the results of a large case-control Norwegian study [65] that showed a significant association between AAD and the *PTPN22* 1858T risk allele. The association of AAD with *PTPN22* 1858T was also supported in the same study [65] by a meta-analysis combining the Norwegian genotype data with those of previously published studies (table 2).

As an extended study of endocrine autoimmunity genetic predisposition, three SNPs, part of a haplotype block in the *programmed death ligand 1 (PD-L1)* gene, showed modest association with UK and Norwegian AAD [66] (table 2). A recessive effect at the most associated alleles was observed.

Similarly, positive disease associations have also been found with the *NACHT leucine-rich-repeat protein 1* gene *(NLRP1/NALP1)* [67], with the *c receptor-like-3* gene *(FCRL3)* [68] and with the *GPR174* gene [69] (table 2).

Recently, a multicentre European study (EURADRENAL Consortium) [62] has analysed the polymorphism of 19 candidate genes for AAD risk and found significant associations with alleles of two *STAT4* markers (rs4274624, p = 0.00016, and rs10931481, p = 0.0007). In the same study, a nominal association of AAD with alleles at *GATA3* was found in three patient cohorts (UK, Norway and Poland; table 2). Furthermore, a nominal association was found at SNPs in both the *NFKB1* and *IL23A* genes in the UK and Italian cohorts, respectively [62] (table 2).

Finally, a genome-wide association analysis demonstrated that 18 SNPs were associated with AAD, including a non-synonymous variant in the *nuclear factor of activated T cells, cytoplasmic, calcineurin-dependent 1 (NFATC1)* gene [70] (table 2).

Implications of Genetic Associations for Pathogenesis of Autoimmune Addison's Disease

Although several genetic markers of AAD have been identified, almost all of them are related to activation and function of T cells. Not surprisingly, all the identified genes are almost invariably associated also with other endocrine and non-endocrine autoimmune diseases, most notably T1DM and thyroid autoimmune diseases. Accordingly, all the genes described must be considered factors that are more predisposing for the development of organ-specific autoimmunity than AAD-specific genes. To date, no AAD-specific gene has been identified.

Nevertheless, the identified genes may be relevant to provide more detailed information on the molecular mechanisms of T cell-mediated adrenal autoimmunity. Indeed, although 21-OH-Ab are the best markers for revealing the adrenal autoimmune process in subjects with clinical or preclinical adrenal insufficiency, the effector cells of the autoimmune-mediated destruction of adrenocortical cells are thought to be T lymphocytes. The involvement of T cells in the pathogenesis of AAD was first stipulated by Nerup et al. [71], who showed that patients with autoimmune adrenal insufficiency have T cells that are reactive against fetal adrenal extracts or adrenal mitochondrial fraction. Subsequently, it was shown that patients with recent-onset AAD have an increased expression of circulating Ia-positive T cells when compared to healthy control subjects [72]. Patients with APS2, but not individuals with isolated Addison's disease, seem to have CD4+CD25+ regulatory T cells with defective suppressive capacity [73]. Taken together, all these studies support the hypothesis of a major role of cellular immunity in the autoimmune destruction of the adrenocortical cells in Addison's disease.

With the aim of better defining the peptide specificity of autoreactive T cells, Husebye et al. [74] immunized BALB/c and SJL mice with recombinant 21-OH and showed a selective significant proliferative response of T cells from lymph nodes against the peptide 342-361 of 21-OH that corresponds to the substrate-binding site of the enzyme.

Recently, the EURADRENAL Consortium published an important study on CD4+ and CD8+ T lymphocytes from AAD patients [75]. The study showed the presence of autoreactive T cells specific for 21-OH in the peripheral blood of AAD patients [75]. These cells were found even 20 years after clinical diagnosis, even though ELISPOT assay showed the highest reactivity to 21-OH within the first 2 years after diagnosis [75]. In addition, the study provided a clear demonstration that these cells were activated by co-culture with the 21-OH-expressing tumour cell line NCI H295 and that they were able to lyse target cells expressing full-length 21-OH protein [75].

There is still a strong need for further studies of cellular immunity in patients with AAD as well as for further studies aimed at identifying AAD-specific gene markers.

References

1 Betterle C, Dal Pra C, Mantero F, Zanchetta R: Autoimmune adrenal insufficiency and autoimmune polyendocrine syndromes: autoantibodies, autoantigens, and their applicability in diagnosis and disease prediction. Endocr Rev 2002;23:327–364.

2 Falorni A, Nikoshkov A, Laureti S, Grenbäck E, Hulting AL, Casucci G, Santeusanio F, Brunetti P, Luthman H, Lernmark A: High diagnostic accuracy for idiopathic Addison's disease with a sensitive radiobinding assay for autoantibodies against recombinant human 21-hydroxylase. J Clin Endocrinol Metab 1995;80:2752–2755.

3 Falorni A, Laureti S, Santeusanio F: Autoantibodies in autoimmune polyendocrine syndrome type II. Endocrinol Metab Clin North Am 2002;31:369–389.

4 Falorni A, Laureti S, Nikoshkov A, Picchio ML, Hallengren B, Vandewalle CL, Gorus FK, Tortoioli C, Luthman H, Brunetti P, Santeusanio F: 21-hydroxylase autoantibodies in adult patients with endocrine autoimmune diseases are highly specific for Addison's disease. Belgian Diabetes Registry. Clin Exp Immunol 1997;107:341–346.

5 Falorni A, Laureti S, De Bellis A, Zanchetta R, Tiberti C, Arnaldi G, Bini V, Beck-Peccoz P, Bizzarro A, Dotta F, Mantero F, Bellastella A, Betterle C, Santeusanio F; SIE Addison Study Group: Update of diagnostic criteria for the etiological classification of primary adrenal insufficiency. J Clin Endocrinol Metab 2004;89:1598–1604.

6 Laureti S, De Bellis A, Muccitelli VI, Calcinaro F, Bizzarro A, Rossi R, Bellastella A, Santeusanio F, Falorni A: Levels of adrenocortical autoantibodies correlate with the degree of adrenal dysfunction in subjects with pre-clinical Addison's disease. J Clin Endocrinol Metab 1998;83:3507–3511.

7 Betterle C, Volpato M, Rees Smith B, Furmaniak J, Chen S, Greggio NA, Sanzari M, Tedesco F, Pedini B, Boscaro M, Presotto F: I. Adrenal cortex and steroid 21-hydroxylase autoantibodies in adult patients with organ-specific autoimmune diseases: markers of low progression to clinical Addison's disease. J Clin Endocrinol Metab 1997;82:932–938.

8 Coco G, Dal Pra C, Presotto F, Albergoni MP, Canova C, Pedini B, Zanchetta R, Chen S, Furmaniak J, Rees Smith B, Mantero F, Betterle C: Estimated risk for developing autoimmune Addison's disease in patients with adrenal cortex autoantibodies. J Clin Endocrinol Metab 2006;91:1637–1645.

9 Nagamine K, Peterson P, Scott HS, Kudoh J, Minoshima S, Heino M, Krohn KJ, Lalioti MD, Mullis PE, Antonarakis SE, Kawasaki K, Asakawa S, Ito F, Shimizu N: Positional cloning of the APECED gene. Nat Genet 1997;17:393–398.

10 Halonen M, Eskelin P, Myhre AG, Perheentupa J, Husebye ES, Kämpe O, Rorsman F, Peltonen L, Ulmanen I, Partanen J: AIRE mutations and human leukocyte antigen genotypes as determinants of the autoimmune polyendocrinopathy-candidiasis-ectodermal dystrophy phenotype. J Clin Endocrinol Metab 2002;87:2568–2574.
11 Laureti S, Vecchi L, Santeusanio F, Falorni A: Is the prevalence of Addison's disease underestimated? J Clin Endocrinol Metab 1999;84:1762.
12 Løvås K, Husebye ES: High prevalence and increasing incidence of Addison's disease in western Norway. Clin Endocrinol (Oxf) 2002;56:787–791.
13 La Marca A, Brozzetti A, Sighinolfi G, Marzotti S, Volpe A, Falorni A: Primary ovarian insufficiency: autoimmune causes. Curr Opin Obstet Gynecol 2010;22:277–282.
14 Ahonen P, Myllärniemi S, Sipilä I, Perheentupa J: Clinical variation of autoimmune polyendocrinopathy-candidiasis-ectodermal dystrophy (APECED) in a series of 68 patients. N Engl J Med 1990;322:1829–1836.
15 Perniola R, Falorni A, Clemente MG, Forini F, Accogli E, Lobreglio G: Organ-specific and non-organ-specific autoantibodies in children and young adults with autoimmune polyendocrinopathy-candidiasis-ectodermal dystrophy (APECED). Eur J Endocrinol 2000;143:497–503.
16 Meloni A, Furcas M, Cetani F, Marcocci C, Falorni A, Perniola R, Pura M, Bøe Wolff AS, Husebye ES, Lilic D, Ryan KR, Gennery AR, Cant AJ, Abinun M, Spickett GP, Arkwright PD, Denning D, Costigan C, Dominguez M, McConnell V, Willcox N, Meager A: Autoantibodies against type I interferons as an additional diagnostic criteria for autoimmune polyendocrine syndrome type I. J Clin Endocrinol Metab 2008;93:4389–4397.
17 Puel A, Döffinger R, Natividad A, Chrabieh M, Barcenas-Morales G, Picard C, Cobat A, Ouachée-Chardin M, Toulon A, Bustamante J, Al-Muhsen S, Al-Owain M, Arkwright PD, Costigan C, McConnell V, Cant AJ, Abinun M, Polak M, Bougnères PF, Kumararatne D, Marodi L, Nahum A, Roifman C, Blanche S, Fischer A, Bodemer C, Abel L, Lilic D, Casanova JL: Autoantibodies against IL-17A, IL-17F, and IL-22 in patients with chronic mucocutaneous candidiasis and autoimmune polyendocrine syndrome type I. J Exp Med 2010;207:291–297.
18 Perniola R, Musco G: The biophysical and biochemical properties of the autoimmune regulator (AIRE) protein. Biochim Biophys Acta 2014;1842:326–337.
19 Cetani F, Barbesino G, Borsari S, Pardi E, Cianferotti L, Pinchera A, Marcocci C: A novel mutation of the autoimmune regulator gene in an Italian kindred with autoimmune polyendocrinopathycandidiasis-ectodermal dystrophy, acting in a dominant fashion and strongly cosegregating with hypothyroid autoimmune thyroiditis. J Clin Endocrinol Metab 2001;86:4747–4752.
20 Su MA, Giang K, Zumer K, Jiang H, Oven I, Rinn JL, Devoss JJ, Johannes KP, Lu W, Gardner J, Chang A, Bubulya P, Chang HY, Peterlin BM, Anderson MS: Mechanisms of an autoimmunity syndrome in mice caused by a dominant mutation in Aire. J Clin Invest 2008;118:1712–1726.
21 Pearce SH, Cheetham T, Imrie H, Vaidya B, Barnes ND, Bilous RW, Carr D, Meeran K, Shaw NJ, Smith CS, Toft AD, Williams G, Kendall-Taylor P: A common and recurrent 13-bp deletion in the autoimmune regulator gene in British kindreds with autoimmune polyendocrinopathy type 1. Am J Hum Genet 1998;63:1675–1684.
22 Rosatelli MC, Meloni A, Meloni A, Devoto M, Cao A, Scott HS, Peterson P, Heino M, Krohn KJ, Nagamine K, Kudoh J, Shimizu N, Antonarakis SE: A common mutation in Sardinian autoimmune polyendocrinopathy-candidiasis-ectodermal dystrophy patients. Hum Genet 1998;103:428–434.
23 Heino M, Peterson P, Kudoh J, Nagamine K, Lagerstedt A, Ovod V, Ranki A, Rantala I, Nieminen M, Tuukkanen J, Scott HS, Antonarakis SE, Shimizu N, Krohn K: Autoimmune regulator is expressed in the cells regulating immune tolerance in thymus medulla. Biochem Biophys Res Commun 1999;257:821–825.
24 Heino M, Peterson P, Sillanpää N, Guérin S, Wu L, Anderson G, Scott HS, Antonarakis SE, Kudoh J, Shimizu N, Jenkinson EJ, Naquet P, Krohn KJ: RNA and protein expression of the murine autoimmune regulator gene (Aire) in normal, RelB-deficient and in NOD mouse. Eur J Immunol 2000;30:1884–1893.
25 Derbinski J, Schulte A, Kyewski B, Klein L: Promiscuous gene expression in medullary thymic epithelial cells mirrors the peripheral self. Nat Immunol 2001;2:1032–1039.
26 Kyewski B, Derbinski J: Self-representation in the thymus: an extended view. Nat Rev Immunol 2004;4:688–698.
27 Ramsey C, Winqvist O, Puhakka L, Halonen M, Moro A, Kämpe O, Eskelin P, Pelto-Huikko M, Peltonen L: Aire deficient mice develop multiple features of APECED phenotype and show altered immune response. Hum Mol Genet 2002;11:397–409.
28 Anderson MS, Venanzi ES, Klein L, Chen Z, Berzins SP, Turley SJ, von Boehmer H, Bronson R, Dierich A, Benoist C, Mathis D: Projection of an immunological self shadow within the thymus by the aire protein. Science 2002;298:1395–1401.
29 Jiang W, Anderson MA, Bronson R, Mathis D, Benoist C: Modifier loci condition autoimmunity provoked by Aire deficiency. J Exp Med 2005;202:805–815.
30 Venanzi ES, Melamed R, Mathis D, Benoist C: The variable immunological self: genetic variation and nongenetic noise in Aire-regulated transcription. Proc Natl Acad Sci USA 2008;105:15860–15865.

31 Pöntynen N, Miettinen A, Arstila TP, Kämpe O, Alimohammadi M, Vaarala O, Peltonen L, Ulmanen I: Aire deficient mice do not develop the same profile of tissue-specific autoantibodies in APECED patients. J Autoimmun 2006;27:96–104.
32 Hubert FX, Kinkel SA, Crewther PE, Cannon PZ, Webster KE, Link M, Uibo R, O'Bryan MK, Meager A, Forehan SP, Smyth GK, Mittaz L, Antonarakis SE, Peterson P, Heath WR, Scott HS: Aire-deficient C57BL/6 mice mimicking the common human 13-base pair deletion mutant present with only a mild autoimmune phenotype. J Immunol 2009;182:3902–3918.
33 Maclaren NK, Riley WJ: Inherited susceptibility to autoimmune Addison's disease is linked to human leukocyte antigens-DR3 and/or DR4, except when associated with type I autoimmune polyglandular syndrome. J Clin Endocrinol Metab 1986;62:455–459.
34 Boehm BO, Manfras B, Seidl S, Holzberger G, Kühnl P, Rosak C, Schöffling K, Trucco M: The HLA-DQ beta non-Asp-57 allele: a predictor of future insulin-dependent diabetes mellitus in patients with autoimmune Addison's disease. Tissue Antigens 1991;37: 130–132.
35 Partanen J, Peterson P, Westman P, Aranko S, Krohn K: Major histocompatibility complex class II and III in Addison's disease. MHC alleles do not predict autoantibody specificity and 21-hydroxylase gene polymorphism has no independent role in disease susceptibility. Hum Immunol 1994;41:135–140.
36 Badenhoop K, Walfish PG, Rau H, Fischer S, Nicolay A, Bogner U, Schleusener H, Usadel KH: Susceptibility and resistance alleles of human leukocyte antigen (HLA) DQA1 and HLA DQB1 are shared in endocrine autoimmune disease. J Clin Endocrinol Metab 1995;80:2112–2117.
37 Betterle C, Volpato M, Rees Smith B, Furmaniak J, Chen S, Greggio NA, Sanzari M, Tedesco F, Pedini B, Boscaro M, Presotto F: I. Adrenal cortex and steroid 21-hydroxylase autoantibodies in adult patients with organ-specific autoimmune diseases: markers of low progression to clinical Addison's disease. J Clin Endocrinol Metab 1997;82:932–938.
38 Yu L, Brewer KW, Gates S, Wu A, Wang T, Babu SR, Gottlieb PA, Freed BM, Noble J, Erlich HA, Rewers MJ, Eisenbarth GS: DRB1*04 and DQ alleles: expression of 21-hydroxylase autoantibodies and risk of progression to Addison's disease. J Clin Endocrinol Metab 1999;84:328–335.
39 Gambelunghe G, Falorni A, Ghaderi M, Laureti S, Tortoioli C, Santeusanio F, Brunetti P, Sanjeevi CB: Microsatellite polymorphism of the MHC class I chain-related (MIC-A and MIC-B) genes marks the risk for autoimmune Addison's disease. J Clin Endocrinol Metab 1999;84:3701–3707.
40 Myhre AG, Undlien DE, Løvås K, Uhlving S, Nedrebø BG, Fougner KJ, Trovik T, Sørheim JI, Husebye ES: Autoimmune adrenocortical failure in Norway autoantibodies and human leukocyte antigen class II associations related to clinical features. J Clin Endocrinol Metab 2002;87:618–623.
41 Wallaschofski H, Meyer A, Tuschy U, Lohmann T: HLA-DQA1*0301-associated susceptibility for autoimmune polyglandular syndrome type II and III. Horm Metab Res 2003;35:120–124.
42 Gambelunghe G, Kockum I, Bini V, De Giorgi G, Celi F, Betterle C, Giordano R, Libè R, Falorni A; Umbria type 1 diabetes registry; Italian Addison Network: Retrovirus-like long terminal repeat DQ-LTR13 and genetic susceptibility to type 1 diabetes mellitus and autoimmune Addison's disease. Diabetes 2005;54:900–905.
43 Baker PR, Baschal EE, Fain PR, Nanduri P, Triolo TM, Siebert JC, Armstrong TK, Babu SR, Rewers MJ, Gottlieb PA, Barker JM, Eisenbarth GS: Dominant suppression of Addison's disease associated with HLA-B15. J Clin Endocrinol Metab 2001;96:2154–2162.
44 Leib-Mösch C, Haltmeier M, Werner T, Geigl EM, Brack-Werner R, Francke U, Erfle V, Hehlmann R: Genomic distribution and transcription of solitary HERV-K LTRs. Genomics 1993;18:261–269.
45 Bieda K, Pani MA, van der Auwera B, Seidl C, Tönjes RR, Gorus F, Usadel KH, Badenhoop K: A retroviral long terminal repeat adjacent to the HLA DQB1 gene (DQ-LTR13) modifies type I diabetes susceptibility on high risk DQ haplotypes. Diabetologia 2002;45: 443–447.
46 Krach K, Badenhoop K, Tönjes RR: The IDDM-associated solitary retroviral promoters DQ-LTR3 and DQ-LTR13 have a distinct impact on the expression of selected DQB1 genes in different cell lines in vitro. Immunogenetics 2003;55:521–529.
47 Bahram S: MIC genes: from genetics to biology. Adv Immunol 2000;76:1–60.
48 Ota M, Katsuyama Y, Mizuki N, Ando H, Furihata K, Ono S, Pivetti-Pezzi P, Tabbara KF, Palimeris GD, Nikbin B, Davatchi F, Chams H, Geng Z, Bahram S, Inoko H: Trinucleotide repeat polymorphism within exon 5 of the MICA gene (MHC class I chain-related gene A): allele frequency data in the nine population groups Japanese, Northern Han, Hui, Uygur, Kazakhstan, Iranian, Saudi Arabian, Greek and Italian. Tissue Antigens 1997;49:448–454.
49 Ricci Vitiani L, Potolicchio I, D'Amato M, Baricordi OR, Sorrentino R: MICA exon 5 microsatellite typing by DNA heteroduplex analysis: a new polymorphism in the transmembrane region. Tissue Antigens 1998;51:309–311.

50 Park YS, Sanjeevi CB, Robles D, Yu L, Rewers M, Gottlieb PA, Fain P, Eisenbarth GS: Additional association of intra-MHC genes, MICA and D6S273, with Addison's disease. Tissue Antigens 2002;60: 155–163.
51 Triolo TM, Baschal EE, Armstrong TK, Toews CS, Fain PR, Rewers MJ, Yu L, Miao D, Eisenbarth GS, Gottlieb PA, Barker JM: Homozygosity of the polymorphism MICA5.1 identifies extreme risk of progression to overt adrenal insufficiency among 21-hydroxylase antibody-positive patients with type 1 diabetes. J Clin Endocrinol Metab 2009;94:4517–4523.
52 Harton JA, Ting JP: Class II transactivator: mastering the art of major histocompatibility complex expression. Mol Cell Biol 2000;20:6185–6194.
53 Ghaderi M, Gambelunghe G, Tortoioli C, Brozzetti A, Jatta K, Gharizadeh B, De Bellis A, Pecori Giraldi F, Terzolo M, Betterle C, Falorni A: MHC2TA single nucleotide polymorphism and genetic risk for autoimmune adrenal insufficiency. J Clin Endocrinol Metab 2006;91:4107–4111.
54 Skinningsrud B, Husebye ES, Pearce SH, McDonald DO, Brandal K, Wolff AB, Løvås K, Egeland T, Undlien DE: Polymorphisms in CLEC16A and CIITA at 16p13 are associated with primary adrenal insufficiency. J Clin Endocrinol Metab 2008;93:3310–3317.
55 Donner H, Braun J, Seidl C, Rau H, Finke R, Ventz M, Walfish PG, Usadel KH, Badenhoop K: Codon 17 polymorphism of the cytotoxic T lymphocyte antigen 4 gene in Hashimoto's thyroiditis and Addison's disease. J Clin Endocrinol Metab 1997;82:4130–4132.
56 Kemp EH, Ajjan RA, Husebye ES, Peterson P, Uibo R, Imrie H, Pearce SH, Watson PF, Weetman AP: A cytotoxic T lymphocyte antigen-4 (CTLA-4) gene polymorphism is associated with autoimmune Addison's disease in English patients. Clin Endocrinol (Oxf) 1998;49:609–613.
57 Vaidya B, Imrie H, Geatch DR, Perros P, Ball SG, Baylis PH, Carr D, Hurel SJ, James RA, Kelly WF, Kemp EH, Young ET, Weetman AP, Kendall-Taylor P, Pearce SH: Association analysis of the cytotoxic T lymphocyte antigen-4 (CTLA-4) and autoimmune regulator-1 (AIRE-1) genes in sporadic autoimmune Addison's disease. J Clin Endocrinol Metab 2000;85: 688–691.
58 Brozzetti A, Marzotti S, Tortoioli C, Bini V, Giordano R, Dotta F, Betterle C, De Bellis A, Arnaldi G, Toscano V, Arvat E, Bellastella A, Mantero F, Falorni A; Italian Addison Network: Cytotoxic T lymphocyte antigen-4 Ala17 polymorphism is a genetic marker of autoimmune adrenal insufficiency: Italian association study and meta-analysis of European studies. Eur J Endocrinol 2010;162:361–369.
59 Wolff AS, Mitchell AL, Cordell HJ, Short A, Skinningsrud B, Ollier W, Badenhoop K, Meyer G, Falorni A, Kampe O, Undlien D, Pearce SH, Husebye ES: CTLA-4 as a genetic determinant in autoimmune Addison's disease. Genes Immun 2015;16: 430–436.
60 Pani MA, Seissler J, Usadel KH, Badenhoop K: Vitamin D receptor genotype is associated with Addison's disease. Eur J Endocrinol 2002;147:635–640.
61 Lopez ER, Zwermann O, Segni M, Meyer G, Reincke M, Seissler J, Herwig J, Usadel KH, Badenhoop K: A promoter polymorphism of the CYP27B1 gene is associated with Addison's disease, Hashimoto's thyroiditis, Graves' disease and type 1 diabetes mellitus in Germans. Eur J Endocrinol 2004;151:193–197.
62 Mitchell AL, Macarthur KD, Gan EH, Baggott LE, Wolff AS, Skinningsrud B, Platt H, Short A, Lobell A, Kämpe O, Bensing S, Betterle C, Kasperlik-Zaluska A, Zurawek M, Fichna M, Kockum I, Nordling Eriksson G, Ekwall O, Wahlberg J, Dahlqvist P, Hulting AL, Penna-Martinez M, Meyer G, Kahles H, Badenhoop K, Hahner S, Quinkler M, Falorni A, Phipps-Green A, Merriman TR, Ollier W, Cordell HJ, Undlien D, Czarnocka B, Husebye E, Pearce SH: Association of autoimmune Addison's disease with alleles of STAT4 and GATA3 in European cohorts. PLoS One 2014;10:e88991.
63 Velaga MR, Wilson V, Jennings CE, Owen CJ, Herington S, Donaldson PT, Ball SG, James RA, Quinton R, Perros P, Pearce SH: The codon 620 tryptophan allele of the lymphoid tyrosine phosphatase (LYP) gene is a major determinant of Graves' disease. J Clin Endocrinol Metab 2004;89:5862–5865.
64 Kahles H, Ramos-Lopez E, Lange B, Zwermann O, Reincke M, Badenhoop K: Sex-specific association of PTPN22 1858T with type 1 diabetes but not with Hashimoto's thyroiditis or Addison's disease in the German population. Eur J Endocrinol 2005;153: 895–899.
65 Skinningsrud B, Husebye ES, Gervin K, Løvås K, Blomhoff A, Wolff AB, Kemp EH, Egeland T, Undlien DE: Mutation screening of PTPN22: association of the 1858T-allele with Addison's disease. Eur J Hum Genet 2008;16:977–982.
66 Skinningsrud B, Husebye ES, Gervin K, Løvås K, Blomhoff A, Wolff AB, Kemp EH, Egeland T, Undlien DE: Programmed death ligand 1 (PD-L1) gene variants contribute to autoimmune Addison's disease and Graves' disease susceptibility. J Clin Endocrinol Metab 2009;94:5139–5145.
67 Magitta NF, Bøe Wolff AS, Johansson S, Skinningsrud B, Lie BA, Myhr KM, Undlien DE, Joner G, Njølstad PR, Kvien TK, Førre Ø, Knappskog PM, Husebye ES: A coding polymorphism in NALP1 confers risk for autoimmune Addison's disease and type 1 diabetes. Genes Immun 2009;10:120–124.

68 Owen CJ, Kelly H, Eden JA, Merriman ME, Pearce SH, Merriman TR: Analysis of the Fc receptor-like-3 (FCRL3) locus in Caucasians with autoimmune disorders suggests a complex pattern of disease association. J Clin Endocrinol Metab 2007;92:1106–1111.
69 Napier C, Mitchell AL, Gan E, Wilson I, Pearce SH: Role of the X-linked gene GPR174 in autoimmune Addison's disease. J Clin Endocrinol Metab 2015; 100:E187–E190.
70 Mitchell AL, Bøe Wolff A, MacArthur K, Weaver JU, Vaidya B; Swedish Addison Registry Study Group, Erichsen MM, Darlay R, Husebye ES, Cordell HJ, Pearce SH: Linkage analysis in autoimmune Addison's disease: NFATC1 as a potential novel susceptibility locus. PLoS One 2015;10:e0123550.
71 Nerup J, Andersen V, Bendixen G: Anti-adrenal, cellular hypersensitivity in Addison's disease. IV. In vivo and in vitro investigations on the mitochondrial fraction. Clin Exp Immunol 1970;6:733–739.
72 Rabinowe SL, Jackson RA, Dluhy RG, Williams GH: Ia-positive T lymphocytes in recently diagnosed idiopathic Addison's disease. Am J Med 1984;77:597–601.
73 Kriegel MA, Lohmann T, Gabler C, Blank N, Kalden JR, Lorenz HM: Defective suppressor function of human CD4+ CD25+ regulatory T cells in autoimmune polyglandular syndrome type II. J Exp Med 2004; 199:1285–1291.
74 Husebye ES, Bratland E, Bredholt G, Fridkin M, Dayan M, Mozes E: The substrate-binding domain of 21-hydroxylase, the main autoantigen in autoimmune Addison's disease, is an immunodominant T cell epitope. Endocrinology 2006;147:2411–2416.
75 Dawoodji A, Chen JL, Shepherd D, Dalin F, Tarlton A, Alimohammadi M, Penna-Martinez M, Meyer G, Mitchell AL, Gan EH, Bratland E, Bensing S, Husebye ES, Pearce SH, Badenhoop K, Kämpe O, Cerundolo V: High frequency of cytolytic 21-hydroxylase-specific CD8+ T cells in autoimmune Addison's disease patients. J Immunol 2014;193:2118–2126.

Prof. Alberto Falorni, MD, PhD
Section of Internal Medicine and Endocrine and Metabolic Sciences
Department of Medicine, University of Perugia
Via E. Dal Pozzo
IT–06126 Perugia (Italy)
E-Mail alberto.falorni@unipg.it

Arvat E, Falorni A (eds): Cortisol Excess and Insufficiency.
Front Horm Res. Basel, Karger, 2016, vol 46, pp 133–145 (DOI: 10.1159/000443872)

From Appearance of Adrenal Autoantibodies to Clinical Symptoms of Addison's Disease: Natural History

Corrado Betterle[a] · Silvia Garelli[b] · Fabio Presotto[b] · Jadwiga Furmaniak[c]

[a]Endocrine Unit, Department of Medicine, University of Padua, Padua, and [b]Unit of Internal Medicine, Ospedale dell'Angelo, Mestre-Venezia, Italy; [c]FIRS Laboratories, RSR Ltd., Cardiff, UK

Abstract

Recent progress in the immunopathology field has greatly improved our understanding of the natural history of autoimmune diseases, particularly of Addison's disease. Addison's disease is known to be a chronic illness characterized by adrenocortical gland insufficiency that develops following a long and mainly asymptomatic period, characterized by the presence of circulating autoantibodies directed to adrenal cortex antigens. In this chapter we describe the groups of subjects at risk of developing Addison's disease, together with the diagnostic tests considered the most appropriate for evaluating adrenal function: determination of basal plasma adrenocorticotropic hormone (ACTH) levels, plasma renin activity, plasma aldosterone and cortisol levels, and cortisol levels after intravenous stimulation with ACTH (ACTH test). The employment of specific clinical, immunological and functional criteria in the subjects with autoantibodies to the adrenal cortex allows identifying those at risk of developing overt disease. The independent risk factors for the progression to adrenal failure have also been identified and they contribute to different risks of developing clinical Addison's disease. Based on the risk level, the subjects should be monitored over time to observe early signs of adrenal dysfunction, and start substitutive treatment as soon as possible. For patients presenting with high risk, prevention strategies and trials might be available.

Organ-specific autoimmune diseases (OSAD) originate when the immune systems attacks a specific organ. These are chronic illnesses characterized by a long preclinical period and their natural history encompasses three distinctive phases: (1) potential, (2) subclinical and (3) clinical. The *potential* phase is characterized by the presence of (1) genetic predisposition (class II HLA, CTLA-4 or *AIRE* gene mutations), (2) organ-specific autoantibodies, (3) minimal or multifocal lymphomonocytic infiltration of the target organ and (4) normal function of the target organ. The *subclinical* phase is characterized by the presence of (1) genetic predisposition, (2) organ-specific autoantibodies, (3) discrete lymphomonocytic infiltration of the target organ and (4) subclinical impairment of target organ function. The *clinical* phase is characterized by the presence of (1) genetic predisposition, (2) organ-specific autoantibodies, (3) diffuse or significant lymphomonocytic infiltration of the target organ and (4) clinical manifestations.

All phases of OSAD are characterized by the presence of high levels of organ-specific autoantibodies. These autoantibodies are in general non-pathogenic markers and in the great majority of OSAD the damage in the target organs is related to the concurrent infiltrating lymphocytes. Because organ-specific autoantibodies usually are not pathogenic, they can also be detected in apparently healthy individuals. However, their presence is associated with the presence of lymphocytic infiltrations in the target organs and consequently they can be considered markers of subsequent development of clinical disease. The value of organ-specific autoantibodies for the prediction of OSAD has been demonstrated in the case of thyroid autoantibodies and autoimmune thyroid disease [1], pancreatic islet cell autoantibodies and type 1 diabetes mellitus [2, 3], and autoantibodies to steroidogenic enzymes and premature ovarian failure [4, 5].

Here we present the current data on the role of adrenal cortex antibodies in predicting Addison's disease (AD).

Adrenal Cortex and 21-Hydroxylase Autoantibodies in Patients with Addison's Disease

Adrenal cortex autoantibodies (ACA) were discovered in 1963 with the indirect immunofluorescence technique on cryostat sections of animal adrenal glands [6]. ACA reacted with a microsomal antigen common to all the three layers of the adrenal cortex, producing a homogenous cytoplasm-staining pattern. In the period from 1963 to 2002, the indirect immunofluorescence technique (IFT) using animal or human normal adrenal cryostat sections was the only method used for detection of ACA, which were found in 61% of evaluated patients with autoimmune AD of different disease duration and in 6.7% of patients with AD caused by tuberculosis [7].

In 1992 it was discovered that the enzyme 21-hydroxylase (21-OH) is the major autoantigen recognized by ACA [8, 9]. Following this discovery, an immunoprecipitation assay using ^{35}S-methionine-labelled 21-OH was introduced into the laboratory practice to detect 21-OH autoantibodies (21-OH-Ab) [10]. Further, a more convenient method to measure 21-OH-Ab based on ^{125}I-labelled recombinant human 21-OH was developed and made available in a kit format [11]. Using specific immunoprecipitation assays, 21-OH-Ab were demonstrated in more than 90% of the patients with recent-onset autoimmune AD [12], but in none with other forms of AD.

Autoantibodies reactive with the adrenal cortex with characteristics different to ACA were subsequently demonstrated in IFT [13]. These autoantibodies, unlike adrenal specific ACA, also showed reactivity to the ovaries, testes and placenta, and were defined as steroid-producing cell autoantibodies. The specific antigens recognized by steroid-producing cell autoantibodies are steroid-producing enzymes, 17α-hydroxylase and the cytochrome p450 side-chain cleavage enzyme [14]. Steroid-producing cell autoantibodies are present in a large proportion of patients with AD (34%) and in 92% of women with premature ovarian failure of less than 5 years' duration [5]. Autoantibodies to steroidogenic enzymes can be considered predictive markers of premature ovarian failure [4, 5], while ACA/21-OH-Ab are strictly adrenal cortex specific and are markers of autoimmune AD (see below).

In 2011, the First International Standardization Program for 21-OH-Ab determination was carried out to compare the measurements from four laboratories using different methods and to assess interlaboratory concordance [15]. This program has shown a very good agreement among the laboratories on reporting 21-OH-Ab-positive/-negative samples. The sensitivity for autoimmune AD was greater than 80% in all four participating laboratories. However, the study highlighted the need to produce an international standard preparation to enable the harmonized expression of the results. With the aim of assessing interlaboratory agreement for 21-OH-Ab measurements, the Euradrenal consortium has performed a Second International Serum Exchange with blindly coded samples from patients with idiopathic primary adrenal insufficiency and from healthy control subjects [16].

The Role of Adrenal Cortex Autoantibodies and 21-Hydroxylase Autoantibodies in the Pathogenesis of Addison's Disease

Preparations of IgG from patients with autoimmune AD positive for 21-OH-Ab were shown to be able to inhibit the activity of 21-OH enzyme in vitro [17]; however, this effect was not evident in in vivo studies [18]. The absence of a pathogenic role in terms of inhibition of 21-OH enzyme activity in vivo was confirmed in a case study of a pregnant woman with autoimmune AD who was positive for ACA/21-OH-Ab. Although ACA/21-OH-Ab passed into the blood stream of the neonate through the placenta and remained detectable for up to 4 months, there was no evidence of the effect of ACA/21-OH-Ab positivity on the adrenal function in the newborn [19].

Adrenal Cortex Autoantibodies and 21-Hydroxylase Autoantibodies in Subjects without Addison's Disease

In the years 1963–2002, ACA and/or 21-OH-Ab have been tested in various groups of patients or individuals without clinical AD and were found to be positive with a mean prevalence of 1.4% in patients with one or more OSAD, of 4.1% in hospitalized patients, in 5% of first-degree relatives of patients with AD, and in 0.6% of healthy individuals [7]. However, the prevalence of ACA/21-OH-Ab was higher in some patients with OSAD such as young patients with chronic hypoparathyroidism, in whom the positivity was up to 47% [20], and patients with premature ovarian failure (positivity of 8–10%) [21, 22].

Natural History of Patients with Adrenal Cortex Autoantibodies and/or 21-Hydroxylase Autoantibodies

The first observation of the predictive role of ACA was reported many years ago in a patient affected by Hashimoto's thyroiditis who developed clinical autoimmune AD several months after detection of ACA positivity [23]. In 1966 it was demonstrated that ACA were present in 4 of 27 (15%) patients with autoimmune polyglandular syndrome type 1, but without AD [24]. Adrenal function was assessed in 3 of the positive patients and one showed a reduced 17-hydroxycorticosteroid response to corticotropin [adrenocorticotropic hormone (ACTH)] stimulation.

Further, in 1978, two identical ACA-positive twins were described. One twin had clinical autoimmune AD while the other had no clinical signs of AD. However, the second twin had elevated basal ACTH levels with cortisol basal levels in the normal range and impaired response of cortisol to synthetic ACTH (Synacthen™) consistent with subclinical AD [25].

Subsequently, two prospective studies were carried out. The first study followed 5 ACA-positive patients with type 1 diabetes mellitus for 2 years [26] and the second study followed 20 ACA-positive hospitalized patients for 6 years [27]. None of the patients developed clinical AD in these limited prospective studies.

In a different study, 30 ACA-positive patients with OSAD were followed for a period of 1–3.5 years and 5 patients had or developed a subclinical AD and were therefore treated with substitutive therapy. However, since they were given treatment, it is difficult to assess if these patients would have certainly progressed to a clinical AD [28].

Greater evidence that a high proportion of ACA-positive patients progress to clinical AD was shown in our study carried out in 1983 [29]. In this study, 4 out of 8 ACA-positive patients with one or more OSAD developed clinical AD within 1–31 months of follow-up. In the subsequent years, many cohorts of ACA and/or 21-OH-Ab-positive patients with OSAD were followed-up in several studies (table 1).

In the first studies in ACA-positive children with OSAD, the positive predictive value of developing AD was very high at 74–90%, and appeared independent of ACA/21-OH-Ab titers, initial adrenal function, HLA status or type of OSAD [4, 20]. In contrast, in ACA-positive adult patients with OSAD, the predictive value of AD was lower (0–42%) and related to high titers of ACA/21-OH-Ab [21, 30], presence of initial adrenal dysfunction, and HLA-DR3 [20] or HLA-DRB1*0404 for patients with type 1 diabetes mellitus [31].

Table 1. Follow-up studies in cohorts of ACA-positive subjects

	Patients		Age range, years	Associated disorders	Mean period of follow-up, months (range)	Cases which developed AD, n	Positive predictive value, %	Annual incidence, %
	n	F/M						
Ahonen et al. [4] 1987	31	23/8	2–34	hypoparathyroidism	100 (14–145)	23	74	n.d.
Betterle et al. [19] 1997	48	45/3	17–69	OSAD	50 (3–163)	10	21	4.9
Betterle et al. [20] 1997	10	5/5	5–12	OSAD	31 (3–121)	9	90	34.6
Peterson et al. [43] 1997	7	5/2	7–15	type 1 diabetes	48	0	0	n.d.
Laureti et al. [30] 1998	19	12/5	18–44	OSAD	12–60	8	42	n.d.
Yu et al. [31] 1999	15	n.d.	8–40	type 1 diabetes	0–36	3	20	n.d.
Coco et al. [32] 2006	100	80/20	4–72	OSAD	3–21	31	47	4.9
All cases (range)	230					84 (0–90)		

n.d. = Not detected.

In a further study of a cohort of 100 ACA/21-OH-Ab-positive patients followed up for a mean period of 3 years (range: 3–121 months), 31 developed clinical AD (15 of 20 children, and 16 of 80 adults) and 9 progressed from normal to subclinical adrenal function. The cumulative risk of clinical AD in ACA/21-OH-Ab-positive patients was 47.5% (95% CI: 39.5–55.5), with an annual incidence of 4.9% (95% CI: 3.4–7.1) [32, 33].

What Is the Best Method to Study Adrenal Function in Adrenal Cortex Autoantibodies/21-Hydroxylase Autoantibody-Positive Patients?

In the majority of studies the evaluation of the adrenocortical function in subjects positive for ACA/21-OH-Ab was performed at the beginning of the study and during follow-up using a high-dose ACTH test (250 μg) [20, 21, 32, 34, 35]. In this test, basal cortisol levels are measured at 8:00 a.m. and then serum cortisol levels are measured 60 min after intravenous injection of ACTH. Overall assessment of adrenal function is based on basal plasma levels of ACTH, plasma levels of aldosterone and plasma renin activity. Combination of these tests allowed identifying 5 different stages of adrenal impairment in the natural history of autoimmune AD in patients positive for ACA/21-OH-Ab (table 2).

Stage 0 is characterized by the presence of ACA and/or 21-OH-Ab only and normal adrenal function tests. There are no clinical manifestations of AD (potential AD).

Stage 1 is characterized by increased plasma renin activity or renin levels with normal or low levels of aldosterone (this observation indicates that the pars glomerulosa of the adrenal cortex is the first area to be affected or at least the most sensitive to the autoimmune aggression). There are no clinical manifestations of AD (subclinical AD with mineralocorticoid deficiency).

Table 2. Stages of adrenal dysfunction detectable by the ACTH test in ACA/21-OH-Ab-positive subjects

Addison's disease	Stage	ACA and/or 21-OH-Ab	Basal plasma renin	Basal plasma aldosterone	Basal ACTH	Basal plasma cortisol	Cortisol 60 min after i.v. ACTH	Clinical mani-festations
Potential	0	+	normal	normal	normal	normal	normal	absent
Subclinical (with mineralocorticoids deficiency)	1	+	increased	normal/ reduced	normal	normal	normal	absent
Subclinical (with mineralocorticoids deficiency and impaired gluco-corticoids reserve)	2	+	increased	reduced	normal	normal	low response	absent
Subclinical (with mineralocorticoids and glucocorticoids deficiency)	3	+	increased	reduced	increased	normal[1]	no response	absent
Clinical	4	+	increased	reduced	very high	low	no response	present

[1] Or within the low limits of normal range.

Stage 2 is characterized, in addition to the previous alterations, by normal levels of basal cortisol and ACTH with a low or no response of cortisol to intravenous ACTH stimulation (this observation indicates that the pars fasciculata of the adrenal cortex is the area affected later or at least more resistant to the autoimmune aggression). There are no clinical manifestations of AD (subclinical AD with mineralocorticoid deficiency and impaired glucocorticoid reserve).

Stage 3 is characterized by increased basal ACTH levels with low basal cortisol and no increase of cortisol levels following intravenous ACTH stimulation. There are no clinical manifestations of AD (subclinical AD with mineralocorticoid and glucocorticoid deficiency).

Stage 4 of adrenal cortex dysfunction is characterized by very high levels of ACTH with markedly low serum cortisol levels and by the presence of clinical manifestations (clinical AD).

These observations suggest that in the natural history of AD, the zona glomerulosa, which produces mineralocorticoids, is the first area involved or the most sensitive to the autoimmune attack, and that the zona fasciculata, which synthetizes cortisol, is the most resistant and is able to protect itself from the autoimmune aggression for many months or even years.

The time of the progression from stages 0 to 4 is quite variable. In some patients, ongoing progression from stages 0 to 4 can be demonstrated, while in some patients not all of the stages are discernible.

It should be noted that contrary to the historical symptomatology, hyperpigmentation is not an early sign of AD and appears many months after the increase of plasma ACTH levels. It has been proposed that an ACTH test with a low dose of ACTH (1 μg) would be more appropriate for the assessment of adrenal function in ACA/21-OH-Ab-positive patients, assuming that the test with high doses might have inadequate sensitivity [36]. However, the low-dose ACTH test did not reveal differences in the cortisol response in either normal controls or patients with ACA/21-OH-Ab in comparison to that obtained with high ACTH doses (250 μg). Although the two tests could be considered equivalent, the high-dose ACTH test has been recommended for diagnostic work-up in the recent European consensus on therapy and management of AD [37].

Is Progression to Addison's Disease Mandatory?

The progression toward AD in autoantibody-positive patients is variable and not mandatory because only a proportion of these patients will develop clinical disease. The clinical onset occurs normally within 10–11 years from the first detection of ACA, and almost never after this period.

We have now re-evaluated the follow-up of 148 patients with ACA/21-OH-Ab positivity followed up for a mean period of 5.8 years (range: 2 months to 27 years; fig. 1a). The cumulative risk of developing overt AD at 11 years is about 30% in this cohort of patients, but it is greatly increased in ACA-positive patients with type 1 autoimmune polyglandular syndrome (up to 78%) compared to patients with other autoimmune associated diseases (22%; fig. 1b). ACA/21-OH-Ab-positive patients without clinical AD for whom more than 11 years of follow-up data were available very rarely developed clinical AD.

The natural history of AD is typically subdivided in three phases: potential, subclinical and clinical (fig. 2). The point of no return for developing clinical AD has been identified as a stage 1, i.e. when renin activity increases. In the subclinical phases of AD, any stress-related event (i.e. trauma, infection, surgery, pregnancy or other) requiring an increase in cortisol secretion may induce an acceleration of adrenocortical failure.

Is It Possible to Predict the Onset of Clinical Adrenal Failure with More Precision?

We have attempted to identify the independent predicting factors for progression to adrenal cortical dysfunction in ACA/21-OH-Ab-positive patients [32]. Using a multivariate analysis we analysed a number of clinical, biochemical and immunological parameters at the start of the follow-up of ACA/21-OH-Ab-positive subjects: (1) age, (2) gender, (3) titers of ACA/21-OH-Ab, (4) adrenal function status, (5) class II HLA haplotype and (6) type of pre-existing autoimmune disease. The study showed that the occurrence of clinical AD was associated with four independent factors: (1) gender (males compared to females, $p < 0.001$), (2) type of autoimmune disease (chronic hypoparathyroidism and/or mucocutaneous candidiasis compared with thyroid autoimmune disease and/or type 1 diabetes mellitus, $p = 0.009$), (3) ACA/21-OH-Ab titers

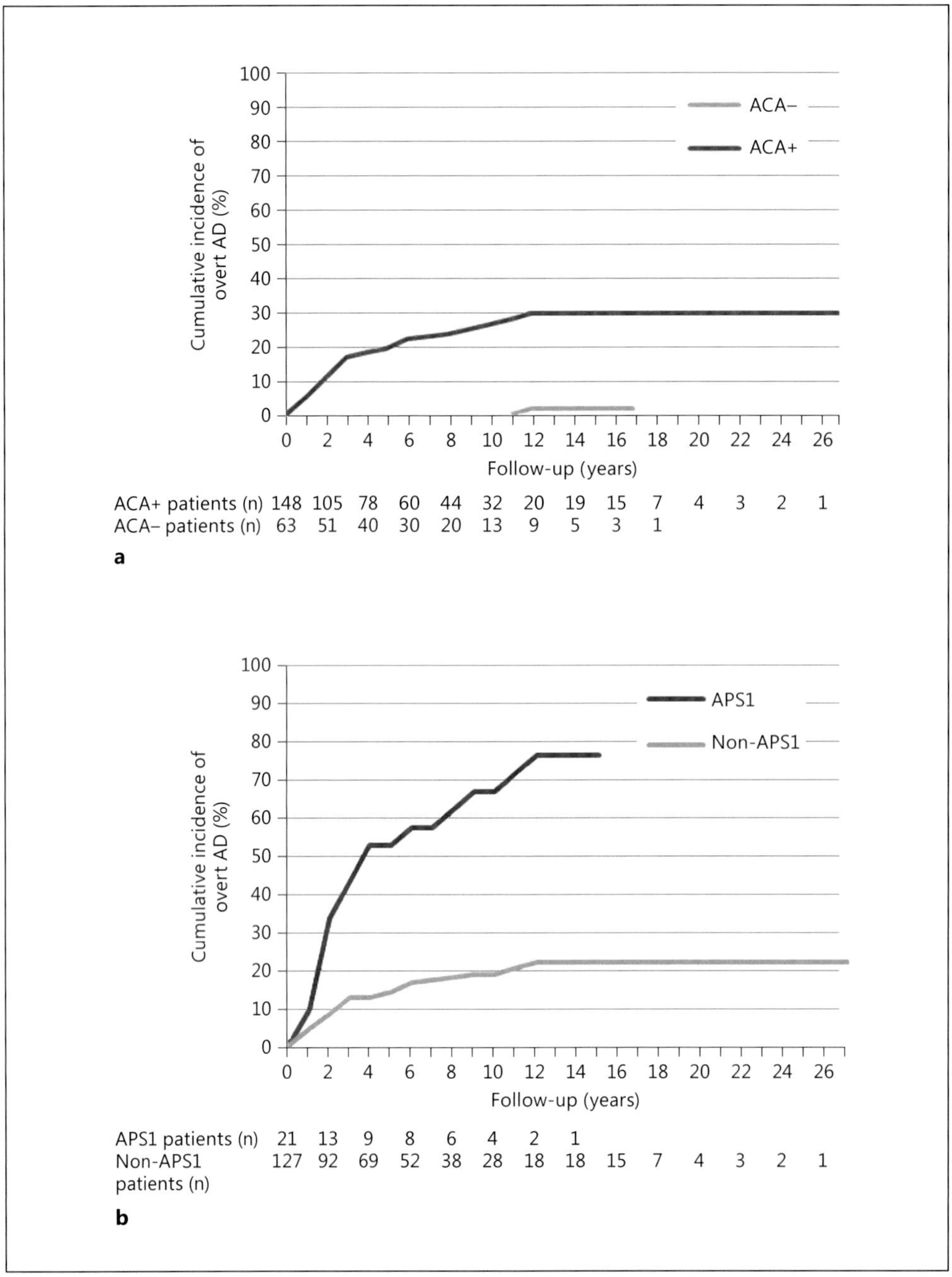

Fig. 1. Cumulative incidence of overt AD in patients with ACA (**a**) and in ACA-positive patients with type 1 autoimmune polyglandular syndrome (APS1) or non-APS1 diseases (**b**).

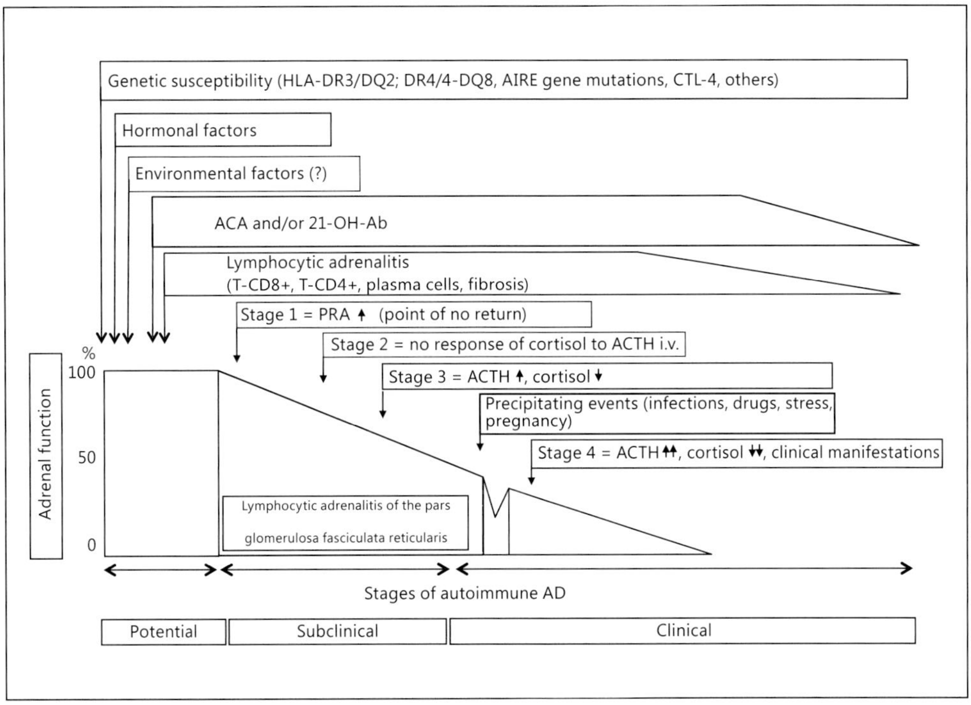

Fig. 2. Natural history of autoimmune AD. PRA = Plasma renin activity.

(high titers compared with medium-low titers, $p = 0.02$) and (4) adrenal function status (impaired adrenal function compared with normal function, $p < 0.0001$). Consequently, the probability of developing AD can be estimated using the logistic regression equation model shown in table 3.

With this equation one individual can be scored. The risk for clinical AD was considered to be low when the score was <0.10, moderate with a score from 0.10 to 0.40, and high when >0.40. The scoring system for a risk may have two practical consequences: (1) it can determine the time intervals for performing biochemical tests according to risk level (table 4), and (2) it can assist in the selection of patients for recruitment to immunointervention trials aimed at preventing the development of the disease.

What Are the Prospects to Modify or Interfere with the Natural History of Addison's Disease?

In 1993 it was reported that some ACA-positive patients with stage 1 or 2 adrenocortical failure had become ACA-negative and recovered adrenal function spontaneously or after 6 months of treatment with high doses of corticosteroid therapy for

Table 3. The logistic regression equation model on the probability of developing AD

Logit P(Y) = –5.1256	
Gender	+0.7911 (if male) +0.0 (if female)
Adrenal function	+2.5737 (if impaired) +0.0 (if normal)
Titer of ACA	+1.7318 (if high) +0.0 (if low-moderate)
Disease	+4.7214 (if hypoparathyroidism or candidiasis) +1.4984 (if type 1 diabetes or thyroid autoimmune disease) +0.0 (if other disease present)

Table 4. Proposed timetable for endocrinological and immunological assessment in subjects with ACA and different risk scores

Risk score	Baseline risk	Time intervals, months
<0.10	low	24–36
0.10–0.40	moderate	12–24
>0.40	high	6–12

Graves' opthalmopathy [35]. In a subsequent study, the same group showed that in one patient the remission of adrenal cortex failure persisted for 100 months of follow-up [38].

Recently, monoclonal antibodies targeting specific molecules involved in the immune responses emerged as effective alternatives for prevention and treatment of autoimmune diseases. In particular rituximab directed against human CD20 antigen expressed on mature B cells showed promising results in type 1 diabetes and Graves' ophthalmopathy [39, 40]. These developments opened new opportunities for AD. In an open-label pilot study of B-lymphocyte depletion therapy, rituximab was given to 6 patients with new-onset idiopathic adrenal failure. Although the benefits of the treatment on adrenal function were not evident in 5 of 6 patients, a single patient showed a remarkable improvement in cortisol and aldosterone secretion for up to 27 months after therapy [41].

Regenerative medical therapy is a different approach for preserving adrenal cortex function. ACTH was used to stimulate self-renewal of adrenal cortex subcapsular progenitor cells for 20 weeks in patients with established AD (i.e. more than 1 year) [42]. The response to the treatment in terms of improvement of cortisol concentrations and withdrawal of corticosteroid replacement was limited to 2/13 patients. However, these observations are encouraging for developing new strategies for prevention or delay of the onset of clinical AD and introducing new opportunities for preserving or even regenerating adrenal function.

Conclusions

Progress in studies on the relationship between adrenal autoantibody positivity and the development of the clinical disease has greatly improved our knowledge about the natural history of AD. AD should be viewed as a chronic disorder with a long preclinical period marked by the presence of ACA. The populations at risk are first-degree relatives of patients with AD and patients with autoimmune diseases, particularly those with chronic hypoparathyroidism or premature ovarian failure. The methods for screening the populations at risk that perform well in international proficiency studies are ACA by indirect immunofluorescence measured in experienced laboratories or 21-OH-Ab by immunoprecipitation assay. However, in order to harmonize the results, international reference preparations for ACA/21-OH-Ab would be very helpful. The recommended method to assess adrenal function in adrenal autoantibody-positive patients is the ACTH test with high doses of ACTH. The risk of progression to AD can be estimated by an equation model where parameters such as age, titer of autoantibodies, adrenal function and associated disease at entry are important factors. Patients with a high risk score would require follow-up every 6 months, and might be ideal candidates for inclusion in prevention trials.

References

1 Walsh JP, Bremner AP, Feddema P, Leedman PJ, Brown SJ, O'Leary P: Thyrotropin and thyroid antibodies as predictors of hypothyroidism: a 13-year, longitudinal study of a community-based cohort using immunoassay techniques. J Clin Endocrinol Metab 2010;95:1095–1104.

2 Betterle C, Spadaccino AC, Presotto F, Zanchetta R, Pedini B, Lai M, Greggio NA, Bottazzo GF: The number of markers of pancreatic autoimmunity is proportional to the risk for type 1 diabetes mellitus in Italian and English patients with organ-specific autoimmune diseases. Ann NY Acad Sci 2002;958:276–280.

3 Sosenko JM, Skyler JS, Palmer JP, Krischer JP, Yu L, Mahon J, Beam CA, Boulware DC, Rafkin L, Schatz D, Eisenbarth G; Type 1 Diabetes TrialNet Study Group; Diabetes Prevention Trial-Type 1 Study Group: The prediction of type 1 diabetes by multiple autoantibody levels and their incorporation into an autoantibody risk score in relatives of type 1 diabetic patients. Diabetes Care 2013;36:2615–620.

4 Ahonen P, Miettinen A, Perheentupa J: Adrenal and steroidal cell antibodies in patients with autoimmune polyglandular disease type I and risk of adrenocortical and ovarian failure. J Clin Endocrinol Metab 1987;64:494–500.

5 Reato G, Morlin L, Chen S, Furmaniak J, Smith BR, Masiero S, Albergoni MP, Cervato S, Zanchetta R, Betterle C: Premature ovarian failure in patients with autoimmune Addison's disease: clinical, genetic, and immunological evaluation. J Clin Endocrinol Metab 2011;96:E1255–E1261.

6 Blizzard RM, Kyle M: Studies of the adrenal antigens and autoantibodies in Addison's disease. J Clin Invest 1963;42:1653–1660.

7 Betterle C: Addison's disease and autoimmune polyglandular syndromes; in Geenen V, Chrousos GP (eds): Immunoendocrinology in Health and Disease. New York, Marcel Dekker, 2004.
8 Winqvist O, Karlsson FA, Kämpe O: 21-hydroxylase, a major autoantigen in idiopathic Addison's disease. Lancet 1992;339:1559–1562.
9 Baumann-Antczak A, Wedlock N, Bednarek J, Kiso Y, Krishnan H, Fowler S, Rees Smith B, Furmaniak J: Autoimmune Addison's disease and 21-hydroxylase. Lancet 1992;340:429–430.
10 Colls J, Betterle C, Volpato M, Rees Smith B, Furmaniak J: A new immunoprecipitation assay for autoantibodies to steroid 21-hydroxylase in Addison's disease. Clin Chem 1995;41:375–380.
11 Tanaka H, Powell M, Chen S, Sawicka S, Asawa T, Betterle C, Volpato M, Rees Smith B, Furmaniak J: Autoimmune adrenal diseases – a new sensitive assay for measurement of steroid 21-hydroxylase autoantibodies. J Clin Endocrinol Metab 1997;82:1440–1446.
12 Betterle C, Scarpa R, Garelli S, Morlin L, Lazzarotto F, Presotto F, Coco G, Masiero S, Parolo A, Albergoni MP, Favero R, Barollo S, Salvà M, Basso D, Chen S, Rees Smith B, Furmaniak J, Mantero F: Addison's disease: a survey on 633 patients in Padova. Eur J Endocrinol 2013;169:773–784.
13 Anderson JR, Goudie RB, Gray K, Stuart-Smith DA: Immunological features of idiopathic Addison's disease: an antibody to cell producing steroid hormones. Clin Exp Immunol 1968;3:107–117.
14 Winqvist O, Gebre-Medhin G, Gustafsson J, Ritzen EM, Lundkvist O, Karlsson FA, Kampe O: Identification of the main gonadal autoantigens in patients with adrenal insufficiency and associated ovarian failure. J Clin Endocrinol Metab 1995;80:1717–1723.
15 Falorni A, Chen S, Zanchetta R, Yu L, Tiberti C, Bacosi ML, Furmaniak J, Bini V, Dotta F, Eisenbarth GS, Rees Smith B, Betterle C: Measuring adrenal autoantibody response: interlaboratory concordance in the first international serum exchange for the determination of 21-hydroxylase autoantibodies. Clin Immunol 2011;140:291–299.
16 Falorni A, Bini V, Betterle C, Brozzetti A, Castaño L, Fichna M, Kämpe O, Mellgren G, Peterson P, Chen S, Rönnelid J, Seissler J, Tiberti C, Uibo R, Yu L, Lernmark Å, Husebye E: Determination of 21-hydroxylase autoantibodies: inter-laboratory concordance in the Euradrenal International Serum Exchange Program. Clin Chem Lab Med 2015;53:1761–1770.
17 Furmaniak J, Kominami S, Asawa T, Wedlock N, Colls J, Smith BR: Autoimmune Addison's disease – evidence for a role of steroid 21-hydroxylase autoantibodies in adrenal insufficiency. J Clin Endocrinol Metab 1994;79:1517–1521.
18 Boscaro M, Betterle C, Volpato M, Fallo F, Furmaniak J, Rees Smith B, Sonino N: Hormonal responses during various phases of autoimmune adrenal failure: no evidence for 21-hydroxylase enzyme activity in vivo. J Clin Endocrinol Metab 1996;81:2801–2804.
19 Betterle C, Dal Pra C, Pedini B, Zanchetta R, Albergoni MP, Chen S, Furmaniak J, Rees Smith B: Assessment of adrenocortical function and autoantibodies in a baby born to a mother with autoimmune polyglandular syndrome type 2. J Endocrinol Invest 2004;27:618–621.
20 Betterle C, Volpato M, Rees Smith B, Furmaniak J, Chen S, Zanchetta R, Greggio NA, Pedini B, Boscaro M, Presotto F: II. Adrenal cortex and steroid 21-hydroxylase autoantibodies in children with organ-specific autoimmune diseases: markers of high progression to clinical Addison's disease. J Clin Endocrinol Metab 1997;82:939–942.
21 Betterle C, Volpato M, Rees Smith B, Furmaniak J, Chen S, Greggio NA, Sanzari M, Tedesco F, Pedini B, Boscaro M, Presotto F: I. Adrenal cortex and steroid 21-hydroxylase autoantibodies in adult patients with organ-specific autoimmune diseases: markers of low progression to clinical Addison's disease. J Clin Endocrinol Metab 1997;82:932–938.
22 Dal Pra C, Chen S, Furmaniak J, Rees Smith B, Pedini B, Moscon A, Zanchetta R, Betterle C: Autoantibodies to steroidogenic enzymes in patients with premature ovarian failure with and without Addison's disease. Eur J Endocrinol 2003;148:565–570.
23 Anderson JR: Auto-antibodies in diseases of man. Br Med Bull 1963;19:251–256.
24 Blizzard RM, Chee D, Davis W: The incidence of parathyroid and other antibodies in the sera of patients with idiopathic hypoparathyroidism. Clin Exp Immunol 1966;1:119–128.
25 Simmonds JP, Lister J: Autoimmune Addison's disease in identical twins. Postgrad Med J 1978;54:552–554.
26 Riley WJ, Maclaren NK, Neufeld M: Adrenal antibodies and Addison's disease in insulin-dependent diabetes mellitus. J Pediatr 1980;97:191–195.
27 Eason RJ, Croxon MS, Perry MC, Somerfield SD: Addison's disease, adrenal autoantibodies and computerized adrenal tomography. NZ Med J 1982;95:569–573.
28 Scherbaum WA, Berg PA: Development of adrenocortical failure in non-Addisonian patients with antibodies to adrenal cortex. A clinical follow-up study. Clin Endocrinol (Oxf) 1982;16:345–352.
29 Betterle C, Zanette F, Zanchetta R, Pedini B, Trevisan A, Mantero F, Rigon F: Complement-fixing adrenal autoantibodies as a marker for predicting onset of idiopathic Addison's disease. Lancet 1983;1:1238–1241.

30 Laureti S, De Bellis AM, Muccitelli VI, Calcinaro F, Bizzaro A, Rossi R, Bellastella A, Santeusanio F, Falorni A: Levels of adrenocortical autoantibodies correlate with the degree of adrenal dysfunction in subjects with preclinical Addison's disease. J Clin Endocrinol Metab 1998;83:3507–3511.
31 Yu L, Brewer, KW, Gates S, Wu A, Wang T, Babu SR, Gottlieb PA, Freed BM, Noble J, Erlich HA, Rewers J, Eisenbarth GS: DRB1*04 and DQ alleles: expression of 21-hydroxylase autoantibodies and risk of progression to Addison's disease. J Clin Endocrinol Metab 1999;84:328–335.
32 Coco G, Dal Pra C, Presotto F, Albergoni MP, Canova C, Pedini B, Zanchetta R, Chen S, Furmaniak J, Rees Smith B, Mantero F, Betterle C: Estimated risk for developing autoimmune Addison's disease in patients with adrenal cortex autoantibodies. J Clin Endocrinol Metab 2006;91:1637–1645.
33 Betterle C, Coco G, Zanchetta R: Adrenal cortex autoantibodies in subjects with normal adrenal function. Best Pract Res Clin Endocrinol Metab 2005;19: 85–89.
34 Betterle C, Scalici C, Presotto F, Pedini B, Moro L, Rigon F, Mantero F: The natural history of adrenal function in autoimmune patients with adrenal autoantibodies. J Endocrinol 1988;117:467–475.
35 De Bellis A, Bizzarro A, Rossi R, Paglionico VA, Criscuolo T, Lombardi G, Bellastella A: Remission of subclinical adrenocortical failure in subjects with adrenal autoantibodies. J Clin Endocrinol Metab 1993; 76:1002–1007.
36 Laureti S, Arvat E, Candeloro P, Di Vito L, Ghigo E, Santeusanio F, Falorni A: Low dose (1 microg) ACTH test in the evaluation of adrenal dysfunction in pre-clinical Addison's disease. Clin Endocrinol (Oxf) 2000;53:107–115.
37 Husebye ES, Allolio B, Arlt W, Badenhoop K, Bensing S, Betterle C, Falorni A, Gan EH, Hulting AL, Kasperlik-Zaluska A, Kämpe O, Løvås K, Meyer G, Pearce SH: Consensus statement on the diagnosis, treatment and follow-up of patients with primary adrenal insufficiency. J Intern Med 2014;275:104–115.
38 De Bellis A, Falorni A, Laureti S, Perrino S, Coronella C, Forini F, Bizzarro E, Bizzarro A, Abbate G, Bellastella A: Time course of 21-hydroxylase antibodies and long-term remission of subclinical autoimmune adrenalitis after corticosteroid therapy: case report. J Clin Endocrinol Metab 2001;86:675–678.
39 Waldron-Lynch F, Herold KC: Immunomodulatory therapy to preserve pancreatic β-cells function in type 1 diabetes. Nat Rev Drug Discov 2011;10:439–452.
40 Salvi M, Vannucchi G, Campi I, Currò N, Simonetta S, Covelli D, Pignataro L, Guastella C, Rossi S, Bonara P, Dazzi D, Ratiglia R, Beck-Peccoz P: Rituximab treatment in a patient with severe thyroid-associated ophthalmopathy: effects on orbital lymphocytic infiltrates. Clin Immunol 2009;131:360–365.
41 Pearce SH, Mitchell AL, Bennett S, King P, Chandran S, Nag S, Chen S, Smith BR, Isaacs JD, Vaidya B: Adrenal steroidogenesis after B lymphocyte depletion therapy in new-onset Addison's disease. J Clin Endocrinol Metab 2012;97:E1927–E1932.
42 Gan EH, MacArthur K, Mitchell AL, Hughes BA, Perros P, Ball SG, James RA, Quinton R, Chen S, Furmaniak J, Arlt W, Pearce SH: Residual adrenal function in autoimmune Addison's disease: improvement after tetracosactide (ACTH1–24) treatment. J Clin Endocrinol Metab 2014;99:111–118.
43 Peterson P, Salmi H, Hyöty H, Miettinen A, Ilonen J, Reijonen H, Knip M, Akerblom HK, Krohn K: Steroid 21-hydroxylase autoantibodies in insulin-dependent diabetes mellitus. Childhood Diabetes in Finland (DiMe) Study Group. Clin Immunol Immunopathol 1997;82:37–42.

Prof. Corrado Betterle, MD
Unit of Endocrinology, Department of Medicine, Azienda Ospedaliera-Università di Padova
Università degli Studi di Padova
Via Ospedale Civile 105
IT–35100 Padova (Italy)
E-Mail corrado.betterle@unipd.it

Arvat E, Falorni A (eds): Cortisol Excess and Insufficiency.
Front Horm Res. Basel, Karger, 2016, vol 46, pp 146–158 (DOI: 10.1159/000443913)

Is Diagnosis and Subclassification of Adrenal Insufficiency as Easy as It Looks?

Lisanne C.C.J. Smans · Pierre M.J. Zelissen

Section of Endocrinology, Department of Internal Medicine, Utrecht University Medical Center, Utrecht, The Netherlands

Abstract

The diagnosis of adrenal insufficiency (AI) is a challenge. Most signs and symptoms are nonspecific and vary considerably depending upon the underlying cause and degree of AI. Identification of AI is crucial because the disease may be life-threatening if left unrecognized. The diagnostic evaluation consists of three steps. The first step is establishing the presence of hypocortisolism. The second step is establishing the level of hypothalamus-pituitary-adrenal axis dysfunction. The third and final step is searching for the exact cause of AI by additional laboratory and imaging techniques. Each diagnostic step can have its own uncertainties. The optimal test in case of intermediate basal cortisol measurements is still a matter of debate. Furthermore, interpretation of the results of the tests is complicated by arbitrary definitions of normal cutoff responses, variability in the analytical accuracy of the cortisol assays used and factors influencing cortisol-binding globulin. This chapter aims to provide a concise stepwise approach for the diagnostic evaluation of AI, taking into account the possible pitfalls associated with the different tests.

Classification of Adrenal Insufficiency

Adrenal insufficiency (AI) results from dysfunction at one or more levels of the hypothalamic-pituitary-adrenal (HPA) axis. Primary adrenal insufficiency (PAI) is caused by dysfunction of the adrenal glands, while central adrenal insufficiency (CAI) results from dysfunction of the hypothalamus or pituitary, also named tertiary (TAI) and secondary adrenal insufficiency (SAI), respectively. Glucocorticoid-induced AI develops after prolonged treatment with exogenous glucocorticoids.

Table 1. Signs and symptoms of AI [22–30]

Signs and symptoms	Type of AI, %	
	PAI	CAI
Weakness and fatigue	74–100	64
Anorexia	53–100	29
Weight loss	25–100	30
Hypotension	55–94	32
Abdominal pain	21–44	5
Nausea, vomiting	36–92	21–24
Diarrhea	6–41	6
Salt-craving	9–78	
Depression	20–58	
Postural symptoms	11–84	
Hyperpigmentation	41–97	
Amenorrhea or reduced libido	25–46	47
Myalgia, joint pain	6–36	28
Headaches	32–44	45
Dry skin	32–34	37
Loss of axillary and pubic hair	24–38	45

Clinical Presentation of Adrenal Insufficiency

The clinical presentation of AI is variable and depends upon the underlying cause and extent of adrenal dysfunction. The most common clinical features of AI are malaise, fatigue, weakness, anorexia, weight loss, (orthostatic) hypotension, nausea, and diffuse myalgia and arthralgia (table 1). Because the onset of AI is often gradual and signs and symptoms are nonspecific, AI may go undetected for a long time [1]. Hyperpigmentation of the skin and mucous membranes is the most classical finding in PAI.

Hyperpigmentation is absent in patients with CAI. Other conditions that can lead to hyperpigmentation are hemochromatosis, porphyria cutanea tarda and ingestion of heavy metals, some antineoplastic agents, antimalarial drugs, tetracyclines, zidovudine, and phenothiazines. Another characteristic feature in PAI is salt-craving, which occurs in up to 78% of patients. Autoimmune destruction of dermal melanocytes, giving rise to areas of depigmented skin (vitiligo), occurs in 10–20% of patients with autoimmune adrenalitis.

AI can also present with acute adrenal crisis (AC), mostly triggered by intercurrent illness or severe stress. The principal manifestation of AC is hypotension or hypovolemic shock, but other symptoms and signs such as weakness, anorexia, nausea, abdominal pain, fever, vomiting, fatigue, electrolyte abnormalities, confusion and coma can also occur. AC should be regarded as a medical emergency. Treatment of patients who present in possible AC should not be delayed and therapy with glucocorticoids should be initiated immediately, after drawing blood for plasma cortisol and ACTH.

Diagnostic Evaluation of Suspected Adrenal Insufficiency

The first step in the diagnostic evaluation of a patient with symptoms and signs compatible with AI is to establish whether hypocortisolism is present by measuring basal morning plasma cortisol concentration, if necessary followed by dynamic testing. The next step is to localize the level of HPA axis dysfunction. The final step is to determine the cause of AI. This is critical because it directs subsequent evaluation, therapy and follow-up (fig. 1).

First Assessment: Hypocortisolism

Several factors are important for the interpretation of plasma cortisol. Cortisol production is pulsatile and has a diurnal pattern with levels being highest in the early morning and declining throughout the day. Cortisol increases in response to physiological and mental stress. The best time to measure plasma cortisol is in the morning between 8.00 and 9.00 h. Cortisol is bound to cortisol-binding globulin (CBG) and albumin, and only around 5% exists in a free state. CBG varies significantly within and between individuals. Decreased and increased CBG can lead to falsely lower or higher plasma cortisol concentrations, respectively [2]. CBG can be influenced by several factors. It is decreased in hyperthyroidism, cirrhosis and the nephrotic syndrome, whereas it is increased in a high estrogen state. For example, CBG increases in women using oral contraceptives, leading to almost a doubling of total plasma cortisol concentration. During pregnancy, cortisol production and secretion increase, its half-life is prolonged due to decreased hepatic clearance and there is a tripling of CBG levels. This leads to increased total plasma cortisol concentrations. These changes underlie the difficulties of the evaluation of AI during pregnancy. Finally, heterophile antibodies in a cortisol immunoassay can lead to falsely lowered plasma cortisol levels [3]. These factors should all be taken into account when interpreting plasma cortisol.

Basal Morning Cortisol

Random plasma cortisol can be best measured early in the morning because overlap between normal and subnormal cortisol levels is the least in the early morning. Basal cortisol is affected by stress, exercise and food intake. Stress and exercise should be minimized as much as possible before a blood sample is taken between 8.00 and 9.00 h after overnight fast. Controversy exists about the level of cortisol indicative of AI. Many patients have intermediate levels and require additional (dynamic) tests. Nonetheless, plasma morning cortisol is a good first assessment of adrenal function. It is easy and quick to perform. Very low (<100 nmol/l) or high (>500 nmol/l) morning cortisol levels obviate the need for dynamic tests.

Alternatives to plasma total cortisol are free plasma cortisol and salivary cortisol measurement in case of suspected increased or decreased CBG. Salivary cortisol is

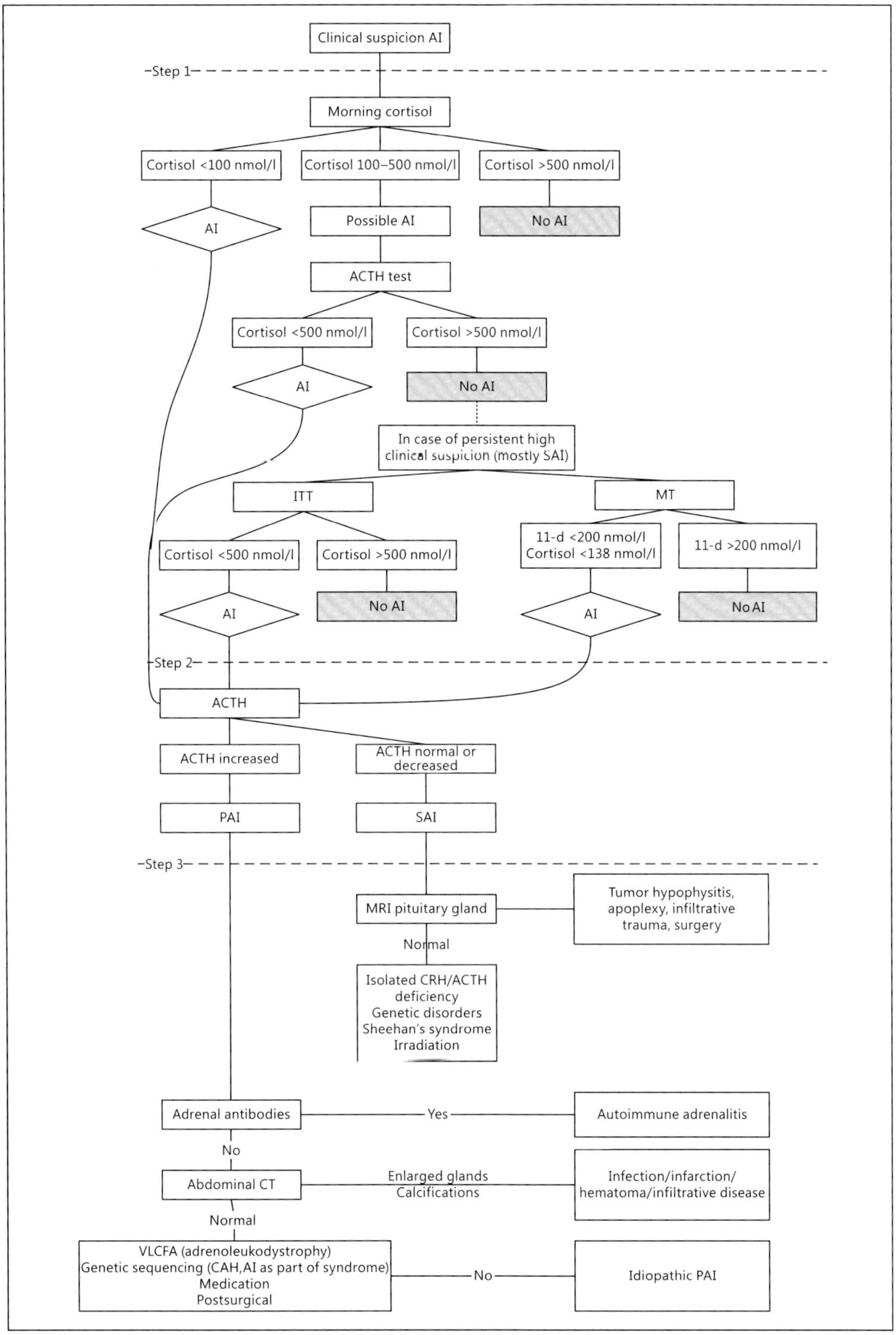

Fig. 1. Flowchart for the diagnostic evaluation of suspected AI. CAH = Congenital adrenal hyperplasia; 11-d = 11-desoxycortisol; VLCFA = very long-chain fatty acids. * Cortisol values not applicable in case of abnormal CBG (see text); ** MT if ITT is contra-indicated (see text).

easy to collect by absorption into a cotton roll (Salivette). It reflects the biologically active free form. The analytical sensitivity varies between immunoassays due to the potential for cross-reactivity with other steroids [4]. A disadvantage of free plasma cortisol and salivary cortisol is that it is not widely available and data on the diagnostic accuracy in AI are limited. Hair cortisol is a new approach and has the potential to provide a retrospective view of cortisol levels over a period of several months [5]. Disadvantages of hair cortisol are that it might not detect AI of relatively short duration. It is not clear if it represents the free cortisol fraction. In addition, it has been shown to correlate with plasma and salivary cortisol in some but not all studies. The diagnostic value of hair cortisol in diagnosing AI is not known.

Dynamic Testing

Different dynamic tests exist for the evaluation of hypocortisolism, such as the ACTH test (Synacthen^{TM}), insulin tolerance test (ITT), metyrapone test (MT) and glucagon stimulation test (GST).

ACTH Test

The ACTH test (Synacthen^{TM}) is a simple, safe and widely used test for AI. The test can be performed on an outpatient basis and side effects are minimal. In addition to directly measuring the functional integrity of the adrenal glands, it also provides an indirect assessment of hypothalamic and pituitary function [6]. When ACTH production is impaired by pituitary or hypothalamic disease, the adrenals atrophy and have less capacity to respond to exogenous stimulation. The test must not be used in AI of suspected short (4–6 weeks) duration (e.g. recent pituitary surgery), when corticotrope damage may have occurred but the adrenals have not yet atrophied [7]. During the ACTH test, cortisol is measured before and after (30 and/or 60 min) administration of ACTH. In the literature there is considerable variation in the choice of the cortisol cutoff value, ranging from 400 nmol/l (14.4 µg/dl) to more than 694 nmol/l (25 µg/dl). However, the majority considers a maximum cortisol value greater than 500 nmol/l (18 µg/dl) acceptable for determining normality. The increase in cortisol following ACTH administration is an unreliable index of adrenal function. It does not distinguish normal patients from those with AI. In PAI, a 250-µg ACTH test is performed. In CAI, however, controversy exists regarding the diagnostic value of the high- (250 µg) versus low-dose (1 µg) ACTH test. The low-dose test has been proposed as a more sensitive test. During the high-dose test, 250 µg of ACTH [60,000 pg/ml (1,320 pmol/l)] is given as compared to 1 µg of ACTH [1,900 pg/ml (41.8 pmol/l)] during the low-dose test. The 250-µg test stimulates maximal secretion and in normal subjects results in a peak plasma ACTH concentration of about twice that during ITT [8]. The low-dose test gives rise to more physiological plasma concentrations of ACTH and possibly provides a more sensitive index of adrenal responsiveness. The low-dose test has a practical disadvantage: the commercially available ACTH (vials of 250 µg) has to be diluted and during intravenous injection it can adhere to the tube, leading to administration of a lower ACTH concentration, possibly giving rise to lower cortisol levels and thus false-positive results. Some studies have reported that the low-dose test is more sensitive, but a meta-analysis comparing the high- and low-dose test found similar sensitivities, concluding that the two tests perform similarly [9–11]. The differences between the studies, such as different populations and cortisol assays, could have led to the discrepant conclusions. It is possible that mild or borderline cases of AI could occasionally be missed by the 250-μg ACTH test. The clinical significance with regard to the risk of AC during intercurrent illness in these cases remains unknown.

Adrenal androgens, secreted by the zona reticularis are regulated primarily by ACTH and thus may be regarded as another parameter of ACTH action on the adrenal cortex. Several studies show that patients with SAI have drastically low serum DHEAS levels, which is also the case in even those who achieved normal cortisol responses to the ACTH test [12, 13]. Furthermore, in SAI a higher cortisol to DHEA molar ratio has been seen. Cortisol is possibly secreted preferentially over DHEA, and this becomes more apparent after low-dose ACTH. The presence of normal DHEA and DHEAS levels could be indicators of normal ACTH secretion and adequate adrenal cortical function [14]. However, interpretation of individual results using age-adjusted references is required. The diagnostic value of this approach in SAI will probably become clearer in future studies.

Insulin Tolerance Test

The ITT is currently considered the gold standard when evaluating patients suspected of having SAI. Hypoglycemic stress stimulates cortisol production by increasing hypothalamic corticotropin-releasing hormone (CRH) and pituitary ACTH secretion. The aim of the ITT is to induce hypoglycemia with a glucose value of <2.2 mmol/l with occurrence of neuroglycopenic symptoms. Short-acting insulin is injected intravenously at doses ranging from 0.1 U/kg in patients highly suspected of having AI to 0.2 U/kg or even more in insulin-resistant states such as acromegaly, obesity and type 2 diabetes mellitus. Cortisol and glucose are measured at different time points. In subjects with no adrenal reserve an AC can occur. A cortisol level greater than 500–550 nmol/l excludes CAI. It has some disadvantages though, namely that it is contraindicated in patients with cardiovascular disease or epilepsy and it requires close observation throughout the test to monitor for adrenergic and neuroglycopenic symptoms. Experience with this test in children and elderly people is limited.

Metyrapone Test

Metyrapone inhibits 11β-hydroxylase, which converts 11-desoxycortisol to cortisol in the final step of adrenal steroidogenesis. 11-Desoxycortisol does not have glucocorticoid activity and therefore does not inhibit ACTH production. Normally when metyrapone is given, the decline in cortisol stimulates ACTH release, and due to the enzyme blockade, causes 11-desoxycortisol to accumulate. In AI, 11-desoxycortisol fails to increase. The test is performed as an overnight test with a single dose of metyrapone administered orally at 23.00 h. Blood is drawn at 8.00 h the next morning for measurement of ACTH, plasma cortisol and 11-desoxycortisol. Adequate adrenal function is confirmed by 11-desoxycortisol >200 nmol/l (>7.0 μg/dl), regardless of the cortisol level. AI is diagnosed if 11-desoxycortisol is <200 nmol/l (<7.0 μg/dl) and plasma cortisol is <138 nmol/l (<5 μg/dl). If 11-desoxycortisol is <200 nmol/l (<7.0 μg/dl) but cortisol >138 nmol/l (>5 μg/dl), the MT is indeterminate because the hypocortisolemia was not adequate to stimulate pituitary production of ACTH. Phenytoin and phenobarbital increase the metabolism of metyrapone, thereby reducing plasma metyrapone levels and decreasing the 11β-hydroxylase blockade. Other drugs which have been found to cause subnormal responses include amitriptyline, chlorpromazine, barbiturates, chlordiazepoxide, estrogens, somatostatin analogues, diclofenac, furosemide, irbesartan, sodium valproate and zidovudine. The MT has been validated against the ITT for the diagnosis of SAI with a specificity of 88–100% and sensitivity of 60–100% [15, 16]. The risk of an AC precipitated by metyrapone should be taken into account during the test.

Glucagon Stimulation Test

The GST is performed by measuring cortisol before and after the administration of 1 mg of glucagon. The GST is used almost exclusively in children. Controversy exists about the diagnostic value of the GST in the evaluation of AI, compared to the ITT, MT and ACTH test. Small studies in healthy controls and pituitary patients initially found that the GST and ITT compared well. These results could not be reproduced by recent larger studies performed in patients after traumatic brain injury and patients following pituitary surgery. These studies found that 30–51% of GST and ITT results were discordant, due to false-positive results of the GST [17, 18]. Cegla et al. [19] showed that against the overnight MT, the GST had a sensitivity of 87.5% and a specificity of 10.5% at a cortisol cutoff level of ≥440 nmol/l, concluding that the GST has inferior diagnostic utility compared to the MT. The GST should not be considered as the test of choice in patients with SAI.

In conclusion, for the diagnosis of hypocortisolism in patients with intermediate cortisol values (100–500 nmol/l), the 250-μg ACTH test is the simplest and safest test showing high specificity in the evaluation of PAI and SAI. The evaluation of SAI after pituitary surgery by means of an ACTH test should not be performed within a period of 4–6 weeks after surgery. Interpretation of the results of the tests and defining normal cutoff responses should be set regarding the analytical accuracy of the cortisol assays used. In case of discrepant results or with persistent high clinical suspicion of SAI, an ITT should be performed. In case an ITT is contraindicated, an MT could be a valuable alternative.

Second Assessment: To Localize the Level of Dysfunction

Once hypocortisolism has been confirmed, the next step is to determine the site of the HPA axis defect. Plasma ACTH level is the best test to distinguish PAI from CAI and glucocorticoid-induced AI. It fails to separate normal patients from those with SAI. In PAI, ACTH is usually >100 pg/ml. ACTH >60 pg/ml (13.2 pmol/l) has a sensitivity of 100% and specificity of 98%. There are additional tests that can help in distinguishing the level of defect. The first evidence of autoimmune AI is an increase in plasma renin activity and normal or low aldosterone concentration, followed by a decreased cortisol response to ACTH stimulation, increased basal ACTH and finally decreased basal serum cortisol concentration. AI becomes clinically manifest after at least 90% of the cortex has been destroyed. Finally, increased potassium (65%) and decreased sodium (85–90%) concentrations can be seen. In SAI and TAI, plasma renin activity and aldosterone concentration are usually normal. Sodium concentration is often decreased due to increased vasopressin levels resulting from decreased inhibition by cortisol. In the past, a CRH stimulation test was proposed to distinguish SAI from glucocorticoid-induced AI or TAI. During this test 1 μg per kg CRH is injected intravenously, followed by sampling of ACTH and cortisol over the subsequent 2 h. In SAI, low or low-normal baseline ACTH was seen, which did not respond to CRH. In glucocorticoid-induced AI and TAI, low baseline ACTH was seen, which showed an exaggerated response to CRH, and remained elevated for a prolonged period of time [20]. However, overlap in ACTH and cortisol results are frequently seen, making the test unsuitable for differentiating between SAI and TAI.

Third Assessment: Determining the Etiology of Adrenal Insufficiency

Primary Adrenal Insufficiency

Autoimmune adrenalitis is the most common cause of PAI. Autoimmune adrenalitis is diagnosed in the presence of positive adrenal antibodies. PAI is characterized by the presence of antibodies against the steroidogenic enzymes, mostly 21-hydroxylase and less frequently side-chain cleavage enzyme and 17α-hydroxylase. Antibodies are present in up to 90% of patients, while they are rarely found in normal subjects. Antibodies against other endocrine glands are commonly seen in patients with autoimmune adrenalitis, possibly leading to autoimmune polyglandular syndrome. PAI can also result from a block in steroid production as in congenital adrenal hyperplasia or be part of a genetic syndrome. In the absence of adrenal antibodies, abdominal CT should be performed in order to detect adrenal calcifications or enlarged glands suggesting an infectious, metastatic, infiltrative or hemorrhagic cause of AI (table 2). The adrenal glands are invariably small in autoimmune adrenalitis. CT-directed percutaneous fine-needle aspiration can ultimately establish the presence of infectious disease or

Table 2. Causes of PAI

Autoimmune adrenalitis Isolated APS type 1 (chronic mucocutaneous candidiasis, hypoparathyroidism, other autoimmune diseases) APS type 2 (thyroid autoimmune disease, type 1 diabetes mellitus, other autoimmune diseases) APS type 4 (autoimmune gastritis, vitiligo, celiac disease, alopecia)
Genetic Congenital adrenal hyperplasia Congenital adrenal hypoplasia Triple A syndrome (Allgrove's syndrome) Adrenoleukodystrophy/adrenomyeloneuropathy Primary generalized glucocorticoid resistance Familial glucocorticoid deficiency or corticotropin insensitivity syndromes Sitosterolemia Wolman's disease Kearns-Sayre syndrome IMAGe syndrome Smith-Lemli-Opitz syndrome
Infectious adrenalitis Tuberculous adrenalitis Fungal (paracoccidioidomycosis, cryptococcosis, histoplasmosis) Syphilis Trypanosomiasis Viral (HIV, CMV, HSV)
Drugs Mitotane, ketoconazole, rifampicin, anticoagulants, tyrosine-kinase inhibitors, aminoglutethimide, fluconazole, etomidate, phenobarbital, phenytoin, metyrapone
Bilateral adrenal hemorrhage or thrombosis Waterhouse-Friderichsen syndrome, antiphospholipid syndrome, DIS
Bilateral adrenal metastases Lung, stomach, breast, colon
Bilateral adrenal infiltration Sarcoidosis, amyloidosis, hemochromatosis
Bilateral adrenalectomy

APS = Autoimmune polyglandular syndrome.

malignancy. In case of hemorrhage in a patient without anticoagulants, measurement of antiphospholipid antibodies should be performed. The presence of adrenoleukodystrophy and adrenomyeloneuropathy should be excluded in case of accompanying neurologic symptoms.

Table 3. Causes of CAI

Tumors
  Adenomas
  Cysts
  Craniopharyngiomas
  Ependymomas
  Meningiomas
  Carcinomas

Surgery or irradiation
Infections

Infiltrative processes
  Lymphocytic hypophysitis
  Hemochromatosis
  Sarcoidosis
  Histiocytosis X
  Wegener's granulomatosis

Pituitary apoplexy
Sheehan's syndrome
Drugs   Antipsychotics

Genetic disorders
  Transcription factors involved in pituitary development (obesity, hyperphagia)
  Congenital pro-opiomelanocortin deficiency
  Prader-Willi syndrome (hypotonia, obesity, mental retardation, hypogonadism)

Trauma
Isolated CRH deficiency

Isolated ACTH deficiency
  Autoimmune
  Triple H syndrome (HPA, hair follicle, hippocampus)
  Mutation prohormone convertase 1 (ACTH deficiency, impairment of memory and alopecia areata)
  DAVID complex (ACTH deficiency and common variable immunodeficiency)

Central Adrenal Insufficiency

Any disease, operation or trauma that affects the hypothalamus or pituitary gland can lead to CAI (table 3). Due to destruction of pituitary tissue, the secretion of other pituitary hormones can be decreased as well, leading to (pan)hypopituitarism. Isolated ACTH deficiency or ACTH deficiency due to genetic pituitary abnormalities are rare. Pituitary MRI should always be performed in order to exclude a tumor or other mass lesion.

Glucocorticoid-Induced Adrenal Insufficiency
Suppression of the HPA axis as a result of treatment with chronic high-dose glucocorticoids is by far the most common cause of AI. However, the true prevalence is not known. Low-dose glucocorticoids can also lead to AI if their metabolism is reduced by drug interactions, for example when inhalation or dermal glucocorticoids and ritonavir are given simultaneously. Glucocorticoids can be taken via various routes, all of which should be considered. Treatment with inhalation and transdermal glucocorticoids as well as glucocorticoid injections are frequently unrecognized causes of glucocorticoid-induced AI. Additionally, glucocorticoids can be present in creams or 'over the counter' preparations. A thorough history regarding supplements, medications and skin care products should be obtained in every patient suspected of having AI. The type of glucocorticoid, route of administration, dose frequency, duration of glucocorticoid therapy and the (cumulative) glucocorticoid dose are related to the risk of HPA axis suppression. Probably, individual sensitivity to glucocorticoids can also play a role. This is hard to predict for the individual patient. The diagnosis of glucocorticoid-induced AI is very difficult. Some commonly used glucocorticoid preparations, especially prednisolone, cortisone, prednisone and to a lesser extent fludrocortisone and methylprednisolone, can potentially cross-react in the cortisol assay, given falsely high cortisol values. Cross-reactivity of dexamethasone, triamcinolone, budesonide and inhalation corticosteroids such as betamethasone, fluticasone and beclomethasone (<1 μg/ml) are unlikely [21]. The only way to get a clear picture of AI is to slowly taper glucocorticoid dosage to less than physiological doses and measure morning cortisol before glucocorticoid ingestion. In addition, dose reduction may allow gradual recovery of the HPA axis when it has been suppressed. This is only possible if the underlying disease, for which the glucocorticoids were given, is in remission. If the glucocorticoid dosage is being tapered to below physiologic replacement, signs and symptoms of AI can occur. These patients should be instructed to double or triple the dose if they suffer from illness or injury. Recovery of the HPA axis from glucocorticoid-induced suppression can take a very long time. If glucocorticoid dosage has been tapered or discontinued, hypocortisolism can be evaluated by measuring morning plasma cortisol, and in case of cortisol values between 100 and 500 nmol/l by performing an ACTH test.

Conclusions

The diagnostic evaluation of AI can be challenging, but by following the three proposed steps it will be straightforward and will lead to a correct diagnosis in most cases, provided that the pitfalls described are taken into account. This method is a fast and reliable diagnostic approach that will help to start treating this potentially life-threatening disease as soon as possible, and avoids unnecessary chronic glucocorticoid replacement with its well-known imperfections and complications in the long run.

References

1 Bleicken B, Hahner S, Ventz M, Quinkler M: Delayed diagnosis of adrenal insufficiency is common: a cross-sectional study in 216 patients. Am J Med Sci 2010;339:525–531.

2 Klose M, Lange M, Rasmussen AK, Skakkebaek NE, Hilsted L, Haug E, Andersen M, Feldt-Rasmussen U: Factors influencing the adrenocorticotropin test: role of contemporary cortisol assays, body composition, and oral contraceptive agents. J Clin Endocrinol Metab 2007;92:1326–1333.

3 Bolland MJ, Chiu WW, Davidson JS, Croxson MS: Heterophile antibodies may cause falsely lowered serum cortisol values. J Endocrinol Invest 2005;28: 643–645.

4 Inder WJ, Dimeski G, Russell A: Measurement of salivary cortisol in 2012 – laboratory techniques and clinical indications. Clin Endocrinol (Oxf) 2012;77: 645–651.

5 Gow R, Koren G, Rieder M, Van Uum S: Hair cortisol content in patients with adrenal insufficiency on hydrocortisone replacement therapy. Clin Endocrinol (Oxf) 2011;74:687–693.

6 Courtney CH, McAllister AS, Bell PM, McCance DR, Leslie H, Sheridan B, Atkinson AB: Low- and standard-dose corticotropin and insulin hypoglycemia testing in the assessment of hypothalamic-pituitary-adrenal function after pituitary surgery. J Clin Endocrinol Metab 2004;89:1712–1717.

7 Nye EJ, Grice JE, Hockings GI, Strakosch CR, Crosbie GV, Walters MM, Jackson RV: Comparison of adrenocorticotropin (ACTH) stimulation tests and insulin hypoglycemia in normal humans: low dose, standard high dose, and 8-hour ACTH-(1–24) infusion tests. J Clin Endocrinol Metab 1999;84:3648–3655.

8 Tordjman K, Jaffe A, Grazas N, Apter C, Stern N: The role of the low dose (1 microgram) adrenocorticotropin test in the evaluation of patients with pituitary diseases. J Clin Endocrinol Metab 1995;80: 1301–1305.

9 Abdu TA, Elhadd TA, Neary R, Clayton RN: Comparison of the low dose short synacthen test (1 microg), the conventional dose short synacthen test (250 microg), and the insulin tolerance test for assessment of the hypothalamo-pituitary-adrenal axis in patients with pituitary disease. J Clin Endocrinol Metab 1999;84:838–843.

10 Zarković M, Ćirić J, Stojanović M, Penezić Z, Trbojević B, Drezgić M, Nesovic M: Optimizing the diagnostic criteria for standard (250-microg) and low dose (1-microg) adrenocorticotropin tests in the assessment of adrenal function. J Clin Endocrinol Metab 1999;84:3170–3173.

11 Dorin RI, Qualls CR, Crapo LM: Diagnosis of adrenal insufficiency. Ann Intern Med 2003;139:194–204.

12 Nasrallah MP, Arafah BM: The value of dehydroepiandrosterone sulfate measurements in the assessment of adrenal function. J Clin Endocrinol Metab 2003;88:5293–5298.

13 Aimaretti G, Baffoni C, Di Vito L, Grottoli S, Gaia D, Gasco V, Giordano R, Zadik Z, Camanni F, Ghigo E, Arvat E: Hypopituitaric patients with corticotropin insufficiency show marked impairment of the cortisol response to ACTH (1–24) independently of the duration of the disease. J Endocrinol Invest 2003;26: 49–55.

14 Sayyed Kassem L, El Sibai K, Chaiban J, Abdelmannan D, Arafah BM: Measurements of serum DHEA and DHEA sulphate levels improve the accuracy of the low-dose cosyntropin test in the diagnosis of central adrenal insufficiency. J Clin Endocrinol Metab 2012;97:3655–3662.

15 Courtney CH, McAllister AS, McCance DR, Hadden DR, Leslie H, Sheridan B, Atkinson AB: The insulin hypoglycaemia and overnight metyrapone tests in the assessment of the hypothalamic-pituitary-adrenal axis following pituitary surgery. Clin Endocrinol (Oxf) 2000;53:309–312.

16 Berneis K, Staub JJ, Gessler A, Meier C, Girard J, Müller B: Combined stimulation of adrenocorticotropin and compound-S by single dose metyrapone test as an outpatient procedure to assess hypothalamic-pituitary-adrenal function. J Clin Endocrinol Metab 2002;87:5470–5475.

17 Agha A, Rogers B, Sherlock M, O'Kelly P, Tormey W, Phillips J, Thompson CJ: Anterior pituitary dysfunction in survivors of traumatic brain injury. J Clin Endocrinol Metab 2004;89:4929–4936.

18 Berg C, Meinel T, Lahner H, Yuece A, Mann K, Petersenn S: Diagnostic utility of the glucagon stimulation test in comparison to the insulin tolerance test in patients following pituitary surgery. Eur J Endocrinol 2010;162:477–482.

19 Cegla J, Jones B, Seyani L, Papadoulou D, Wynne K, Martin NM, Meeran K, Chapman R, Donaldson M, Goldstone AP, Tan T: Comparison of the overnight metyrapone and glucagon stimulation tests in the assessment of secondary hypoadrenalism. Clin Endocrinol (Oxf) 2013;78:738–742.

20 Schulte HM, Chrousos GP, Avgerinos P, Oldfield EH, Gold PW, Cutler GB Jr, Loriaux DL: The corticotropin-releasing hormone stimulation test: a possible aid in the evaluation of patients with adrenal insufficiency. J Clin Endocrinol Metab 1984;58: 1064–1067.

21 Stokes F, Bailey L, Ganguli A, Davison A: Assessment of endogenous, oral and inhaled steroid cross-reactivity in the Roche cortisol immunoassay. Ann Clin Biochem 2013;51:503–506.
22 Zelissen PMJ: Addison Patients in the Netherlands: Medical Report of the Survey. The Hague, Dutch Addison Society, 1994.
23 Dunlop D: Eighty-six cases of Addison's disease. Br Med J 1963;2:887–891.
24 Irvine WJ, Barnes EW: Adrenocortical insufficiency. Clin Endocrinol Metab 1972;1:549–594.
25 Nerup J: Addison's disease – clinical studies. A report of 108 cases. Acta Endocrinol (Copenh) 1974; 76:127–141.
26 Rosa de G, Corsello SM, Cecchini L, Della Casa S, Testa A: A clinical study of Addison's disease. Exp Clin Endocrinol 1987;90:232–242.
27 Bleicken B, Hahner S, Ventz M, Quinkler M: Delayed diagnosis of adrenal insufficiency is common: a cross-sectional study in 216 patients. Am J Med Sci 2010;339:525–531.
28 Charmandari E, Nicolaides NC, Chrousos GP: Adrenal insufficiency. Lancet 2014;383:2152–2156.
29 Ross IL, Levitt NS: Addison's disease symptoms – a cross sectional study in urban South Africa. PLoS One 2013;8:e53526.
30 Quinkler M, Beuschlein F, Hahner S, Meyer G, Schöfl C, Stalla GK: Adrenal cortical insufficiency – a life threatening illness with multiple etiologies. Dtsch Arztebl Int 2013;110:882–888.

Prof. Lisanne C.C.J. Smans
Section of Endocrinology, Department of Internal Medicine
Utrecht University Medical Center
NL–3508 Utrecht (The Netherlands)
E-Mail L.C.C.J.Smans@umcutrecht.nl

Arvat E, Falorni A (eds): Cortisol Excess and Insufficiency.
Front Horm Res. Basel, Karger, 2016, vol 46, pp 159–170 (DOI: 10.1159/000443915)

Secondary Adrenal Insufficiency: Where Is It Hidden and What Does It Look Like?

Federica Guaraldi[a] · Ioannis Karamouzis[a] · Rita Berardelli[b] · Valentina D'Angelo[b] · Alessia Rampino[c] · Clizia Zichi[b] · Ezio Ghigo[a] · Roberta Giordano[c]

[a]Division of Endocrinology, Diabetes and Metabolism, Department of Medical Science, [b]Division of Oncological Endocrinology, Department of Medical Science, and [c]Department of Clinical and Biological Science, University of Turin, Turin, Italy

Abstract

Adrenal failure secondary to hypothalamic-pituitary disease is a common although underestimated and underdiagnosed condition, with serious consequences. Corticotropin deficiency can be isolated or more frequently occur in association with other pituitary hormones deficiencies. The most frequent endogenous cause of secondary adrenal insufficiency (SAI) is a tumor of the hypothalamic-pituitary region, usually associated with panhypopituitarism secondary to tumor growth or to its treatment with surgery or irradiation. Less commonly, SAI is due to nontumoral disorders including infiltrative lesions, infective processes, vascular alterations, traumatic brain injury, empty sella or genetic disorders. Finally, long-term administration of exogenous glucocorticoids can determine secondary and/or tertiary hypoadrenalism acting at the hypothalamic level and leading to prolonged suppression of the hypothalamic-pituitary-adrenal axis. It is essential to perform validated diagnostic procedures in order to promptly diagnose hypoadrenalism so as to prevent an adrenal crisis. At the same time, diagnosis is complex as no single test has sufficient sensitivity to identify all patients with SAI. Therefore, clinical judgment and follow-up are crucial for the assessment of corticotropin deficiency. Patients with persisting suggestive symptoms and/or a clinical history of higher risk for adrenal insufficiency deserve careful subsequent reassessments.

Secondary adrenal insufficiency (SAI) may result from any disease that involves the hypothalamic-pituitary unit and be secondary to a defect in corticotropin [adrenocorticotropic hormone (ACTH)] release or the lack of adrenal gland responsiveness to ACTH. Corticotropin deficiency can be isolated or occur in association with other pituitary hormone defects [1].

F. Guaraldi and I. Karamouzis contributed equally to this work.

There is generally a specific sequential failure of pituitary hormones that starts with growth hormone (GH) and is followed by gonadotropins (FSH and LH) and, finally, by thyrotropin-stimulating hormone (TSH) and ACTH [1]. The fact that ACTH is usually the last hormone to be lost may teleologically reflect its need for survival. However, in some patients with pituitary disorders (i.e. lymphocytic hypophysitis or genetic defects), ACTH deficiency can occur as a first and/or isolated hormone deficiency [1].

SAI is more common than primary adrenal deficiency, with an estimated prevalence of 150–280 cases per million, a predominance in women and a peak of age at diagnosis in the sixth decade [1].

Where Is It Hidden?

All hypothalamic-pituitary disorders can potentially lead to SAI, which can be isolated or occur in the context of multiple hormone deficiency, up to panhypopituitarism if both the anterior and posterior pituitaries are involved [1]. Tumors of the hypothalamic-pituitary region are the most frequent cause of endogenous SAI [1].

Isolated ACTH deficiency is rare and has been described in association with a great variety of conditions. An underlying immunological dysregulation has been hypothesized on the basis of the frequent association with extrapituitary autoimmune disorders and the identification of autoantibodies directed against the hypothalamus and pituitary, although the etiology remains to be elucidated [2].

Pituitary Tumors

Pituitary adenomas account for about 10% of all intracranial tumors with a peak incidence between 30 and 60 years of age (females are usually younger at diagnosis than men, with the majority of the cases presenting in women between 20 and 45 years of age and in men between 35 and 60 years of age) [3]. Loss of pituitary function represents one of their major clinical manifestations, particularly in patients with large tumors. A high incidence of SAI has been reported in large series of patients with nonfunctioning pituitary adenomas [4]. In prolactinomas – the most prevalent pituitary adenomas (45–66% of the cases; prevalence of 62 cases/100,000 individuals) – SAI is more frequent in patients with macro- than in patients with microadenomas, with an overall prevalence of 14–23% [5]. About 30% of the patients with GH-producing adenomas present insufficiency of at least one pituitary axis, with SAI reported in 12–35% of them [6]. GH secretion appears to be a risk factor for the development of SAI per se, independently from adenoma size [6].

Transsphenoidal surgery (TSS), the treatment of choice in patients with symptomatic nonfunctioning pituitary macroadenomas and functioning adenomas, is another common cause of SAI. Particularly, data from the few available studies demonstrate that hypothalamic-pituitary-adrenal (HPA) axis function usually does not recover after surgery and affects 13–60% of the patients (vs. 19–62% preoperatively), depending both on the number of patients included in the study and the time of hormonal assessment [7]. The prevalence of new-onset SAI after successful TSS of a GH-producing pituitary adenoma appears to largely depend on the timing of evaluation of HPA axis function. Indeed, the incidence rates 1 year after surgery and in the long term are comparable and lower than the incidence in the immediate postoperative period (about 14%) [8]. Retrospective data from cohorts of patients with ACTH-secreting adenomas show a prevalence of postoperative SAI of about 25–30% during remission, which appears to be secondary to the presurgical functional suppression of ACTH-producing cells induced by hypercortisolism [1, 9].

Several factors have been demonstrated in the etiopathogenesis of postsurgical SAI in patients with ACTH-secreting adenomas, including hypothalamic corticotropin-releasing factor suppression, corticotroph resistance to corticotropin-releasing factor and lower ACTH potency in the adrenal gland [1]. The time for HPA axis recovery is largely variable and appears to depend on individual cortisol sensitivity, disease severity and duration, together with study population characteristics, surgical outcomes, type and doses of glucocorticoid (GC) replacement therapy, and diagnostic tests [1]. It is noticeable that the rate of the SAI is inversely proportional to the number of surgical interventions needed for disease cure [9].

SAI can also be secondary to radiotherapy (RT), which plays an integral role in the management of pituitary adenomas, especially in cases with residual or recurrent disease after TSS [10, 11]. Fractionated stereotactic conformal RT, stereotactic radiosurgery (SRS), Gamma Knife and linear accelerator have been recently developed as more accurate techniques allowing more precise tumor localization and irradiation, with a consequent reduction of irradiation in the surrounding tissues and long-term toxicity. The risk of pituitary function defect is both a dose- and time-dependent phenomenon. Impairment of HPA axis function is reported in up to 60% of patients after 10 years from pituitary fractionated irradiation with doses of 30–50 Gy [11]. Studies in patients with acromegaly treated with conventional RT (mean dose of about 50 Gy) after unsuccessful pituitary surgery show a 35% prevalence of SAI with a mean onset at 6.5 years after treatment. SRS (mean dose of about 25 Gy) is associated with a drastic reduction in SAI occurrence (up to 14% after 2–4 years) [11]. Furthermore, after a second Gamma Knife irradiation, new-onset ACTH deficiency occurs with the same prevalence as the first time [11]. Post-RT SAI occurs less frequently in nonfunctioning pituitary adenomas treated with similar doses of RT (about 15% of the cases), especially in patients treated with SRS [11]. Post-RT data for Cushing's disease recurrence after TSS show a very low corticotroph deficiency (about 3%) during a 3.5-year biochemical remission period, while its rate is significantly higher when RT is the first-line treatment (15% of the cases with conventional RT, 12% with SRS) [11]. SRS was associated with an approximate 11% prevalence of SAI in patients with Cushing's disease during a 3.5-year disease-free period [11].

RT is rarely required in prolactinomas, and is mainly used as a third-line treatment. A low incidence of SAI (0–14%) has been reported in patients who underwent RT after medical therapy failure, usually occurring at least 3 years after treatment [11]. Finally, the HPA axis appears to be relatively radioresistant in patients irradiated for nonpituitary disorders, as clinically apparent ACTH deficiency is uncommon (around 3%) in those receiving total radiation doses <50 Gy, while the incidence dramatically increases (27–35%) after intensive irradiation (50–70 Gy) [11].

Extrapituitary Tumors

SAI – isolated or associated to other pituitary deficiencies – is a well-known complication of nonadenomatous pituitary tumors (i.e. craniopharyngiomas, Rathke's cleft cysts and meningiomas), with variable pre- and postoperative prevalence depending also on the type of tumor.

Patients with craniopharyngioma present the highest risk, with SAI present in 24–36% of the cases at diagnosis and in up to 90% after TSS [1]. Improvements in the HPA axis after craniopharyngioma removal are relatively uncommon (resolution rate: 0–22%) [12].

Surgery is the mainstay of treatment for symptomatic Rathke's cleft cysts, with transsphenoidal resection the preferred approach. Preoperative loss of adrenal function ranges from 6 to 46%. Postoperative resolution or improvement of adrenal insufficiency occurs frequently; permanent hypocortisolism may result while attempting to resect a cyst's capsule, which can be quite adherent to the pituitary lobes [12].

Very few studies have investigated HPA axis function in patients with parasellar meningiomas. Overall, preoperative loss of corticotroph function ranges from 6 to 15%; postoperatively, onset of hypocortisolism is relatively uncommon, while up to 30% of preexisting cases improve [12].

Nontumoral Disorders

According to a recent multicenter study performed in more than 700 patients with hypopituitarism [13], nontumoral diseases, traditionally considered rare causes of hypopituitarism, account for the majority of cases (49.2%), especially in women (57.5%), with SAI the third most frequent defect after gonadotropic and thyreotropic defects. Increased prevalence can be largely attributed to the widespread use of head magnetic resonance imaging (MRI) and computed tomography (CT) imaging and improved clinician awareness.

Long-term administration of exogenous GC represents a very common cause of secondary and/or tertiary hypoadrenalism, associated with prolonged suppression of the HPA axis starting at the hypothalamic level [1].

Infiltrative Lesions

Infiltrative lesions can be classified into primary and secondary hypophysitis (i.e. sarcoidosis, Langerhans' cell histiocytosis or histiocytosis X, Wegener's granulomatosis, hemochromatosis, Takayasu's disease, and Cohan's syndrome) depending on the intra- or extrapituitary origin of the disease, respectively [14, 15].

Lymphocytic hypophysitis is the most common form of primary disease (incidence: 1 case/9 million persons/year; less than 400 reported cases). According to the affected pituitary portion, we can distinguish adenohypophysitis, which is more common in younger women (F:M ratio 6:1) especially during or shortly after pregnancy, and infundibolo-neurohypophysitis and panhypophysitis, which tend to occur in older subjects and have a less remarkable predilection for females [14, 15].

Patients may be pauci- or asymptomatic for a long period of time and then manifest with overt neurological (i.e. headache, impaired vision and nausea) and systemic symptoms secondary to pituitary insufficiency. SAI is the most common (about 40% of the cases) and earliest defect in adeno- and panhypophysitis, followed by hyperprolactinemia (30%), hypothyroidism (20%), hypogonadism (15%) and GH deficiency (10%) [14]. Diabetes insipidus is almost invariably present in neuro- and panhypopituitarism, but only in about 20% of the patients with adenohypophysitis, who in turn typically present with visual disturbances and anterior pituitary dysfunction [14]. The disease typically progresses from inflammation to fibrosis, with subsequent atrophy of pituitary and empty sella. Spontaneous remission is rare [14].

The pathogenic and diagnostic role of antipituitary and antihypothalamic antibodies remains debated [14, 16]. Moreover, these antibodies are poorly specific, as they have been detected in many extrapituitary autoimmune and nonautoimmune disorders, and their prevalence is also highly variable, depending on the study and the diagnostic technique applied [14, 16].

Secondary hypophysitis typically presents with multiple hormone deficiency, irreversible in most of the cases and sometimes associated with hyperprolactinemia and neurological symptoms, while isolated ACTH deficiency is uncommon [15].

Infective Processes

Pituitary infections are very rare but potentially life-threatening disorders, commonly affecting people from developing countries or immunocompromised patients. Although microorganisms of all species (i.e. bacteria, viruses, parasites and fungi) can spread to the pituitary, tuberculous hypophysitis, pyogenic abscess, aspergillosis and coccidioidomycosis are the most common infections [15].

Typical presentation includes neurological (i.e. headache, visual and cognitive disturbances) and endocrinological symptoms due to concomitant panhypopituitarism, and more rarely hyperprolactinemia. Isolated ACTH deficiency is uncommon. Acute adrenal insufficiency can be precipitated by antitubercular drugs. Other diseases' pathognomonic signs and symptoms or evidence of systemic infection can (but not invariably) be present [15]. Diagnosis is suggested by MRI features, but can be confirmed only by surgical exploration or histological exam on surgical biopsy [15].

Vascular Alterations

Pituitary apoplexy is caused by a sudden increase in pituitary size secondary to hemorrhagic infarction, typically occurring in patients with pituitary macroadenomas or in the postpartum period (Sheehan's syndrome). Increased vulnerability to ischemia secondary to estrogen-induced pituitary enlargement and hypervascularization, small sella size, disseminated intravascular coagulopathy and autoimmunity have been hypothesized in the pathogenesis of Sheehan's syndrome [1, 14].

GH deficiency is the most common alteration affecting almost all patients, and is associated with TSH, gonadotropin, prolactin and ACTH deficiency in more than 80% of the cases, with a positive correlation between antipituitary and hypothalamic antibodies and the number of affected pituitary axes [1, 14, 16].

Subarachnoid hemorrhage typically affects patients aged 40–60 years, with an estimated yearly incidence of 6/100,000. Pituitary dysfunction is reported in 0–68% of the patients, varying according to the evaluation timing and diagnostic criteria [17]. Delayed-onset hypogonadism and SAI (0–33% of the cases) are typical. The etiology is complex and includes increased intracranial pressure, pituitary ischemia secondary to arterial vasospasm or microinfarctions, venous stasis, surgical procedures, neuroinflammatory responses, autoimmunity, and genetic predisposition [17].

Very rarely, ACTH deficiency has been reported in association with intracranial aneurism, sickle cell anemia [1] and hemorrhagic fever with renal syndrome (a severe systemic infection presenting with hypovolemic shock and renal failure caused by hantavirus) [18].

Traumatic Brain Injury

In the last decade, pituitary insufficiency has been increasingly reported in patients with traumatic brain injury (TBI). For this reason, several authoritative authors have outlined the importance of defining the burden of pituitary disorders in TBI patients, and of criteria for the early identification of high-risk patients deserving systematic screening [19].

Reported prevalence of TBI-induced hypopituitarism differs considerably among reported studies ranging from 5 to 90%, similarly to the prevalence of SAI ranging from 5 to 13%. This variability could be attributed to the different timing of evaluation, severity of the trauma, diagnostic criteria, methods and assays to test endocrine function [19].

Transient hypopituitarism has been almost exclusively reported in the first 6 months after TBI. Therefore, an early assessment of pituitary function after the event could lead to overestimate the prevalence of pituitary dysfunction in these patients, especially if patients with a more severe trauma are included. Indeed, the chance to develop hypopituitarism is directly related to the severity of trauma [19].

Empty Sella

Empty sella is defined as the herniation of the subarachnoid space within the sella turcica associated with elongated pituitary stalk and flattened pituitary. It can be partial (<50% of the sella is filled with cerebrospinal fluid) or total. According to the etiology, it can be classified into: *primary*, of unknown origin, and *secondary*, resulting from spontaneous or treatment-induced pituitary adenoma shrinkage, pituitary apoplexy

Table 1. Genetic causes of SAI

Gene	Chromosome	Inheritance mode	Endocrinological manifestation in addition to adrenal insufficiency	MRI findings	Associated malformations
Transcription factors					
HESX homeobox 1	3p21	Recessive	Panhypopituitarism, short stature, delayed puberty	Hypoplastic/hyperplastic anterior pituitary	Cognitive changes, septo-optic dysplasia
Orthodentical (OTX) homeobox 2	1q23	Dominant/ negative	Panhypopituitarism	Hypoplastic anterior pituitary, ectopic posterior pituitary	Eye malformations
LIM homeobox 4	1q25	Dominant	Panhypopituitarism	Hypoplastic anterior pituitary, ectopic posterior pituitary	–
PROP paired-like homeobox 1	3p11	Recessive	Panhypopituitarism	Normal, hypoplastic, hyperplastic or cystic anterior pituitary	–
POMC					Severe obesity, hyperphagia, red hair pigmentation
Sex-determining region Y (SOX-3)	Xq27	X-linked recessive	Panhypopituitarism	Hypoplasia anterior pituitary, infundibular hypoplasia, ectopic posterior pituitary; severe hypoglycemia and jaundice (neonates with T-box mutations)	Mental retardation
Prader-Willi syndrome					
Deletion of the paternal copies of the small nuclear riboprotein polypeptide N, NDN gene and clusters of snoRNAs	15q11-13	Deletion or silencing of genes in imprinting center	Hypogonadism		Hypotonia, obesity, mental retardation

or hypophysitis. In the majority of the cases, it is asymptomatic and incidentally discovered during head CT or MRI; less frequently, patients present with neurological, visual or endocrinological signs secondary to liquor-induced compression on the pituitary gland and stalk and nearby structures. Some degrees of pituitary deficiency – typically GH and less frequently other hormones – have been reported in 8–60% of the cases, often in association with hyperprolactinemia [20].

Genetic Disorders

Very rarely, SAI can be secondary to mutations of genes involved in pituitary development, POMC (proopiomelanocortin) synthesis and processing, and sex-determining region Y, or develop in the context of Prader-Willi syndrome [1]. Diagnosis is usually performed during childhood; in the majority of the cases, patients present with multiple pituitary hormone deficiencies (except for POMC mutations), sometimes associated with other physical or cognitive disorders (table 1) [1].

Table 2. Biochemical diagnosis of SAI

Test	Procedure	High probability of adrenal insufficiency	Adrenal insufficiency excluded
Early morning cortisol	Serum cortisol (07.00–09.00 h)	<80–110 nmol/l (30–50 μg/l)	>400-500 nmol/l (150–180 μg/l)
ITT	Serum glucose and cortisol every 30 min for 90 min after insulin i.v. (0.1–0.15 U/kg)	Peak cortisol <500 nmol/l (180 μg/l)	Peak cortisol >500–550 nmol/l (200 μg/l)
MET	Serum 11-DOC and ACTH at 08.00 h after MET 30 mg/kg p.o. at 23.00 h the night before	11-DOC <200 nmol/l (7–9 μg/dl) and/or ACTH <16.5-44 pmol/l (75–200 pg/ml)	11-DOC >200–260 nmol/l (7–9 μg/dl) and/or ACTH >16.5–44 pmol/l (75–200 pg/ml)
CRH	Serum cortisol and plasma ACTH at 0, every 15 min to 1 h and every 30 min to 2 h after CRH i.v. (1 μg/kg, up to a maximum of 100 μg)	Peak ACTH >33 pmol/l (100 pg/ml); peak cortisol >500–550 nmol/l (180–200 μg/l)	Peak ACTH >33 pmol/l (100 pg/ml); peak cortisol >500–550 nmol/l (180–200 μg/l)
ACTH test	Serum cortisol at 0 and 30 or 60 min after ACTH 1–24 i.v.	Peak cortisol <500 nmol/l (180 μg/l)	Peak cortisol >500 nmol/l (180 μg/l)

Exogenous Glucocorticoid Administration

Chronic GC administration inhibits HPA axis function at the hypothalamic-pituitary level by negative feedback, which can induce adrenal insufficiency and, eventually, adrenal atrophy [1, 21, 22]. Because of the large diffusion of GC treatments, they represent one of the most frequent causes of SAI [1, 21, 22].

HPA suppression has been traditionally reported to occur after systemic administration of 20 mg of prednisone (or equivalent dose of other steroids) per day for more than 3 weeks. Indeed, HPA axis suppression is uncommon after sudden cessation of therapy in patients treated with any dose of steroids for shorter periods, although some authors have demonstrated that patients receiving 20–30 mg/day of prednisone (or equivalent dose of other steroids) for more than 5 days are at risk for SAI [23]. Inhaled and topical GC can also cause adrenal suppression in a dose-dependent fashion [1].

According to a recent meta-analysis [22], 1,190 out of the 3,753 (31%) patients treated with GC from the included studies were diagnosed with adrenal insufficiency, with the risk associated with the route of administration (oral higher than inhalation, topical and nasal), dose and duration of treatment. Because of the considerable inter-individual variability in response to GC, there are no absolute cutoff values for type of GC, dose, route of administration or duration of treatment [1]. Moreover, symptoms are often absent or nonspecific and, although not frequent, the coadministration of drugs that affect GC metabolism (i.e. CYP3A4 inhibitors and GC receptor agonists) has to be considered [1]. For all these reasons, SAI cannot be safely excluded a priori in any patient treated with GC [1, 22]. Finally, although prevalence of adrenal insufficiency after GC discontinuation declines over time, a considerable number of patients were still affected after 6 months [1, 22].

How Does It Look?

Clinical Presentation
Differently from primary adrenal insufficiency, clinical manifestations of SAI result only from GC deficiency, as aldosterone and adrenal androgens secretion is preserved. Moreover, SAI rarely manifests with an acute adrenal crisis, although acute presentation can be precipitated by stress like surgery, trauma or infection [24].

At the same time, patients can present with some signs (i.e. hyponatremia and volume expansion) typical of primary adrenal insufficiency caused by the so-called 'inappropriate increase in arginine vasopressin secretion' [1]. Symptoms and signs secondary to deficiency of other anterior pituitary hormones as well as neurological signs can coexist.

Endocrinological Evaluation (table 2)
Diagnosis of SAI is often delayed because of unspecific symptoms and diagnostic issues [25]. Indeed, despite more than 50 years of clinical research, the choice of the most appropriate test for the assessment of HPA axis alterations in patients with hypothalamus-pituitary disorders remains largely debated [1].

Currently available tests measure *total cortisol* concentration and not the biologically active free cortisol, leading to false-normal results in the presence of high concentrations of cortisol-binding globulin (e.g. women receiving oral estrogens or in pregnancy), and falsely hypocortisolism in the presence of low cortisol-binding globulin (e.g. patients with cirrhosis) [1]. *Salivary cortisol* concentration might be a useful alternative, although the normal cutoff is not fully validated [1].

On the contrary, urinary free cortisol concentrations are not helpful for diagnosis of adrenal insufficiency mainly because the lower reference range levels are not contributory; the same is true for measurement of basal plasma ACTH concentration, which is required only for differential diagnosis with primary forms [1].

A morning serum cortisol concentration below 80–110 nmol/l (30–50 μg/l; blood drawing between 7.00 h and 9.00 h) is strongly suggestive of adrenal insufficiency, whereas values more than 400–500 nmol/l (150–180 μg/l) are consistent with an intact HPA axis. For values between 80–110 and 400–500 nmol/l, adrenal insufficiency cannot be excluded and dynamic tests are required [1].

The insulin tolerance test has been conventionally used as the reference gold standard test for the diagnosis of ACTH insufficiency, as it examines the integrity of the whole HPA axis by stimulating corticotropin-releasing hormone (CRH), ACTH and, subsequently, cortisol release [1]. Insulin (0.10–0.15 U/kg) is given to induce hypoglycemia (<2.2 mmol/l), and cortisol concentrations are measured every 30 min for at least 90 min; a peak serum cortisol >500–550 nmol/l (180–200 μg/l) is considered a normal response [1]. However, this test is labor-intensive, presents several limitations and is contraindicated in patients with cardiovascular and cerebrovascular disease or who have a history of seizures [26]. Therefore, alternative tests have been proposed over the years, namely the overnight metyrapone, CRH and ACTH stimulation tests.

The overnight metyrapone test has so far been considered a convenient and sensitive method, with a good correlation with the insulin tolerance test [26]. The metyrapone test (30 mg/kg administered orally with a snack at midnight) inhibits adrenal 11β-hydroxylase and the conversion of 11-deoxycortisol (11-DOC) to cortisol. The diagnostic accuracy of this test has been shown to depend on the ACTH and/or 11-DOC cutoff used [27]. Shortcomings of the metyrapone test are the limited availability of reliable 11-DOC assays and the fact that the drug is not widely available due to local restrictions [27].

The CRH test is used to differentiate secondary from tertiary adrenal insufficiency. It entails intravenous administration of CRH (dose of 1 μg/kg, up to a maximum of 100 μg) and measurement of serum cortisol and plasma ACTH concentrations at baseline, every 15 min to 1 h, then every 30 min up to 2 h after stimulation. Patients with SAI present a little or no ACTH response, whereas response is exaggerated in patients with tertiary forms. However, this test is not of great diagnostic help because individual responses to exogenous CRH are highly variable, while cutoffs and ranges of normal reference values have not been univocally defined yet [28].

The ACTH test at the standard dose of 250 μg has been used over the years as an alternative tool to diagnose SAI, providing an indirect assessment of the integrity of corticotroph function in chronic ACTH deficiency [29]. It is based on stimulation of the adrenal glands by pharmacological doses of exogenous ACTH 1–24 peptide, administered intravenously or intramuscularly. Serum cortisol levels are measured at baseline and at 30 and 60 min after stimulation. A peak cortisol concentration above 500 nmol/l (180 μg/l) is generally considered a normal response, although different cutoffs have been proposed [29].

Although the ACTH test is considered to be safe, reliable and accurate, it has been suggested that the dose of 250 μg is largely supraphysiological, so it would elicit very high circulating ACTH levels and induce many false-normal responses, especially in patients with mild or recent-onset SAI [28]. Therefore, several studies have explored the use of low-dose (1.0 μg) ACTH, in the attempt to increase ACTH test sensitivity, with controversial results. In fact, the 1.0-μg ACTH test has been indicated as a more useful tool for the evaluation of SAI by some authors, while others have shown that even this test lacks diagnostic sensitivity and does not give real advantages in comparison with the standard dose test [29]. Moreover, technical issues – caused by the need to dilute the commercially available dose ampule of 250 μg of ACTH 1–24 to 1 μg, and the potential binding of such a small hormone amount to the surface of injection devices – can impair test accuracy [30].

For all the abovementioned reasons, it has to be emphasized that no single test is able to correctly identify all patients with SAI: mild SAI can be missed, while even healthy individuals might show abnormal values. Therefore, clinical judgment remains important and follow-up is crucial for assessment of ACTH deficiency. Patients with persisting suggestive symptoms or risk factors for adrenal insufficiency deserve careful, sometimes subsequent, reassessment [31].

Imaging

Head MRI should be performed to exclude tumors and other lesions of the sellar and parasellar region once SAI has been confirmed [1–4]. Typical MRI features of primary hypophysitis include symmetrical pituitary enlargement with homogeneous contrast enhancement, a parasellar dark signal on T2-weighted sections, a thickened (rarely displaced) pituitary stalk and loss of posterior pituitary T1 hyperintensity when neurohypophysis is involved [32]. Diagnosis of secondary hypophysitis is suggested by MRI features, i.e. sellar mass associated with pituitary stalk's thickening and nodularity in tuberculous hypophysitis, and round cystic lesions with peripheral gadolinium enhancement in pituitary abscess [14, 32]. Traumatic damage can present with pituitary stalk deviation, associated with hemorrhage, infraction, or empty sella [32].

Conclusions

SAI is an underestimated and underdiagnosed condition, which can be isolated or occur in association with other pituitary hormone defects, that has potentially severe clinical consequences. Diagnosis is complex as no single hormonal evaluation is able to correctly identify all patients with this condition, and mild SAI can be missed. Therefore, clinical judgment and follow-up are crucial for the assessment of corticotropin deficiency, in order to avoid an adrenal crisis.

References

1 Crowley RK, Argese N, Tomlinson JW, Stewart PM: Central hypoadrenalism. J Clin Endocrinol Metab 2014;99:4027–4036

2 Hannon MJ, O'Halloran DJ: Isolated acquired ACTH deficiency and primary hypothyroidism: a short series and review. Pituitary 2011;14:358–361.

3 Davis JR, Farrell WE, Clayton RN: Pituitary tumours. Reproduction 2001;121:363–371.

4 Greenman Y, Stern N: Non-functioning pituitary adenomas. Best Pract Res Clin Endocrinol Metab 2009; 23:625–638.

5 Tirosh A, Benbassat C, Lifshitz A, Shimon I: Hypopituitarism patterns and prevalence among men with macroprolactinomas. Pituitary 2015;18:108–115.

6 Sherlock M, Reulen RC, Alonso AA, Ayuk J, Clayton RN, Sheppard MC, Hawkins MM, Bates AS, Stewart PM: ACTH deficiency, higher doses of hydrocortisone replacement, and radiotherapy are independent predictors of mortality in patients with acromegaly. J Clin Endocrinol Metab 2009;94:4216–4223.

7 Dekkers OM, Pereira AM, Romijn JA: Treatment and follow-up of clinically nonfunctioning pituitary macroadenomas. J Clin Endocrinol Metab 2008;93:3717–3726.

8 Burgers AM, Kokshoorn NE, Pereira AM, Roelfsema F, Smit JW, Biermasz NR, Romijn JA: Low incidence of adrenal insufficiency after transsphenoidal surgery in patients with acromegaly: a long-term follow-up study. J Clin Endocrinol Metab 2011;96:E1163–E1170.

9 Aranda G, Enseñat J, Mora M, Puig-Domingo M, Martínez de Osaba MJ, Casals G, Verger E, Ribalta MT, Hanzu FA, Halperin I: Long-term remission and recurrence rate in a cohort of Cushing's disease: the need for long-term follow-up. Pituitary 2015;18:142–149.

10 Darzy KH: Radiation-induced hypopituitarism after cancer therapy: who, how and when to test. Nat Clin Pract Endocrinol Metab 2009;5:88–99.

11 Fernandez A, Brada M, Zabuliene L, Karavitaki N, Wass JA: Radiation-induced hypopituitarism. Endocr Relat Cancer 2009;16:733–772.

12 Dusick JR, Fatemi N, Mattozo C, McArthur D, Cohan P, Wang C, Swerdloff RS, Kelly DF: Pituitary function after endonasal surgery for nonadenomatous parasellar tumors: Rathke's cleft cysts, craniopharyngiomas, and meningiomas. Surg Neurol 2008; 70:482–490.
13 Tanriverdi F, Dokmetas HS, Kebapci N, Kilicli F, Atmaca H, Yarman S, Ertorer ME, Erturk E, Bayram F, Tugrul A, Culha C, Cakir M, Mert M, Aydin H, Taskale H, Ersoz N, Canturk Z, Anaforoglu I, Ozkaya M, Oruk G, Hekimsoy Z, Kelestimur F, Erbas T: Etiology of hypopituitarism in tertiary care institutions in Turkish population: analysis of 773 patients from Pituitary Study Group database. Endocrine 2014;47: 198–205.
14 Caturegli P, Newschaffer C, Olivi A, Pomper MG, Burger PC, Rose NR: Autoimmune hypophysitis. Endocr Rev 2005;26:599–614.
15 Carpinteri R, Patelli I, Casanueva FF, Giustina A: Inflammatory and granulomatous expansive lesions of the pituitary. Best Pract Res Clin Endocrinol Metab 2009;23:639–650.
16 De Bellis A, Sinisi AA, Pane E, DelloIacovo A, Bellastella G, Di Scala G, Falorni A, Giavoli C, Gasco V, Giordano R, Ambrosio MR, Colao A, Bizzarro A, Bellastella A; Italian Hypophysitis Network Group: Involvement of hypothalamus autoimmunity in patients with autoimmune hypopituitarism: role of antibodies to hypothalamic cells. J Clin Endocrinol Metab 2012;97:3684–3690.
17 Karaca Z, Tanriverdi F, Dagli AT, Selcuklu A, Casanueva FF, Unluhizarci K, Kelestimur F: Three years prospective investigation of pituitary functions following subarachnoid haemorrhage. Pituitary 2013; 16:76–82.
18 Stojanovic M, Pekic S, Cvijovic G, Miljic D, Doknic M, Nikolic-Djurovic M, Micic D, Hrvacevic R, Nesic V, Popovic V: High risk of hypopituitarism in patients who recovered from hemorrhagic fever with renal syndrome. J Clin Endocrinol Metab 2008;93: 2722–2728.
19 Lauzier F, Turgeon AF, Boutin A, Shemilt M, Côté I, Lachance O, Archambault PM, Lamontagne F, Moore L, Bernard F, Gagnon C, Cook D: Clinical outcomes, predictors, and prevalence of anterior pituitary disorders following traumatic brain injury: a systematic review. Crit Care Med 2014;42:712–721.

Roberta Giordano, MD
Division of Endocrinology, Diabetology and Metabolism, Department of Medical Science, University of Turin
Corso Dogliotti 14
IT–10126 Turin (Italy)
E-Mail roberta.giordano@unito.it

20 Guitelman M, Garcia Basavilbaso N, Vitale M, Chervin A, Katz D, Miragaya K, Herrera J, Cornalo D, Servidio M, Boero L, Manavela M, Danilowicz K, Alfieri A, Stalldecker G, Glerean M, FainsteinDay P, Ballarino C, Mallea Gil MS, Rogozinski A: Primary empty sella (PES): a review of 175 cases. Pituitary 2013;16:270–274.
21 Schlaghecke R, Kornely E, Santen RT, Ridderskamp P: The effect of long-term glucocorticoid therapy on pituitary-adrenal responses to exogenous corticotropin-releasing hormone. N Engl J Med 1992;326:226–230.
22 Broersen LH, Pereira AM, Jørgensen JO, Dekkers OM: Adrenal insufficiency in corticosteroids use: systematic review and meta-analysis. J Clin Endocrinol Metab 2015;100:2171–2180.
23 Axelrod L: Perioperative management of patients treated with glucocorticoids. Endocrinol Metab Clin North Am 2003;32:367–383.
24 Hahner S, Loeffler M, Bleicken B, Drechsler C, Milovanovic D, Fassnacht M, Ventz M, Quinkler M, Allolio B: Epidemiology of adrenal crisis in chronic adrenal insufficiency: the need for new prevention strategies. Eur J Endocrinol 2010;162:597–602.
25 Bleicken B, Hahner S, Ventz M, Quinkler M: Delayed diagnosis of adrenal insufficiency is common: a cross-sectional study in 216 patients. Am J Med Sci 2010;339:525–531.
26 Jones SL, Trainer PJ, Perry L, Wass JA, Bessser GM, Grossman A: An audit of the insulin tolerance test in adult subjects in an acute investigation unit over one year. Clin Endocrinol (Oxf) 1994;41:123–128.
27 Fiad TM, Kirby JM, Cunningham SK, McKenna TJ: The overnight single-dose metyrapone test is a simple and reliable index of the hypothalamic-pituitary-adrenal axis. Clin Endocrinol (Oxf) 1994;40:603–609.
28 Schmidt IL, Lahner H, Mann K, Petersenn S: Diagnosis of adrenal insufficiency: evaluation of the corticotropin-releasing hormone test and basal serum cortisol in comparison to the insulin tolerance test in patients with hypothalamic-pituitary-adrenal disease. J Clin Endocrinol Metab 2003;88:4193–4198.
29 Ospina NS, Al Nofal A, Bancos I, Javed A, Khalid B, Kapoor E, Lteif AN, Natt N, Murad MH: ACTH stimulation tests for the diagnosis of adrenal insufficiency: systematic review and meta-analysis. J Clin Endocrinol Metab 2015, Epub ahead of print.
30 Wade M, Baid S, Calis K, Raff H, Sinaii N, Nieman L: Technical details influence the diagnostic accuracy of the 1 microg ACTH stimulation test. Eur J Endocrinol 2010;162:109–113.
31 Dickstein G: Hypothalamo-pituitary-adrenal axis testing: nothing is sacred and caution in interpretation is needed. Clin Endocrinol (Oxf) 2001;54:15–16.
32 Buchfelder M, Schlaffer S: Imaging of pituitary pathology. Handb Clin Neurol 2014;124:151–166.

Arvat E, Falorni A (eds): Cortisol Excess and Insufficiency.
Front Horm Res. Basel, Karger, 2016, vol 46, pp 171–183 (DOI: 10.1159/000443918)

Quality of Life and Life Expectancy in Patients with Adrenal Insufficiency: What Is True and What Is Urban Myth?

Stephanie Burger-Stritt · Alina Pulzer · Stefanie Hahner

Department of Medicine I, Endocrinology and Diabetology, University Hospital Würzburg, Würzburg, Germany

Abstract

For a long time it has been assumed that patients with chronic adrenal insufficiency under established replacement therapy have a normal life expectancy and a normal everyday life. Recent studies now indicate both an impairment of quality of life (QoL) with a negative impact on daily life and increased mortality in a significant number of patients. The clinical presentation of patients varies considerably. While some neither suffer from reduced QoL nor from adrenal crisis, others are significantly more affected by the disease. Long-term management of patients is thus more challenging and goes far beyond identification of the correct maintenance dose of corticosteroids. The mortality from adrenal crisis is still high and prevention should be a top priority for endocrinologists. Concepts of replacement therapy as well as patient education and emergency equipment are currently being reassessed. Developments to improve patient care and treatment comprise novel glucocorticoid preparations that are closer to the physiological circadian cortisol profile, a uniform European emergency card and more standardized crisis prevention measures.

Adrenal insufficiency (AI) was mostly fatal until the description of corticosteroids by Edward Kendall and Tadeus Reichstein and the subsequent availability of glucocorticoid preparations more than 70 years ago. Initiation of glucocorticoid replacement in newly diagnosed AI usually leads to rapid recovery of the patients, which is often experienced as a miracle cure of a long-standing unexplained sickness. For a long time it was assumed that patients under established replacement therapy have a normal life expectancy and a normal everyday social and work life. However, this presumption has been disproved by several recent studies indicating an impairment of quality of life (QoL) and life expectancy in chronic AI [1–4]. In daily practice, counseling of patients may often be a balancing act between creating hope for a normal or near-normal life and provision of understanding and explanations in case of persistent impairment of a patient's clinical condition. The clinical presentation of patients with chronic AI under established hormone replacement is highly variable. While some patients complete marathons or may have successful professional careers, others show significant impairment in their QoL and vitality, resulting in inability to deal with the demands of daily and work life. Furthermore, recent data indicate increased mortality in patients with AI. These observations have led to a reassessment of treatment concepts that have been applied for several decades. Furthermore, the so far unanswered question arises of whether subgroups of patients may be defined as particularly being at risk of impairment in their subjective health status or of premature death.

Quality of Life in Chronic Adrenal Insufficiency

In general, it needs to be taken into account that QoL is defined differently and that it is investigated by various instruments. The World Health Organization defines QoL as 'individuals' perception of their position in life in the context of the culture and value systems in which they live and in relation to their goals, expectations, standards and concerns'. Different terms are used like 'quality of life', 'general well-being', 'health-related quality of life' and 'subjective health status' focusing on QoL in general or in the context of a specific disease. QoL is subjective. It may be associated with health but always involves multiple physical and mental dimensions and reflects the subjective perception of health and well-being in a single individual. Thus, similar conditions may be differently judged by an individual person.

The first evidence regarding impaired QoL in chronic AI derives from a Norwegian observational study in 79 patients with Addison's disease performed by Løvås et al. [1] investigating a large patient cohort in comparison to a background population. General health perception and vitality were consistently impaired and fatigue was increased in the patients. Comparable results were obtained in a German cohort of patients with primary and secondary AI with slightly higher impairment in secondary AI compared to primary AI. However, even after exclusion of patients with a concomitant disease, QoL parameters remained significantly impaired for most subscales [2]. Interestingly, age was inversely correlated with several QoL subscales, with the highest difference to age-matched controls in young patients (fig. 1b), suggesting a kind of dilution effect by further complaints emerging with increasing age. Several subsequent studies focusing on QoL in AI have confirmed these observations, revealing a combined impairment of physical and emotional health with particularly reduced vitality and increased exhaustion tendency, fatigue and anxiety [3–9]. In addition, an increased incidence of affective and depressive disorders has been reported [10, 11].

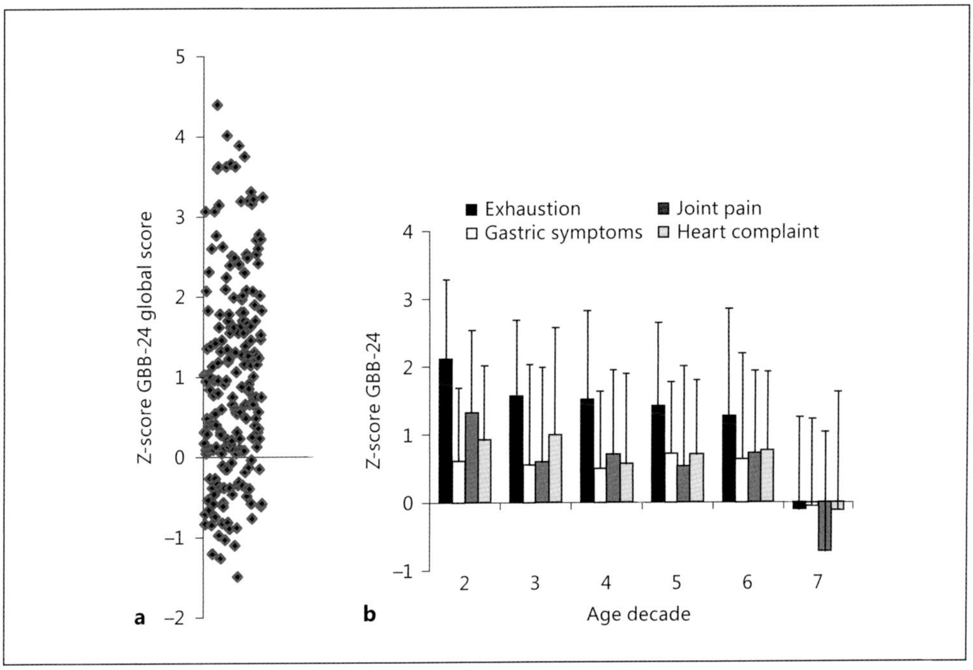

Fig. 1. Giessen Complaint List (GBB-24). Data from 210 patients with primary and secondary AI (data drawn from [2]). Higher scores indicate stronger QoL impairment. **a** Age- and sex-matched Z-scores of the GBB-24 global score demonstrating a broad scattering of Z-scores. **b** Age- and sex-matched Z-scores of the four GBB-24 subscales. Distribution over the respective age decades demonstrating the largest difference between age-matched controls in younger patients.

Remarkably, high interindividual variability of QoL scores was consistently observed in the different patient cohorts, indicating that a subgroup of patients exists that may be particularly vulnerable while others do not differ from age- and sex-matched controls (fig. 1a).

Taken together, using standardized tools for assessment of subjective health status, several studies similarly demonstrate a significant QoL impairment in patients with AI compared to the general population. The reasons for this observation are so far unclear. Suffering from a chronic disease per se seems to be of minor impact as other patient groups with chronic disease show less or even no impairment. Delayed diagnosis and the need for life-long replacement therapy have been demonstrated to be associated with impaired QoL in AI [4, 12, 13]. It has further been speculated that nonphysiological mineralocorticoid replacement and autoimmunity in Addison's disease may be contributing factors, which, however, has so far not been investigated in detail. Furthermore, the pattern of impairment in secondary nonautoimmune AI is highly similar to that of primary AI, suggesting that factors which are prevalent in both groups may be more relevant. Accordingly, the lack of DHEA and epinephrine and particularly the nonphysiological glucocorticoid replacement associated with slight overreplacement and noncircadian cortisol profiles are regarded as important contributing factors.

Impact of Adrenal Insufficiency on Daily and Work Life

Observing significant differences in QoL scores compared to the general population does not necessarily entail a relevant impact on daily life. However, 40–80% of patients from different cohorts reported restriction in their daily life and leisure time activities, which was attributed to their AI [1, 2, 14]. Correspondingly, the number of patients reporting working disability was up to four times higher than observed in the general population [1, 2].

Patients with chronic AI have a high prevalence of further endocrine and nonendocrine comorbidities with potential further impact on both QoL and treatment. In a prospective study following 423 patients with AI (primary AI = 221; secondary AI = 202) for 2 years [15], the mean number of days of missed work per year in employed patients was more than twice as high as was reported in the general German population during the same time period (unpubl. data). In a French survey of 94 patients with primary and secondary AI, 38% reported absence from work or school during the previous 3 months [14].

Thus, the impaired health status observed in a large number of patients appears to compromise work life, characterized by an increased number of patients out of work and a higher average number of sick-days as compared to the general population.

New Glucocorticoid Replacement Strategies for Improvement of Quality of Life and Outcome in Adrenal Insufficiency

In the light of the observed impairment of QoL, current treatment concepts have been revisited. Special attention has been paid to the nonphysiological glucocorticoid profile achieved by the available standard replacement therapy. The short half-life of oral hydrocortisone requires repeated dosing with peaks and troughs of cortisol levels during the day and mostly slight overdosing over time. In retrospective analyses, it could be demonstrated that the daily glucocorticoid dose is negatively correlated with QoL parameters [2, 9, 12].

Hypercortisolism has a severe and lasting negative impact on QoL, mood and cognitive function as has been shown in patients with Cushing's syndrome. The mechanisms determining QoL by glucocorticoids are largely unknown. Prolonged exposure to elevated glucocorticoids attenuates serotonin responses in the hippocampus and increases the effects of excitatory amino acids causing cell damage. Furthermore, decreased glucose uptake in the brain and atrophy of brain regions like the hippocampus have been observed. Glucocorticoids may furthermore reduce the synthesis of brain neurotrophic factors [16].

Due to the retrospective nature of the abovementioned analyses in patients with AI, it may, however, not be finally clarified if the observation of reduced QoL in patients receiving high glucocorticoid doses is due to negative effects of higher glucocorticoid exposure or rather reflects that treatment doses are more likely to be increased in patients complaining of impaired health status. However, these data show that after a dose increase, replacement doses need to be carefully reassessed at follow-up.

Dosing regimens of conventional hydrocortisone have been compared in a few very small interventional studies, but have provided conflicting results. Dose distribution and weight-adjusted dosing generally result in a better approximation of the physiological cortisol profiles. Outcome data on potential long-term complications of glucocorticoid replacement are so far missing. Several years ago, Riedel et al. [17] found that twice-daily glucocorticoid dosage was superior to once-daily dosing in 14 patients with primary AI. Ekman et al. [18] evaluated 2 versus 4 daily hydrocortisone doses in 15 females with primary AI. QoL tended to be improved with the 4-dose regimen which was preferred by the study participants. In contrast, other small studies did not detect differences regarding the number of doses.

In an attempt to improve oral hydrocortisone treatment, new preparations have been developed in recent years. A once-daily dual-release (modified release) hydrocortisone tablet (Plenadren®) has recently gained market access for the indication of replacement therapy in AI [3, 19]. Taken as a single morning dose, cortisol levels during the day better resemble the physiological profile. However, the circadian profile is not fully restored due to the lack of the early morning rise. Favorable effects on metabolic parameters and QoL could be demonstrated in the initial 12-week trial in 64 patients with Addison's disease. As the modified-release hydrocortisone preparation results in about 20% lower serum cortisol area under the curves than reached by conventional therapy, switching the dose from conventional hydrocortisone to modified-release hydrocortisone would result in a decrease of cortisol exposure which may at least partly explain some of the observed favorable metabolic effects. In an open-label study [20] of patients with chronic AI from different origins, 30 patients on overall lower daily hydrocortisone doses were switched to the same dose of modified-release hydrocortisone. They again showed significant decreases in BMI and HbA1c. No change in QoL scores assessed by AddiQoL (Addison's Disease-Specific Quality of Life Questionnaire) was seen. In patients remaining on conventional hydrocortisone, a significant decrease in AddiQoL scores was documented, leading to the conclusion that modified-release hydrocortisone seems to stabilize health-related QoL over time. However, taking into account the open-label character of this trial, AddiQoL scores may have been influenced by additional factors.

The relevance of the early morning rise of cortisol is a matter of debate. In a pilot study, Løvås and Husebye [21] reestablished physiological cortisol profiles in 7 patients with Addison's disease by administration of hydrocortisone as a continuous subcutaneous infusion (CSHI) via an insulin pump. The total hydrocortisone dose could be reduced in most patients and significant improvements in SF-36 scores for physical functioning and vitality could be achieved after 3 months of treatment. Two patients wished to continue subcutaneous treatment. This study was recently followed by larger studies assessing CSHI. In 33 patients with Addison's disease, physiological circadian cortisol profiles, normalization of ACTH levels and more physiological glucocorticoid metabolites were achieved [22]. The effect on QoL assessed by standardized questionnaires was less pronounced than in the initial study by Løvås and Husebye [21]. However, several dimensions of QoL showed significant improvement while no effect on sleep quality as a further end point was detected [22]. In an Australian double-blind, placebo-controlled multicenter study of 10 patients with Addison's disease comparing CSHI with oral hydrocortisone, subcutaneous hydrocortisone again restored a circadian cortisol profile [23]. No improvement was observed regarding QoL scores. However, patients already presented with a good baseline subjective health status which was similar to an Australian reference cohort and could not be further improved by CSHI. Interestingly, 50% of patients preferred pump treatment despite being invasive compared to oral hydrocortisone. Taken together, CSHI has been shown to be a feasible and safe method to restore circadian cortisol profiles. The particular impact on QoL and the identification of subgroups of patients significantly profiting from this kind of treatment remains to be further elucidated by subsequent studies.

The Role of DHEA Replacement

DHEA and DHEAS are highly abundant in humans with normal adrenal function, but are generally lacking in chronic AI. Indirect DHEA effects result from conversion to androgens and estrogens in the adrenal glands, the gonads and in peripheral target cells. Furthermore, direct DHEA effects have been observed. DHEA functions as a neurosteroid exerting neuroprotective, neurotrophic and anti-inflammatory effects within the brain.

Lack of neuroprotective action and, in females, clinical signs and symptoms of androgen deficiency may impact QoL in different aspects. Accordingly, several studies have shown that DHEA replacement has antidepressive and anxiolytic activity, and positively influences mood, QoL and sexuality. In a meta-analysis of 10 eligible trials, the positive effects on general well-being and depressive symptoms were rated as mild [24]. In general, beneficial effects of DHEA show high interindividual variation. Retrospective data comparing patients receiving DHEA treatment with patients not receiving DHEA showed more impaired QoL scores in the patients under DHEA treatment [2]. As DHEA does not belong to the standard treatment protocol, it is highly likely that this observation is based on a selection bias as patients complaining most will more frequently receive DHEA as an additional treatment. However, in combination with only moderate effects on QoL in other interventional studies, it can be assumed that the impairment of QoL may not simply be explained by the lack of DHEA. Nevertheless, in individual patients, initiation of replacement therapy leads to significant and clinically relevant improvement of general well-being, depression and symptoms of androgen deficiency, justifying a trial of DHEA replacement for selected patients.

Adrenomedullary Insufficiency in Chronic Adrenal Insufficiency

Patients with AI also present impaired adrenomedullary function and decreased epinephrine levels [25]. High local glucocorticoid levels are required for the synthesis of phenylethanolamine-N-methyltransferase, the enzyme catalyzing the last step in epinephrine synthesis. Whether the observed deficit in epinephrine is of any clinical relevance, or whether it is largely compensated by increased norepinephrine activity is unknown. However, reported neuroglycopenic symptoms and increased fatigue may potentially be attributed to the lacking epinephrine action [4, 26].

Mortality and Risk of Adrenal Crisis in Chronic Adrenal Insufficiency

In both primary and secondary AI, mortality is increased compared to the general population [27–29]. A retrospective analysis of 1,675 patients with primary AI from Sweden revealed a risk ratio for all-cause mortality of 2.19 (95% CI: 1.91–2.51) in men and 2.86 (95% CI: 2.54–3.20) in women [27]. Death risk from cardiovascular, malignant, endocrine and infectious disease were particularly high with the highest risk ratio for infectious disease [5.57 (95% CI: 2.04–12.13) in females and 6.57 (95% CI: 2.56–15.17) in males]. It has been hypothesized that the increased mortality from cardiovascular disease and cancer is caused by an oversubstitution of glucocorticoids, but so far evidence supporting this concept is missing [27]. The observational periods comprise several decades and replacement doses have been lowered in recent years; therefore, it might be of interest to reassess whether this observation still holds true for current treatment concepts. Particularly in young patients, AI was identified as being associated with increased mortality due to adrenal failure, infections and sudden death [6]. In support of this, Bensing et al. [29] documented the highest death risk for patients diagnosed in childhood.

Deciphering the contributing role of ACTH deficiency to mortality in secondary AI is more difficult due to the frequent prevalence of further hormone deficiencies. Two recent studies assessing the mortality in patients suffering from hypopituitarism identified an increased risk of death from infectious disease in the subgroup of patients with ACTH deficiency [30, 31]. In a Swedish analysis of patients with hypopituitarism, the standard mortality ratio for death from infectious disease was particularly high in the subgroup of patients with secondary AI (8.9; 95% CI: 4.7–15.2). This was frequently associated with signs and symptoms of adrenal crisis and particularly affected young males [30].

Patients with AI are at risk of a life-threatening adrenal crisis. How far adrenal crisis has contributed to death in the available analyses from Norway and Sweden is difficult to determine. In the study by Erichsen et al. [28], AI accounted for 15% of deaths in patients with Addison's disease, most likely reflecting adrenal crisis. In the Swedish analyses by Bergthorsdottir et al. [27] and Bensing et al. [29] 'endocrine causes' were reported as the cause of death in 12.6 and 8.3%, respectively. As an adrenal crisis is usually triggered by additional factors like infectious disease or other intercurrent illnesses, one might speculate that insufficient glucocorticoid coverage and a subsequent adrenal crisis explains the excess mortality from infectious disease and potentially also cardiovascular disease observed in the respective cohorts.

The incidence rate of adrenal crisis in different studies ranges between 5 and 17 adrenal crises per 100 patient-years, depending on the investigated cohort and the definition of adrenal crisis used. It has to be noted that so far no general definition of adrenal crisis exists. In a retrospective analysis of 444 patients with primary or secondary AI, we observed a frequency of 6.3 adrenal crises/100 patient-years [32]. Similar results were obtained from a large postal survey conducted by the UK Addison's Disease Self-Help Group in 841 patients from the UK, Canada, Australia and New Zealand, revealing an incidence of 8 adrenal crises per 100 patient-years [33]. Patients with congenital adrenal hyperplasia are also at risk of an adrenal crisis, with a reported frequency of 5.7 crises/100 patient-years in adult congenital adrenal hyperplasia patients. In this context, the transition period was revealed as a particularly vulnerable phase [34]. As expected, a higher frequency was found in patients after bilateral adrenalectomy for Cushing's syndrome (9.3 crises/100 patient-years) [35]. An analysis of health insurance data from the years 2008–2012 revealed an even higher frequency of adrenal crisis of 14–17/100 patient-years in patients with primary AI due to Addison's disease [36]. In a first prospective study following 423 patients over a 2-year period, we observed 64 adrenal crises in 767.5 patient-years (8.3 crises/100 patient-years).

The main precipitating factors of adrenal crises are gastrointestinal infections [15, 32–34]. Interestingly, emotional stress was also identified as a trigger of adrenal crises in the prospective trial. While retrospective analyses indicate comorbidity, female sex and diabetes insipidus in secondary AI as additional risk factors [32, 33], in the prospective analysis, a previous adrenal crisis was seen as the only risk factor (odds ratio = 2.85; 95% CI: 1.5–5.5) [15]. In addition, insufficient education of patients in dose adaption is a major risk factor for the development of an adrenal crisis, as in 42% of cases, in which vomiting was reported, only oral dose adjustment or even no change in replacement therapy had been indicated by the participants. Four out of 10 deaths in the patient population could be ascribed to an adrenal crisis, strongly suggesting the requirement of an improvement of existing prevention strategies. Interestingly, patients who experienced an adrenal crisis during the prospective study were more proactive in dose adjustments of glucocorticoids, indicating that adrenal crises cannot only be explained by the lack of dose adjustments [15]. Again, the distribution in the occurrence of adrenal crises is variable, suggesting thus far unknown factors influencing susceptibility. However, it is important to note that 2 patients died from an adrenal crisis, without previously having suffered from one. Four patients died from an adrenal crisis during 2 years of follow-up, leading to a mortality rate from adrenal crises of 0.5 per 100 patient-years (table 1).

How Can We Prevent Adrenal Crisis and Premature Death in Adrenal Insufficiency Patients?

Assuming that patients with AI are at a high risk of suffering from a life-threatening adrenal crisis, the prevention of adrenal crisis is of key importance. Basically, all patients suffering from AI should regularly obtain patient education in dose adjustment in situations of physical and psychological stress. Furthermore, patients should be equipped with an emergency card and an emergency set consisting of 100 mg of hydrocortisone for parenteral administration. Recent data revealing a high incidence of adrenal crises in a patient population under stable replacement therapy imply that more than occasional patient education is needed to prevent an adrenal crisis. A Dutch clinical study from 2013, involving 246 patients suffering from AI showed that a glucocorticoid educational group meeting is highly supportive to improve the self-management and to prevent adrenal crises. Six months after a 3-hour educational meeting, significantly more patients gave the right answers when testing the knowledge of patients on self-management [37]. Annual and standardized follow-up patient education, including a 'didactic success control' could further improve the training status of patients. Patients should be educated in dose adjustment and parenteral glucocorticoid administration. Preferentially, family members should also join patient education courses to be able to help patients in emergency situations.

It is of high importance that patients are well informed in dealing with their disease, in particular as long lag times between contacting a physician and receiving medical help in terms of parenteral hydrocortisone application have been repeatedly reported [38]. Recent data investigating the current management time lines in adrenal crises of 46 patients suffering from AI showed that the initiation of glucocorticoid administration was delayed in 46% of the patients. In this context, self-injection of glucocorticoids seems to be a valuable tool to improve self-management and prevent adrenal crises [38]. Moreover, self-injection of hydrocortisone is a very valuable tool in case of bridging time until sufficient medical treatment can be obtained, such as in the case of vomiting or diarrhea. So far, intramuscular administration of hydrocortisone is permitted for the use in emergency situations. Recent data from our group indicate that subcutaneous administration of hydrocortisone represents a safe and

Table 1. Studies reporting on adrenal crisis in patients with AI

Reference	Patients investigated	Crisis frequency	Further outcome data
Omori et al. [40], 2003	Primary AI (n = 22) Secondary AI (n = 115)	29% of patients had experienced at least 1 AC	Patients with untreated hypogonadism had a significantly higher relative risk compared to those without hypogonadism or with treated hypogonadism
White and Arlt [33], 2010	Addison's disease (n = 841)	8 ACs/100 patient-years About 55% of women and 52% of men reported one or more AC since diagnosis, at an average of 12.8 years since diagnosis for women and 11.4 years for men	Gastric infection was the most important factor predicting the likelihood of adrenal crisis Concomitant diabetes and/or asthma increase the frequency of ACs
Hahner et al. [32], 2010	Primary AI (n = 254) Secondary AI (n = 190)	6.3 ACs/100 patient-years (6.6 in primary AI, 5.8 in secondary AI) 384 ACs in 6,092 patient-years were documented 42% (PAI 47% and SAI 35%) reported at least 1 AC	Main precipitating causes: gastrointestinal infection and fever (45%), but also other stressful events Patients with PAI reported more frequent emergency glucocorticoid administration In PAI, patients with concomitant nonendocrine disease were at higher risk of crisis; in SAI, female sex and diabetes insipidus were associated with higher crisis incidence
Reisch et al. [34], 2012	CAH (n = 122)	Questionnaire based: 5.8 ACs/100 patient-years (257 ACs in 4,456 patient-years) Patient chart based: 4.9 ACs/100 patient-years (106 ACs in 2,181 patient-years)	ACs mostly occurred during childhood; gastrointestinal infections (29%) and salt-wasting crisis (18%) were the main causes of AC No difference in the overall frequency of AC in males and females
Ritzel et al. [35], 2013	Bilateral adrenalectomy due to Cushing's disease (n = 203)	9.3 ACs/100 patient-years 6 studies comprising 203 patients	–
Meyer et al. [36], 2014	Addison's disease (n = 2,477)	14–17 ACs/100 patient-years	–
Hahner et al. [15], 2015	Primary AI (n = 221) Secondary AI (n = 202)	8.3 ACs/100 patient-years 64 ACs in 767.5 patient-years were documented	Precipitating causes: gastrointestinal infection, fever and emotional stress, but also other stressful events (e.g. major pain, surgery, strenuous physical activity, heat, pregnancy) or unexplained sudden onset of AC Patients with a previous AC were at higher risk of crisis; no further risk factors could be identified 10 patients died during the 2-year follow-up; in 4 cases death was associated with AC (0.5 AC -related deaths per 100 patient-years)

AC = Adrenal crisis; CAH = congenital adrenal hyperplasia; PAI = primary AI; SAI = secondary AI.

efficient alternative for intramuscular self-injection in the prevention of adrenal crises. Most importantly, the subcutaneous application of hydrocortisone was preferred by patients over intramuscular injection [39]. A higher patient acceptance of subcutaneous over intramuscular injection suggests more frequent administration of hydrocortisone self-injection to prevent adrenal crises. Only patients with an elevated

BMI showed a delayed increase in cortisol levels after subcutaneous injection, suggesting that in some cases of massive overweight, intramuscular injection should be preferred over subcutaneous injection.

Conclusions

Despite standard treatment, a substantial number of patients suffer from reduced QoL, which has a direct impact on daily life. Current efforts are already being made to optimize hormone replacement therapy. Elimination of mortality from adrenal crisis by increasing awareness of the risk of adrenal crises among health professionals and patients and improving tools for crisis prevention and treatment is of utmost importance. Regular, repeated and standardized patient education as well the emergency card and emergency kit represent the three central pillars in the prevention of adrenal crises. Understanding both the mechanisms leading to impaired QoL and the pathophysiology of an adrenal crisis will be particularly helpful to optimize clinical management of our patients with chronic AI.

References

1 Løvås K, Loge JH, Husebye ES: Subjective health status in Norwegian patients with Addison's disease. Clin Endocrinol (Oxf) 2002;56:581–588.

2 Hahner S, Loeffler M, Fassnacht M, Weismann D, Koschker AC, Quinkler M, Decker O, Arlt W, Allolio B: Impaired subjective health status in 256 patients with adrenal insufficiency on standard therapy based on cross-sectional analysis. J Clin Endocrinol Metab 2007;92:3912–3922.

3 Forss M, Batcheller G, Skrtic S, Johannsson G: Current practice of glucocorticoid replacement therapy and patient-perceived health outcomes in adrenal insufficiency – a worldwide patient survey. BMC Endocr Disord 2012;12:8.

4 Meyer G, Hackemann A, Penna-Martinez M, Badenhoop K: What affects the quality of life in autoimmune Addison's disease? Horm Metab Res 2013;45: 92–95.

5 Løvås K, Husebye ES, Holsten F, Bjorvatn B: Sleep disturbances in patients with Addison's disease. Eur J Endocrinol 2003;148:449–456.

6 Erichsen MM, Lovas K, Skinningsrud B, Wolff AB, Undlien DE, Svartberg J, Fougner KJ, Berg TJ, Bollerslev J, Mella B, Carlson JA, Erlich H, Husebye ES: Clinical, immunological, and genetic features of autoimmune primary adrenal insufficiency: observations from a Norwegian registry. J Clin Endocrinol Metab 2009;94:4882–4890.

7 Kluger N, Matikainen N, Sintonen H, Ranki A, Roine RP, Schalin-Jantti C: Impaired health-related quality of life in Addison's disease – impact of replacement therapy, comorbidities and socio-economic factors. Clin Endocrinol (Oxf) 2014;81:511–518.

8 Tiemensma J, Andela CD, Kaptein AA, Romijn JA, van der Mast RC, Biermasz NR, Pereira AM: Psychological morbidity and impaired quality of life in patients with stable treatment for primary adrenal insufficiency: cross-sectional study and review of the literature. Eur J Endocrinol 2014;171:171–182.

9 Ragnarsson O, Mattsson AF, Monson JP, Filipsson Nystrom H, Akerblad AC, Koltowska-Haggstrom M, Johannsson G: The relationship between glucocorticoid replacement and quality of life in 2737 hypopituitary patients. Eur J Endocrinol 2014;171: 571–579.

10 Thomsen AF, Kvist TK, Andersen PK, Kessing LV: The risk of affective disorders in patients with adrenocortical insufficiency. Psychoneuroendocrinology 2006;31:614–622.

11 Warmuz-Stangierska I, Baszko-Blaszyk D, Sowinski J: Emotions and features of temperament in patients with Addison's disease. Endokrynol Pol 2010;61:90–92.

12 Bleicken B, Hahner S, Loeffler M, Ventz M, Decker O, Allolio B, Quinkler M: Influence of hydrocortisone dosage scheme on health-related quality of life in patients with adrenal insufficiency. Clin Endocrinol (Oxf) 2010;72:297–304.

13 Tiemensma J, Andela CD, Pereira AM, Romijn JA, Biermasz NR, Kaptein AA: Patients with adrenal insufficiency hate their medication: concerns and stronger beliefs about the necessity of hydrocortisone intake are associated with more negative illness perceptions. J Clin Endocrinol Metab 2014;99:3668–3676.

14 Touraine P, Chenuc G, Colin C: Self-perceived health status of patients with adrenal insufficiency receiving glucocorticoid replacement therapy – French data from a worldwide patient survey. Ann Endocrinol (Paris) 2015;76:9–12.

15 Hahner S, Spinnler C, Fassnacht M, Burger-Stritt S, Lang K, Milovanovic D, Beuschlein F, Willenberg HS, Quinkler M, Allolio B: High incidence of adrenal crisis in educated patients with chronic adrenal insufficiency: a prospective study. J Clin Endocrinol Metab 2015;100:407–416.

16 Pivonello R, Simeoli C, De Martino MC, Cozzolino A, De Leo M, Iacuaniello D, Pivonello C, Negri M, Pellecchia MT, Iasevoli F, Colao A: Neuropsychiatric disorders in Cushing's syndrome. Front Neurosci 2015;9:129.

17 Riedel M, Wiese A, Schurmeyer TH, Brabant G: Quality of life in patients with Addison's disease: effects of different cortisol replacement modes. Exp Clin Endocrinol 1993;101:106–111.

18 Ekman B, Bachrach-Lindstrom M, Lindstrom T, Wahlberg J, Blomgren J, Arnqvist HJ: A randomized, double-blind, crossover study comparing two- and four-dose hydrocortisone regimen with regard to quality of life, cortisol and ACTH profiles in patients with primary adrenal insufficiency. Clin Endocrinol (Oxf) 2012;77:18–25.

19 Nilsson AG, Marelli C, Fitts D, Bergthorsdottir R, Burman P, Dahlqvist P, Ekman B, Engstrom BE, Olsson T, Ragnarsson O, Ryberg M, Wahlberg J, Lennernas H, Skrtic S, Johannsson G: Prospective evaluation of long-term safety of dual-release hydrocortisone replacement administered once daily in patients with adrenal insufficiency. Eur J Endocrinol 2014;171:369–377.

20 Quinkler M, Miodini Nilsen R, Zopf K, Ventz M, Oksnes M: Modified-release hydrocortisone decreases BMI and HbA1c in patients with primary and secondary adrenal insufficiency. Eur J Endocrinol 2015;172:619–626.

21 Løvås K, Husebye ES: Continuous subcutaneous hydrocortisone infusion in Addison's disease. Eur J Endocrinol 2007;157:109–112.

22 Oksnes M, Björnsdottir S, Isaksson M, Methlie P, Carlsen S, Nilsen RM, Broman JE, Triebner K, Kämpe O, Hulting AL, Bensing S, Husebye ES, Løvås K: Continuous subcutaneous hydrocortisone infusion versus oral hydrocortisone replacement for treatment of Addison's disease: a randomized clinical trial. J Clin Endocrinol Metab 2014;99:1665–1674.

23 Gagliardi L, Nenke MA, Thynne TR, von der Borch J, Rankin WA, Henley DE, Sorbello J, Inder WJ, Torpy DJ: Continuous subcutaneous hydrocortisone infusion therapy in Addison's disease: a randomized, placebo-controlled clinical trial. J Clin Endocrinol Metab 2014;99:4149–4157.

24 Alkatib AA, Cosma M, Elamin MB, Erickson D, Swiglo BA, Erwin PJ, Montori VM: A systematic review and meta-analysis of randomized placebo-controlled trials of DHEA treatment effects on quality of life in women with adrenal insufficiency. J Clin Endocrinol Metab 2009;94:3676–3681.

25 Merke DP, Chrousos GP, Eisenhofer G, Weise M, Keil MF, Rogol AD, Van Wyk JJ, Bornstein SR: Adrenomedullary dysplasia and hypofunction in patients with classic 21-hydroxylase deficiency. N Engl J Med 2000;343:1362–1368.

26 Klement J, Hubold C, Cords H, Oltmanns KM, Hallschmid M, Born J, Lehnert H, Peters A: High-calorie glucose-rich food attenuates neuroglycopenic symptoms in patients with Addison's disease. J Clin Endocrinol Metab 2010;95:522–528.

27 Bergthorsdottir R, Leonsson-Zachrisson M, Oden A, Johannsson G: Premature mortality in patients with Addison's disease: a population-based study. J Clin Endocrinol Metab 2006;91:4849–4853.

28 Erichsen MM, Lovas K, Fougner KJ, Svartberg J, Hauge ER, Bollerslev J, Berg JP, Mella B, Husebye ES: Normal overall mortality rate in Addison's disease, but young patients are at risk of premature death. Eur J Endocrinol 2009;160:233–237.

29 Bensing S, Brandt L, Tabaroj F, Sjoberg O, Nilsson B, Ekbom A, Blomqvist P, Kampe O: Increased death risk and altered cancer incidence pattern in patients with isolated or combined autoimmune primary adrenocortical insufficiency. Clin Endocrinol (Oxf) 2008;69:697–704.

30 Burman P, Mattsson AF, Johannsson G, Hoybye C, Holmer H, Dahlqvist P, Berinder K, Engstrom BE, Ekman B, Erfurth EM, Svensson J, Wahlberg J, Karlsson FA: Deaths among adult patients with hypopituitarism: hypocortisolism during acute stress, and de novo malignant brain tumors contribute to an increased mortality. J Clin Endocrinol Metab 2013;98:1466–1475.

31 Gaillard RC, Mattsson AF, Akerblad AC, Bengtsson BA, Cara J, Feldt-Rasmussen U, Koltowska-Haggstrom M, Monson JP, Saller B, Wilton P, Abs R: Overall and cause-specific mortality in GH-deficient adults on GH replacement. Eur J Endocrinol 2012;166:1069–1077.
32 Hahner S, Loeffler M, Bleicken B, Drechsler C, Milovanovic D, Fassnacht M, Ventz M, Quinkler M, Allolio B: Epidemiology of adrenal crisis in chronic adrenal insufficiency: the need for new prevention strategies. Eur J Endocrinol 2010;162:597–602.
33 White K, Arlt W: Adrenal crisis in treated Addison's disease: a predictable but under-managed event. Eur J Endocrinol 2010;162:115–120.
34 Reisch N, Willige M, Kohn D, Schwarz HP, Allolio B, Reincke M, Quinkler M, Hahner S, Beuschlein F: Frequency and causes of adrenal crises over lifetime in patients with 21-hydroxylase deficiency. Eur J Endocrinol 2012;167:35–42.
35 Ritzel K, Beuschlein F, Mickisch A, Osswald A, Schneider HJ, Schopohl J, Reincke M: Clinical review: outcome of bilateral adrenalectomy in Cushing's syndrome: a systematic review. J Clin Endocrinol Metab 2013;98:3939–3948.
36 Meyer G, Neumann K, Badenhoop K, Linder R: Increasing prevalence of Addison's disease in German females: health insurance data 2008–2012. Eur J Endocrinol 2014;170:367–373.
37 Repping-Wuts HJ, Stikkelbroeck NM, Noordzij A, Kerstens M, Hermus AR: A glucocorticoid education group meeting: an effective strategy for improving self-management to prevent adrenal crisis. Eur J Endocrinol 2013;169:17–22.
38 Hahner S, Hemmelmann N, Quinkler M, Beuschlein F, Spinnler C, Allolio, B: Timelines in the management of adrenal crisis – targets, limits and reality. Clin Endocrinol (Oxf) 2015;82:497–502.
39 Hahner S, Burger-Stritt S, Allolio B: Subcutaneous hydrocortisone administration for emergency use in adrenal insufficiency. Eur J Endocrinol 2013;169: 147–154.
40 Omori K, Nomura K, Shimizu S, Omori N, Takano K: Risk factors for adrenal crisis in patients with adrenal insufficiency. Endocr J 2003;50:745–752.

Prof. Stefanie Hahner, MD
Department of Medicine I, Endocrinology and Diabetology, University Hospital Würzburg
Oberdürrbacher Strasse 6
DE–97080 Würzburg (Germany)
E-Mail hahner_s@ukw.de

Arvat E, Falorni A (eds): Cortisol Excess and Insufficiency.
Front Horm Res. Basel, Karger, 2016, vol 46, pp 184–195 (DOI: 10.1159/000443919)

Congenital Adrenal Hyperplasia: Unresolved Issues

Mabel Yau[a] · Ahmed Khattab[a] · Dix Poppas[b] · Lucia Ghizzoni[c] · Maria New[a]

[a]Adrenal Steroid Disorders Group, Department of Pediatrics, Icahn School of Medicine at Mount Sinai, and [b]Institute of Pediatric Urology, Department of Urology, Komansky Center for Children's Health, New York Presbyterian Hospital, Weill Cornell Medical School, New York, N.Y., USA; [c]Division of Endocrinology, Diabetology and Metabolism, Department of Medical Sciences, University of Turin, Turin, Italy

Abstract

Congenital adrenal hyperplasia (CAH) describes a family of disorders that comes from enzymatic deficiencies in cortisol production, with 21-hydroxylase deficiency causing ~90% of cases. Distinction is made between the severe classical form and milder nonclassical form of CAH. Molecular genetic analysis is used to confirm the hormonal diagnosis. A high rate of genotype-phenotype discordance has been found in 21-hydroxylase deficiency. The goal of treatment is to replace with synthetic glucocorticoids and mineralocorticoids and suppress adrenal androgen production. The treatment of patients affected with nonclassical CAH, particularly males, remains controversial. Variable synthetic glucocorticoids are used and new modes of glucocorticoid delivery are under investigation. To improve height, growth hormone and other adjuvant therapies are employed. Long-term outcomes of genital surgery using modern techniques in females affected with classical CAH continue to be investigated. Prenatal treatment with dexamethasone is available to avoid ambiguous genitalia in these females. Although studies have shown its safety to mother and fetus, prenatal treatment is still regarded as experimental. Currently, prenatal diagnosis of CAH can only be obtained through invasive methods. Recently, the detection of cell-free fetal DNA in maternal plasma has made it possible to make this diagnosis earlier and noninvasively.

Congenital adrenal hyperplasia (CAH) refers to a group of autosomal recessive disorders in which genetic enzyme deficiencies lead to impaired steroid synthesis. The production of cortisol from cholesterol occurs in the zona fasciculata of the adrenal cortex through five major enzymatic conversions. Impaired cortisol synthesis, which is common to all forms of CAH, leads to elevation of adrenocorticotropic hormone

(ACTH) and overstimulation of the adrenal cortex. Impaired enzyme function at each step of adrenal cortisol biosynthesis leads to an increase in precursors and deficient products [1].

A distinction is made between classical and nonclassical (NC) forms of the disorder. The classical forms, salt-wasting and simple virilizing, are defined by significantly reduced enzyme activity with impaired cortisol production manifesting clinically at birth with genital ambiguity and adrenal insufficiency. The salt-wasting form is differentiated from the simple virilizing form by mineralocorticoid deficiency.

NC forms are caused by less severe enzyme defects. Symptoms are generally milder and present postnatally [1]. NC-CAH has variable presentations ranging from premature adrenarche in childhood to decreased fecundity or infertility in adults [2]. Similar to classical CAH, NC-CAH may cause premature development of pubic hair, acne, secondary polycystic ovarian syndrome, advanced bone age with accelerated linear growth velocity, and short stature. In adult males, early balding, acne, infertility or short stature may prompt the diagnosis of NC-CAH. Females with NC-CAH do not have virilized genitalia at birth.

The most common enzymatic defect is 21-hydroxylase deficiency (21-OHD) encoded by the CYP21A2 gene, which accounts for over 90% of CAH cases. Worldwide data from nearly 6.5 million newborn screens for 21-OHD indicate that classical CAH occurs in approximately 1:15,000 live births [3]. NC-21-OHD CAH is more common. The incidence of NC-21-OHD CAH in the heterogeneous population of New York City is 1 in 100, making NC-21-OHD CAH one of the most frequent recessive disorders in humans [4]. NC-21-OHD CAH is particularly frequent in Ashkenazi Jews, in whom 1 in 3 are carriers of the allele, and 1 in 27 are affected with NC-21-OHD CAH [4–6]. Steroid 11β-hydroxylase deficiency is the second most common cause of CAH, accounting for 5–8% of all cases [7]. It occurs in 1 in 100,000 live births in the general population and is more common in some populations of North African origin [8–10]. In Moroccan Jews, for example, the disease incidence of 11β-hydroxylase deficiency was initially estimated to be 1 in 5,000 live births [11]; subsequently, it was shown to occur less frequently [12], but remains more common in Moroccan Jews than in other populations.

Genotype-Phenotype Disconcordance

The gold standard for hormonal diagnosis of 21-OHD is the ACTH stimulation test (250-μg ACTH intravenously), measuring levels of 17-hydroxyprogesterone and Δ4 androstenedione at baseline and at 60 min. The values of 17-hydroxyprogesterone can then be plotted in a nomogram (fig. 1) and correlate strongly with disease severity and presentation [13].

Establishment of a genetic diagnosis is important for genetic counseling of parents for future offspring and for genetic counseling of the patient concerning his/her re-

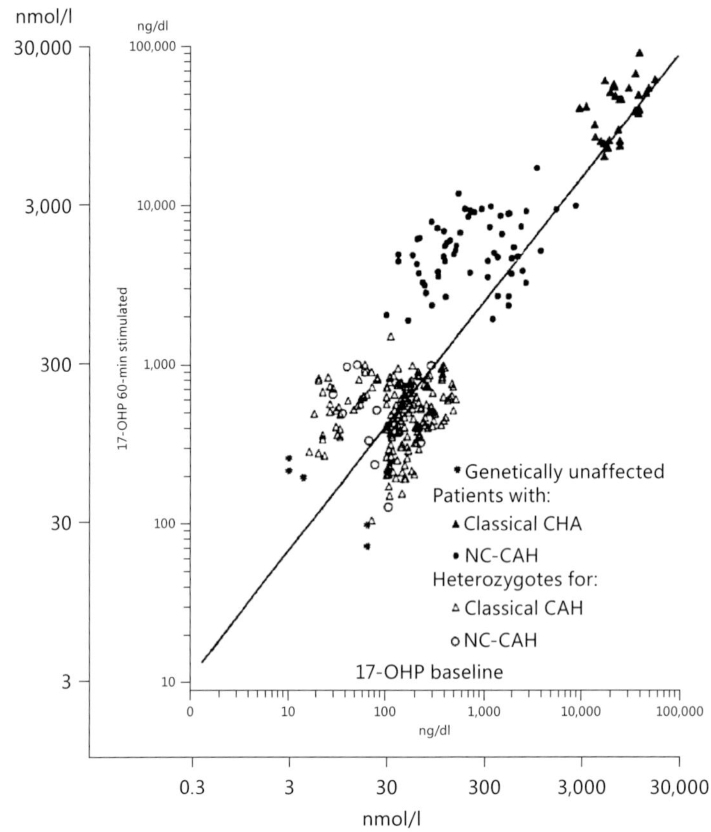

Fig. 1. 17-hydroxyprogesterone (17-OHP) nomogram for the diagnosis of steroid 21-OHD 60-min Cortosyn stimulation test. Nomogram relating baseline to ACTH-stimulated serum concentrations of 17-OHP. The scales are logarithmic. A regression line for all data points is shown. Data points cluster as shown into three nonoverlapping groups: classic and NC forms of 21-OHD are readily distinguished from each other and from those that are heterozygotes and unaffected. Distinguishing unaffected from heterozygotes is difficult. Adapted from New et al. [52]; permission obtained.

productive options. Genetic testing for common mutations in the CYP21A2 gene is widely available commercially and can be useful in confirming the hormonal diagnosis. Patients with NC-CAH frequently are compound heterozygotes with a severe mutation and a mild mutation [14].

At least 100 mutations causing 21-OHD have been identified [14]. The majority of mutations causing 21-OHD are the result of recombination events between the active coding gene, CYP21A2, and the pseudogene, CYP21P. During meiosis, misalignment of homologous chromosomes leads to unequal crossover, resulting in large gene deletions. Gene conversion can result from misalignment of sister chromatids during mitosis in which a sequence of the CYP21P pseudogene may be transferred to the CYP21A2 gene. Transfer of a mutation from the CYP21P pseudogene to the CYP21A2 active gene leads to an enzymatic defect. Deletions and gene conversion events may be common findings in 21-OHD, owing to the chromosomal arrangement of the gene and pseudogene (i.e. homologous genes in a tandem array) [15]. In silico studies of these gene mutations have shown functional enzymatic impairments [16]. Mutations affecting important functions such as membrane anchoring or substrate binding lead to the severe classical forms of disease.

The severity of the mutation predicts the degree of enzymatic deficiency, and is thus expected to correlate with clinical presentation [14, 16]. However, in a study of 1,507 families with CAH due to 21-OHD, genotype-phenotype nonconcordance occurred in approximately 50% of genotypes [14]. For example, one single-nucleotide mutation altering the splicing of an intron (I2G) is particularly common and is associated with both simple virilizing and salt-wasting phenotypes. This high rate of nonconcordance has yet to be explained. In the future, studies of nonconcordance cases, evaluating for undetected rare mutations and gene modifiers, should be considered. Only 5% of the CYP21A2 mutations are de novo mutations that arise independently of the pseudogene; these mutations are often unique to single families [17]. Structural and functional analysis of mutant enzymes in silico are required to determine the severity of enzymatic impairment from novel or rare mutations in which no clinical information are available and the phenotype cannot be predicted from the genotype [16, 17].

Glucocorticoid Treatment and Investigational Treatments

The goal of therapy in CAH is to both correct the deficiency in cortisol secretion and to suppress ACTH overproduction. Proper treatment with glucocorticoids reduces stimulation of the androgen pathway, thus preventing further virilization and allowing normal growth and development [18]. The most widely used dosage of hydrocortisone (or its equivalent) for the treatment of pediatric patients with classical CAH is about 10–15 mg/m^2/day divided into 2 or 3 doses per day, and for pediatric patients with NC-CAH it is 5–8 mg/m^2/day divided into 2 or 3 doses per day [18]. Long-acting glucocorticoids traditionally have been reserved for adult patients due to concerns about growth suppression with long-acting glucocorticoids [19]. Glucocorticoid regimens for adult patients with classical CAH can be converted from hydrocortisone to bioequivalent doses of dexamethasone. A small dose of dexamethasone at bedtime (0.25–0.5 mg) is usually adequate for androgen suppression in NC adult patients. Overtreatment should be avoided because it can lead to Cushing's syndrome.

Dexamethasone at a dose of 0.25 mg/m^2/day has been used in infants [20] and growing children [21] by Rivkees and colleagues with normal growth and bone age advancement during the follow-up period. This dosing is based on a dexamethasone potency to suppress adrenal androgen production of 80- to 100-fold that of hydrocortisone [22].

As current regimens of glucocorticoid therapy are unable to simulate the normal cortisol circadian rhythm, new modes of glucocorticoid delivery are being studied. Continuous subcutaneous hydrocortisone infusion via pump technology used in diabetes mellitus has been successfully demonstrated in one patient [23]. A delayed and extended release form of hydrocortisone, Chronocort, has been designed to approximate physiological cortisol secretion and is in clinical trials [24].

Management of NC-CAH

Difficulty with fertility in females with CAH may be due to anovulatory menstrual cycles, secondary polycystic ovarian syndrome, nonsuppressible serum progesterone levels or an inadequate vaginal introitus [25]. Fertility is reduced in poorly treated salt-wasting CAH. NC-CAH is an important and frequently unrecognized form of infertility in males and females [2]. Males with CAH, particularly if poorly treated, may have reduced sperm counts and low testosterone as a result of high androstenedione concentrations produced by the adrenal glands. Androstenedione is converted to testosterone which is then converted to estradiol, which suppresses secretion of gonadotropins. Although benign, testicular adrenal rest tumors may interfere with spermatogenesis. Regular testicular examination and periodic testicular ultrasonography are not recommended for early detection of adrenal rest tumors of the testes in males with NC-CAH [18].

Adjuvant Therapies

Without appropriate postnatal treatment with glucocorticoids, excessive adrenal androgen production can lead to progressive phallic (penile or clitoral) enlargement, premature adrenarche, acne and frontal baldness in both males and females [1]. The mean age at onset of puberty in both males and females is slightly younger than the general population [26]. In those who are inadequately treated, central precocious puberty can occur. Following the onset of puberty, in a majority of successfully treated patients, the milestones of further development of secondary sex characteristics in general appear to be normal [26]. In female adolescents and adults, signs of hyperandrogenism may include male-pattern alopecia (temporal balding), acne, hirsutism, menstrual irregularities and impaired fertility [1, 2]. Although the expected age of menarche may be delayed in females with classical CAH, when adequately treated many have regular menses after menarche [27]. In males, short stature and impaired fertility are the frequent signs of NC-CAH [1].

Women with both classical and nonclassical CAH frequently develop concurrent androgen excess as a result of polycystic ovarian syndrome. The precise interaction of the gonads and adrenal cortex via serum steroids remains to be determined. Several interesting schemas for the development of polycystic ovarian syndrome have been proposed, but the mechanism remains unresolved [28]. Persistent hyperandrogenism despite adequate adrenal suppression with glucocorticoids is indicative of concurrent polycystic ovarian syndrome and may be treated with oral contraceptives to suppress ovarian androgen production [29]. Spironolactone, an androgen antagonist, may be used in conjunction with glucocorticoids and oral contraceptives [29].

Advanced somatic and epiphyseal development occurs with an exaggerated and early growth spurt. Estrogens produced from excessive adrenal androgens result in bone age advancement [30]. Following an early growth spurt, the epiphyses mature and close prematurely, resulting in a final adult height that is significantly below that expected from parental heights. Excess glucocorticoid treatment can also lead to poor growth.

Even in the setting of good adrenal control on glucocorticoid treatment, final height may be compromised and below the target height. Analysis of 47 patients with classic CAH due to 21-OHD, who were separated into two groups defined by the degree of hormonal control, failed to show a normal height outcome with the use of standard treatment [31]. Adjunctive therapies have been used in children with poor height predictions. Gonadotropin-releasing hormone (GnRH) analogue treatment suppresses central puberty to prevent premature epiphyseal closure. Growth hormone treatment counters the deceleration in growth velocity that accompanies GnRH analogue treatment. Recombinant growth hormone alone or in combination with a GnRH analogue has been shown to improve final adult height in CAH patients [32].

In patients at risk of compromised adult height due to bone age advancement, growth hormone therapy has been shown to be effective in improving final adult height. Growth hormone therapy can be combined with GnRH analogues. In a study of 34 patients treated with growth hormone therapy for 5.6 ± 1.8 years in males and 4.5 ± 1.6 years in females, the mean gain in height was 9.2 ± 6.7 cm in males and 10.5 ± 3.7 cm in females [32].

Aromatase inhibitors, originally developed for the treatment of estrogen receptor-positive breast cancer, have been used to improve adult height in children with CAH without an FDA-approved indication [33]. Aromatase is the enzyme which converts testosterone to estradiol and androstenedione to estrone. The conversion of the excessive androgens as a result of 21-hydroxylase or 11β-hydroxylase deficiency to estrogens is blocked by aromatase inhibitors [33]. Thus, the advancement of bone age can be slowed or halted by aromatase inhibitors without suppressing pubertal development. No clinical trials of aromatase inhibitors in patients with CAH have been performed.

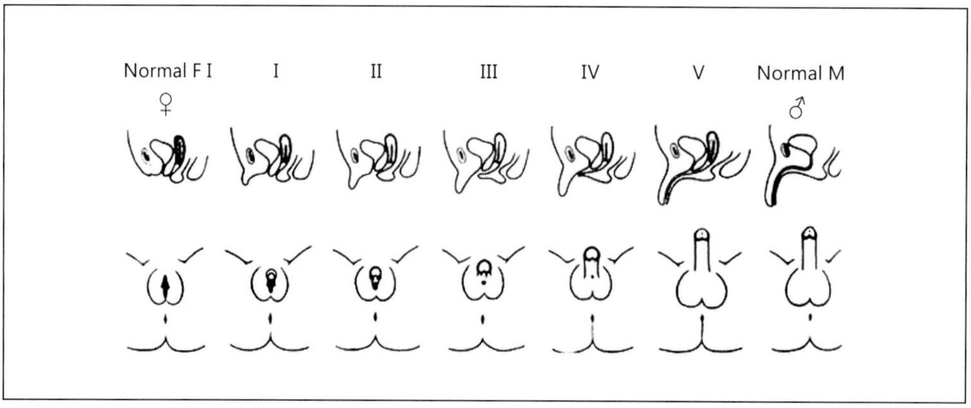

Fig. 2. Different degrees of virilization according to the scale developed by Prader [34]. Stage I: clitoromegaly without labial fusion. Stage II: clitoromegaly and posterior labial fusion. Stage III: greater degree of clitoromegaly, single perineal urogenital orifice, and almost complete labial fusion. Stage IV: increasingly phallic clitoris, urethra-like urogenital sinus at base of clitoris, and complete labial fusion. Stage V: penile clitoris, urethral meatus at tip of phallus and scrotum-like labia (appears like males without palpable gonads).

Surgical Intervention in Females with Classical CAH

Females with classical CAH owing to 21-OHD and 11β-hydroxylase deficiency present at birth with virilization of their genitalia. Adrenocortical function begins around the 7th week of gestation; thus, a female fetus with classical CAH is exposed to adrenal androgens at the critical time of genital organogenesis that begins around the 9th week of gestation. Exposure of the female fetus to fetal adrenal androgens leads to clitoral enlargement, fusion and scrotalization of the labial folds, and rostral migration of the urethral/vaginal perineal orifice, placing the phallus in the male position [1]. Degrees of genital virilization are classified into five Prader stages (fig. 2) [34]. The internal female reproductive organs, including the uterus, fallopian tubes and ovaries, develop normally. Thus, females with classical CAH maintain the potential for fertility.

Vaginoplasty and clitoroplasty is suggested for severely virilized females affected with CAH (Prader stage III or greater) [18]. However, there is no consensus on the timing of these procedures. Long-term studies of women with CAH who underwent genitoplasty in infancy or early childhood disclose impaired genital sensitivity, sexual difficulties, decreased intercourse frequency and stress urinary leakage [35, 36]. There are reports of complications resulting from genitoplasty such as strictures, fistulas, urinary infection, fibrosis and scarring, which have caused stress and depression in patients, especially with regard to their sexual relationships [36]. However, the vast majority of these findings come from patients whose surgery was performed prior to the advances in surgical techniques that have developed over the past 2 decades. Our current knowledge of clitoral neurovascular anatomy has recently led to more refined surgical techniques [37]. In addition, uretheral and vaginal reconstructive surgery has changed significantly since 1996 with the introduction of urogenital sinus mobilization procedures [38]. The long-term outcomes resulting from these modern surgical techniques are just now being evaluated. The stigmas attached to ambiguous genitalia and impaired fertility may result in emotional distress in patients who require repeated surgical procedures and genital examinations that reinforce their genitourinary ambiguity [39].

Prenatal Treatment

As genital organogenesis begins at ~9 weeks of gestation, the excess fetal androgen production due to 21-hydroxylase or 11β-hydroxylase deficiency prior to 9 weeks of gestation causes female genitals to become virilized. For the fetus at risk of these forms of CAH, dexamethasone treatment must be initiated before 9 weeks of gestation to prevent genital ambiguity or reduce the degree of clitoromegaly in female fetuses [40, 41]. Dexamethasone is not metabolized by the placenta and crosses the maternal-fetal barrier. Therefore, it can be used to suppress fetal androgen production in fetuses affected by CAH. The current recommendation is dexamethasone at 20 μg/kg of maternal prepregnancy weight, given in 2–3 divided doses.

New et al. [42] reported a study of prenatal diagnoses between 1978 and 2002 that confirms the efficacy of this treatment protocol. Of 595 pregnancies evaluated, 126 fetuses were found to be affected, 108 of these with classic forms and 64 of which were female. Female newborns in this cohort were highly virilized at birth, with a mean Prader score of 3.77. Of 51 pregnant women who received treatment, 27 began dexamethasone early (before 9 weeks of gestation) and continued to term. Female newborns in this group were only mildly virilized, with a mean Prader score of 1.04. The remaining 13 pregnant women began treatment late or were treated only partially. Female newborns in this group had an intermediate degree of virilization, with a mean Prader score of 3 [42]. Statistically significant adverse effects of dexamethasone treatment (relative to the untreated group) included an excess weight gain of 7.1 lb (3.2 kg) and the presence of edema and striae in mothers. No correlation was noted between prenatal dexamethasone treatment and fetal demise, birth weight, hypertension or gestational diabetes mellitus [42]. Normal birth weight and length and normal physical and psychological development were also reported in treated fetuses (affected and unaffected) in a French multicenter study [43].

There are some concerns regarding behavioral and developmental effects of prenatal dexamethasone treatment. Although a Swedish follow-up study of 40 children to a mean age of 11 years showed good general adaptation, psychological well-being and school performance, concerns regarding memory and gender behavior led to a hold on enrollment [44]. An impaired verbal working memory and increased social anxiety were noted in children unaffected with CAH who were treated short term with prenatal dexamethasone [44]. A larger follow-up study of cognitive outcomes in children exposed to prenatal dexamethasone did not show impaired working memory which was previously reported [45]. This study demonstrated slower mental procession in females with CAH treated prenatally with dexamethasone compared to controls [45].

The Swedish study also noted more gender-neutral behaviors in boys exposed to prenatal dexamethasone [44]. Further, research on the prenatal dexamethasone protocol was misconstrued as an unethical prevention of benign behavioral sex variations such as tomboyism and lesbianism [46]. This claim has been dispelled by the Office for Human Research Protections [47].

Prenatal Diagnosis

Modern prenatal diagnosis of CAH is made with the use of molecular genetics. Previously, diagnosis was dependent on hormonal evaluation of amniotic fluid [48]. CAH is now diagnosed prenatally by molecular genetic studies obtained from amniocentesis at 16–20 weeks of gestation or chorionic villus sampling at 10–12 weeks of gestation. Specific probes for 21-hydroxylase mutations allow direct and rapid identification of known mutations through the use of polymerase chain reaction (i.e. allele specific). Panels of oligonucleotide probes currently available for use in prenatal diagnosis are expected to identify well more than 95% of current 21-hydroxylase mutations [49]. A genetic diagnosis of CAH can be made reliably when the genotype of both parents is known. However, the phenotype is less reliably predicted as there is a high prevalence of genotype/phenotype nonconcordance [14].

Of the invasive prenatal diagnostic methods, CAH is diagnosed prenatally by amniocentesis at 16–20 weeks of gestation, or earlier, by chorionic villus sampling at 10–12 weeks of gestation. Chorionic villus sampling is currently advocated over amniocentesis to permit diagnosis in the first trimester and to allow discontinuation of unnecessary steroid treatment in the case of a male fetus or an unaffected female fetus. The earliest possible prenatal diagnosis of CAH using these invasive methods is much later than 9 weeks, which means that both male and unaffected female fetuses are also exposed to unnecessary dexamethasone treatment. Further, both amniocentesis and chorionic villus sampling are invasive procedures, with a risk to the mother and fetus. Thus, there is an acute need for diagnosing CAH before genital organogenesis begins at around 9 weeks, so that steroid therapy will be administered solely to mothers pregnant with an affected female fetus and unnecessary treatment of male and unaffected female fetuses will be avoided [42].

Research on noninvasive prenatal diagnosis for some of these disorders, especially the 21-hydroxylase form of CAH, is promising, and this may become the new standard treatment in years to come. Prenatal sex determination by SRY can be determined as early as 4 weeks and 5 days [50]. However, sex determination only eliminates the need for unnecessary treatment in males and not in unaffected females. For female fetuses, the genetic diagnosis is required to avoid unnecessary treatment in unaffected female fetuses. In 2014, the development and validation of targeted massive parallel sequencing by New et al. [51] for the noninvasive prenatal diagnosis of CAH using maternal plasma was reported. In this study, 14 families, each with a child affected with classical CAH (proband), and parents with at least one mutant CYP21A2 gene were recruited for noninvasive prenatal diagnosis. The fetal CAH status and sex were correctly deduced using this noninvasive prenatal diagnostic method. Seven pregnancies had CAH, 5 were carriers and 2 were normal. Invasive prenatal diagnostic methods of chorionic villus sampling and amniocentesis were used to validate the diagnosis in 7 cases. The CAH status of the remaining cases was confirmed postnatally. In one family, CAH status was deduced from maternal plasma drawn as early as 5 weeks and 6 days [51]. This new noninvasive technique of prenatal diagnosis will avoid unnecessary invasive antenatal surgical diagnostic procedures (amniocentesis and chorionic villus sampling), which carry a minimal but clinically significant risk. Further, with this noninvasive prenatal diagnostic method, only the affected female fetus receives prenatal treatment with low-dose dexamethasone and unnecessary treatment to the male fetus and unaffected female fetus is avoided [51].

Finally, poor developing countries do not conduct prenatal diagnosis as they rarely have sterile facilities for the surgical procedures of amniocentesis and chorionic villus sampling. As drawing blood in the method of noninvasive prenatal diagnosis does not require sterile facilities, we can now offer prenatal diagnosis of CAH and other monogenic disorders to poor developing countries. However, the difficulty with the cost of noninvasive prenatal diagnosis for poor developing countries has yet to be resolved.

References

1 New MI, Lekarev O, Mancenido D, Parsa P, Yuen T: Congenital adrenal hyperplasia owing to 21-hydroxylase deficiency; New MI (ed): Genetic Steroid Disorders. San Francisco, Elsevier, 2014, pp 29–52.
2 New MI: Extensive clinical experience: nonclassical 21-hydroxylase deficiency. J Clin Endocrinol Metab 2006;91:4205–4214.
3 Pang SY, Wallace MA, Hofman L, Thuline HC, Dorche C, Lyon IC, Dobbins RH, Kling S, Fujeda K, Suwa S: Worldwide experience in newborn screening for classical congenital adrenal hyperplasia due to 21-hydroxylase deficiency. Pediatrics 1988;81: 866–874.
4 Speiser PW, Dupont B, Rubinstein P, Piazza A, Kastelan A, New MI: High frequency of nonclassical steroid 21-hydroxylase deficiency. Am J Hum Genet 1985;37:650–667.
5 Sherman SL, Aston CE, Morton NE, Speiser PW, New MI: A segregation and linkage study of classical and nonclassical 21-hydroxylase deficiency. Am J Hum Genet 1988;42:830–838.
6 Zerah M, Ueshoba H, Wood E, Speiser PW, Crawford C, McDonald T, Pareira J, Gruen D, New MI: Prevalence of nonclassical steroid 21-hydroxylase deficiency based on a morning salivary 17-hydroxyprogesterone screening test: a small sample study. J Clin Endocrinol Metab 1990;70:1662–1667.
7 Zachmann M, Tassinari D, Prader A: Clinical and biochemical variability of congenital adrenal hyperplasia due to 11 beta-hydroxylase deficiency. A study of 25 patients. J Clin Endocrinol Metab 1983;56:222–229.

8 Curnow KM, Slutsker L, Vitek J, Cole T, Speiser PW, New MI, White PC, Pascoe L: Mutations in the CYP11B1 gene causing congenital adrenal hyperplasia and hypertension cluster in exons 6, 7, and 8. Proc Natl Acad Sci USA 1993;90:4552–4556.

9 White PC, Obeid J, Agarwal AK, Tannin GM, Nikkila H: Genetic analysis of 11 beta-hydroxysteroid dehydrogenase. Steroids 1994;59:111–115.

10 Khemiri M, Ridane H, Bou YO, Matoussi N, Khaldi F: 11 beta hydroxylase deficiency: a clinical study of seven cases (in French). Tunis Med 2006;84:106–113.

11 Rösler A, Leiberman E, Cohen T: High frequency of congenital adrenal hyperplasia (classic 11 beta-hydroxylase deficiency) among Jews from Morocco. Am J Med Genet 1992;42:827–834.

12 Paperna T, Gershoni-Baruch R, Badarneh K, Kasinetz L, Hochberg Z: Mutations in CYP11B1 and congenital adrenal hyperplasia in Moroccan Jews. J Clin Endocrinol Metab 2005;90:5463–5465.

13 New MI, Lorenzen F, Lerner AJ, Kohn B, Oberfield SE, Pollack MS, Dupont B, Stoner E, Levy DJ, Pang S, Levine LS: Genotyping steroid 21-hydroxylase deficiency: hormonal reference data. J Clin Endocrinol Metab 1983;57:320–326.

14 New MI, Abraham M, Gonzales B, Dumic M, Razzaghy-Azar M, Chitayat D, Sun L, Zaidi M, Wilson RC, Yuen T: Genotype-phenotype correlation in 1,507 families with congenital adrenal hyperplasia owing to 21-hydroxylase deficiency. Proc Natl Acad Sci USA 2013;110:2611–2616.

15 Harada F, Kimura A, Iwanaga T, Shomizawa K, Yata J, Sasazuki T: Gene conversion-like events cause steroid 21-hydroxylase deficiency in congenital adrenal hyperplasia. Proc Natl Acad Sci USA 1987;84:8091–8094.

16 Haider S, Islam B, D'Atri V, Sgobba M, Poojari C, Sun L, Yuen T, Zaidi M, New MI: Structure-phenotype correlations of human CYP21A2 mutations in congenital adrenal hyperplasia. Proc Natl Acad Sci USA 2013;110:2605–2610.

17 Massimi A, Malaponti M, Federici L, Vinciguerra D, Manca Bitti ML, Vottero A, Ghizzoni L, Maccarrone M, Cappa M, Bernardini S, Porzio O: Functional and structural analysis of four novel mutations of CYP21A2 gene in Italian patients with 21-hydroxylase deficiency. Horm Metab Res 2014;46:515–520.

18 Speiser PW, Azziz R, Baskin LS, Ghizzoni L, Hensle TW, Merke DP, Meyer-Bahlburg HF, Miller WL, Montori VW, Oberfield SE, Ritzen M, White PC; Endocrine Society: Congenital adrenal hyperplasia due to steroid 21-hydroxylase deficiency: an Endocrine Society clinical practice guideline. J Clin Endocrinol Metab 2010;95:4133–4160.

19 Bonfig W, Bechtold S, Schmidt H, Knorr D, Schwarz HP: Reduced final height outcome in congenital adrenal hyperplasia under prednisone treatment: deceleration of growth velocity during puberty. J Clin Endocrinol Metab 2007;92:1635–1639.

20 Rivkees SA, Stephenson K: Low-dose dexamethasone therapy from infancy of virilizing congenital adrenal hyperplasia. Int J Pediatr Endocrinol 2009;2009:274682.

21 Rivkees SA, Crawford JD: Dexamethasone treatment of virilizing congenital adrenal hyperplasia: the ability to achieve normal growth. Pediatrics 2000;106:767–773.

22 Rivkees SA: Dexamethasone therapy of congenital adrenal hyperplasia and the myth of the 'growth toxic' glucocorticoid. Int J Pediatr Endocrinol 2010;2010:569680.

23 Hindmarsh PC: The child with difficult to control congenital adrenal hyperplasia: is there a place for continuous subcutaneous hydrocortisone therapy. Clin Endocrinol (Oxf) 2014;81:15–18.

24 Verma S, Vanryzin C, Sinaii N, Kim SM, Nieman LK, Ravindran S, Calis KA, Arlt W, Ross RJ, Merke DP: A pharmacokinetic and pharmacodynamic study of delayed- and extended-release hydrocortisone (Chronocort) vs. conventional hydrocortisone (Cortef) in the treatment of congenital adrenal hyperplasia. Clin Endocrinol (Oxf) 2010;72:441–447.

25 Reichman DE, White PC, New MI, Rosenwaks Z: Fertility in patients with congenital adrenal hyperplasia. Fertil Steril 2014;101:301–309.

26 Trinh L, Nimkarn S, New MI, Lin-Su K: Growth and pubertal characteristics in patients with congenital adrenal hyperplasia due to 21-hydroxylase deficiency. J Pediatr Endocrinol Metab 2007;20:883–891.

27 Premawardhana LD, Hughes IA, Read GF, Scanlon MF: Longer term outcome in females with congenital adrenal hyperplasia (CAH): the Cardiff experience. Clin Endocrinol (Oxf) 1997;46:327–332.

28 New MI: Nonclassical congenital adrenal hyperplasia and the polycystic ovarian syndrome. Ann NY Acad Sci 1993;687:193–205.

29 Auchus RJ, Arlt W: Approach to the patient: the adult with congenital adrenal hyperplasia. J Clin Endocrinol Metab 2013;98:2645–2655.

30 Jaaskelainen J, Voutilainen R: Growth of patients with 21-hydroxylase deficiency: an analysis of the factors influencing adult height. Pediatr Res 1997;41:30–33.

31 New MI, Gertner JM, Speiser PW, del Balzo P: Growth and final height in classical and nonclassical 21-hydroxylase deficiency. Acta Paediatr Jpn 1988;30(suppl):79–88.

32 Lin-Su K, Harbison MD, Lekarev O, Vogiatzi MG, New MI: Final adult height in children with congenital adrenal hyperplasia treated with growth hormone. J Clin Endocrinol Metab 2011;96:1710–1717.

33 Wit JM, Hero M, Nunez SB: Aromatase inhibitors in pediatrics. Nat Rev Endocrinol 2012;8:135–147.
34 Prader A: Genital findings in the female pseudo-hermaphroditism of the congenital adrenogenital syndrome; morphology, frequency, development and heredity of the different genital forms (in German). Helv Paediatr Acta 1954;9:231–248.
35 Crouch NS, Liao LM, Woodhouse CR, Conway GS, Creighton SM: Sexual function and genital sensitivity following feminizing genitoplasty for congenital adrenal hyperplasia. J Urol 2008;179:634–638.
36 Nordenstrom A, Frisen L, Falhammar H, Filipsson H, Holmdahl G, Janson PO, Thoren M, Hagenfeldt K, Nordenskjold A: Sexual function and surgical outcome in women with congenital adrenal hyperplasia due to CYP21A2 deficiency: clinical perspective and the patients' perception. J Clin Endocrinol Metab 2010;95:3633–3640.
37 Poppas DP, Hochsztein AA, Baergen RN, Loyd E, Chen J, Felsen D: Nerve sparing ventral clitoroplasty preserves dorsal nerves in congenital adrenal hyperplasia. J Urol 2007;178:1802–1806; discussion 1806.
38 Rink RC, Metcalfe PD, Cain MP, Meldrum KK, Kaefer MA, Casale AJ: Use of the mobilized sinus with total urogenital mobilization. J Urol 2006;176:2205–2211.
39 Zainuddin AA, Grover SR, Shamsuddin K, Mahdy ZA: Research on quality of life in female patients with congenital adrenal hyperplasia and issues in developing nations. J Pediatr Adolesc Gynecol 2013;26: 296–304.
40 David M, Forest MG: Prenatal treatment of congenital adrenal hyperplasia resulting from 21-hydroxylase deficiency. J Pediatr 1984;105:799–803.
41 Speiser PW, Laforgia N, Kato K, Pareira J, Khan R, Yang SY, et al: First trimester prenatal treatment and molecular genetic diagnosis of congenital adrenal hyperplasia (21-hydroxylase deficiency). J Clin Endocrinol Metab 1990;70:838–848.
42 New MI, Abraham M, Yuen T, Lekarev O: An update on prenatal diagnosis and treatment of congenital adrenal hyperplasia. Semin Reprod Med 2012;30: 396–399.
43 Forest MG, David M, Morel Y: Prenatal diagnosis and treatment of 21-hydroxylase deficiency. J Steroid Biochem Mol Biol 1993;45:75–82.
44 Hirvikoski T, Nordenstrom A, Wedell A, Ritzen M, Lajic S: Prenatal dexamethasone treatment of children at risk for congenital adrenal hyperplasia: the Swedish experience and standpoint. J Clin Endocrinol Metab 2012;97:1881–1883.
45 Meyer-Bahlburg HF, Dolezal C, Haggerty R, Silverman M, New MI: Cognitive outcome of offspring from dexamethasone-treated pregnancies at risk for congenital adrenal hyperplasia due to 21-hydroxylase deficiency. Eur J Endocrinol 2012;167:103–110.
46 Dreger A, Feder EK, Tamar-Mattis A: Prenatal dexamethasone for congenital adrenal hyperplasia: an ethics canary in the modern medical mine. J Bioeth Inq 2012;9:277–294.
47 New MI: Vindication of prenatal diagnosis and treatment of congenital adrenal hyperplasia with low-dose dexamethasone. Am J Bioeth 2010;10:67–68.
48 Mancenido D, New MI: The history of prenatal diagnosis of congenital adrenal hyperplasia; in New MI (ed): Genetic Steroid Disorders. San Francisco, Elsevier, 2014, pp 53–62.
49 Speiser PW, Dupont J, Zhu D, Serrat J, Buegeleisen M, Tusie-Luna MT, Lesser M, New MI, White PC: Disease expression and molecular genotype in congenital adrenal hyperplasia due to 21-hydroxylase deficiency. J Clin Invest 1992;90:584–595.
50 Tardy-Guidollet V, Menassa R, Costa JM, David M, Bouvattier-Morel C, Baumann C, Houang M, Lorenzini F, Philip N, Odent S, Guichet A, Morel Y: New management strategy of pregnancies at risk of congenital adrenal hyperplasia using fetal sex determination in maternal serum: French cohort of 258 cases (2002–2011). J Clin Endocrinol Metab 2014;99: 1180–1188.
51 New MI, Tong YK, Yuen T, Jiang P, Pina C, Chan KC, Khattab A, Liao GJ, Yau M, Kim SM, Chiu RW, Sun L, Zaidi M, Lo YM: Noninvasive prenatal diagnosis of congenital adrenal hyperplasia using cell-free fetal DNA in maternal plasma. J Clin Endocrinol Metab 2014;96:E1022–E1030.

Prof. Maria New, MD, PhD
Icahn School of Medicine at Mount Sinai
One Gustave L. Levy Place, Box 1198
New York, NY 10029 (USA)
E-Mail maria.new@mssm.edu

Arvat E, Falorni A (eds): Cortisol Excess and Insufficiency.
Front Horm Res. Basel, Karger, 2016, vol 46, pp 196–210 (DOI: 10.1159/000443920)

Adrenal Insufficiency Therapy: How to Keep the Balance between Good Quality of Life and Low Risk for Long-Term Side Effects?

Katerina Simunkova · Eystein S. Husebye

Department of Clinical Science, University of Bergen, Bergen, Norway

Abstract

Glucocorticoid treatment in adrenal insufficiency remains a challenge since many patients complain of fatigue, reduced health-related quality of life and working ability. Moreover, there is a fear of increased mortality and morbidity related to adrenal crises and chronic overexposure to glucocorticoids. In order to counter these negative effects on daily life and future health, recent recommendations speak for lower replacement doses and administration forms that attempt to mimic the circadian variation in cortisol. At the same time, low replacement doses should not put the patient at an increased risk of an adrenal crisis. This chapter provides an overview of current state-of-the-art approaches to treatment and follow-up of adrenal insufficiency aimed at avoiding over- and undertreatment.

Without treatment, 80% of patients with primary adrenal insufficiency (PAI) die within 2 years, and all die within 5 years after diagnosis [1]. This was the situation until Kendall and Reichstein introduced hydrocortisone (HC) and later fludrocortisone in 1950s. Since then, replacement therapy in PAI has been virtually unchanged until the recent introduction of long-acting HC (Plenadren) [2]. Its development was prompted by the appreciation that health-related subjective health status (HRQoL) and working ability was reduced in PAI patients [3], and that current replacement therapy did not mimic the circadian variation in cortisol secretion very well.

Diagnostic procedures, treatment and management of PAI vary considerably within Europe [4]. Still, untimely mortality in adrenal crisis, reduced subjective health status and diminished working capacity are major issues [5, 6]. Being a rare disease,

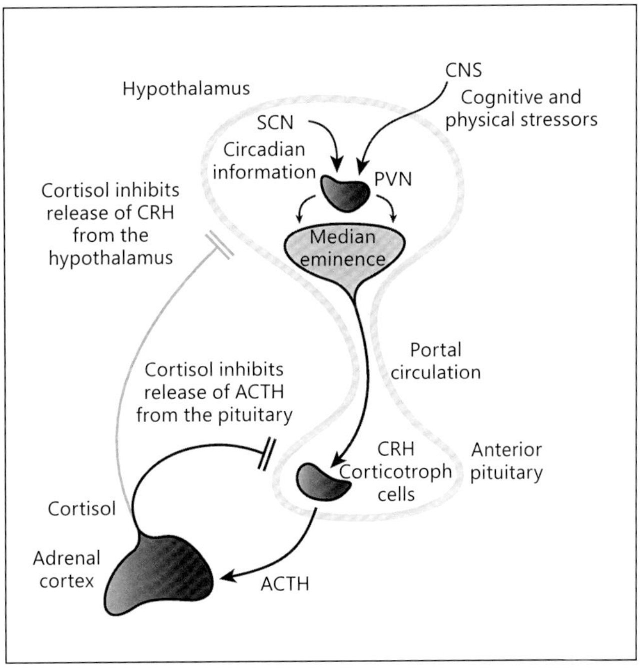

Fig. 1. Regulation of the HPA axis (from [17]). CRH = Corticotrophin-releasing hormone; SCN = Suprachiasmatic nucleus; PVN = paraventricular nucleus

there is a lack of controlled studies addressing the natural course of PAI and its treatment. Those available are generally small and short-term [7], and not double-blind [8, 9]. Only general recommendations are available regarding stress doses of glucocorticoids, based mostly on empirical knowledge [4]. Likewise, follow-up routines and patient education is often not performed according to any standardized scheme.

Studies on the physiology of the hypothalamic-pituitary-adrenal axis (HPA) in rats and humans have shown that cortisol secretion occurs in pulses. This ultradian pulsing superimposed on the circadian wave directly influences glucocorticoid-mediated gene transcription [10, 11]. Abrogation of these finely tuned rhythms by shift work and frequent travelling through time zones can lead to sleep disturbances and even predispose to cardiovascular disease and cancer [12–14]. These findings hint to the need for near-physiological replacement therapy in PAI both in terms of doses and how and when they are administered.

The Hypothalamic-Pituitary-Adrenal Axis

Cortisol is produced and secreted by the adrenal glands under strict control by the pituitary gland and hypothalamus [15]. The HPA axis works as a feedback loop mechanism with a natural inbuilt delay [16]. The pituitary gland may be activated by several stimuli and releases corticotrophin-releasing hormone (CRH) and vasopressin

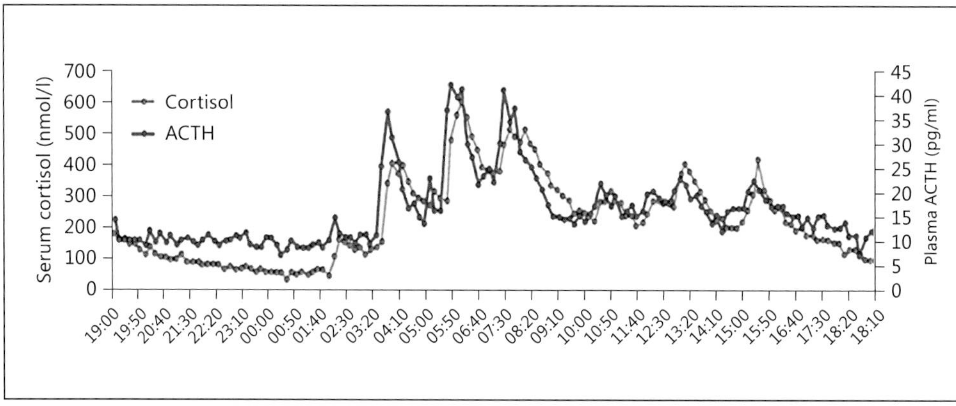

Fig. 2. Circadian and ultradian variation of human cortisol and ACTH in blood samples (from [21]).

into the hypothalamic-pituitary portal circulation. Acting on the corticotroph cells in the pituitary gland, CRH and vasopressin releases adrenocorticotropic hormone (ACTH) into the circulation, which acts on the adrenal cortex to produce and secrete glucocorticoids, including cortisol. By feeding back on the pituitary gland, cortisol inhibits ACTH and CRH release and thus its own production [17] (fig. 1). Under normal circumstances serum cortisol begins to rise in the latter part of the night and reaches a peak between 7:00 and 9:00 a.m. in the morning. Levels then fall during the day, reaching a nadir in the late evening at bedtime [18]; however, these levels are influenced by stressful events and stress intensity, and show large individual variation [19, 20].

Superimposed on this circadian rhythm is an ultradian oscillation of ACTH and cortisol, producing a series of pulses of varying amplitude at a frequency of approximately 1 pulse/h (fig. 2) [21]. Monitoring the cortisol production rate by deconvolution analysis has revealed that production rates of cortisol are between 5.7 and 9.9 mg/m^2 per day [22], which is the equivalent of a daily dose of 15–20 mg of HC.

At the cellular level, glucocorticoid ultradian oscillations induce 'gene pulsing' through rapid, transient binding of glucocorticoids to their receptors, thereby regulating gene transcription [10, 23, 24]. This dynamic and versatile transcriptional system enables cells to rapidly detect and respond to changes in circulating glucocorticoid levels and provides a sensitive mechanism for the maintenance of homeostasis by differential regulation of hundreds of genes in response to either high or low concentrations of cortisol [21]. Glucocorticoid receptor activity can be tuned to different doses of glucocorticoids in a tissue-specific manner, potentially in order to regulate expression of specific genes at different points in the circadian cycle. When the glucocorticoid rhythm is the result of pharmacological replacement, abnormal gene expression could be the consequence, leading to desensitization of physiological and behavioural responses to stress [25]. For example, administering cortisol in the evening instead of the morning decreases insulin sensitivity [26].

Taken together, the HPA axis is a highly dynamic and versatile regulatory system with the ability to rapidly fine-tune cortisol levels to current challenges, which is difficult to mimic by replacement therapy.

Quality of Life

Earlier it was considered that patients with adrenal insufficiency did fairly well once they were diagnosed and treated. Løvås et al. [3] did the first systematic assessment of HRQoL in PAI using the generic questionnaire Short-Form Health Survey (SF-36) and a fatigue questionnaire. The results revealed reduced general health and vitality, as well as reduced physical function in females. While many patients scored normally, a substantial group had reduced HRQoL. The vitality scores placed PAI patients somewhere between patients with congestive heart failure and type 2 diabetes mellitus [3]. Polyendocrinopathy was associated with lower scores. In addition, it was found that working ability was reduced as the number of persons receiving disability pension was 2.5 times higher. These findings have been replicated and expanded in a number of populations with very similar findings [6, 27–30]. Bleicken et al. [31] found that the reduced HRQoL was independent of type of medication regardless of whether HC, cortisone acetate (CA) or prednisolone was used. Changes in number of daily doses attempting to closely mimic the diurnal rhythm provided only short improvement [32]. Patients preferred 3 over 2 daily doses and 4 daily doses over 3, but a higher number of doses increased non-compliance. Those on daily doses of HC above 30 mg had significantly impaired HRQoL [32, 33], which could reflect a negative effect of HC per se or the fact that an increased dose was prescribed to try to amend symptoms of adrenal insufficiency. High replacement doses are associated with psychological morbidity and maladaptive personality traits [33]. However, HRQoL in patients on relatively low replacement doses according to current recommendations are also reduced, indicating that the quality of the treatment, and not the dosing, is a major reason [34]. Delayed diagnosis also seemed to be a factor adversely affecting HRQoL in adrenal insufficiency [30].

There are several potential explanations for the reduced HRQoL. The leading hypothesis has been that current replacement regimens are unable to mimic the dynamics in cortisol secretion. This is supported by observations of some improvement in HRQoL when more physiological treatment modalities such as extended-release HC were used [2, 35, 36] (see below). Another explanation is the lack of dehydroepiandrosterone (DHEA) [37], which could explain why HRQoL is lower in women compared to men [3]. Disappointingly, studies of DHEA treatment in PAI have only had small effects or none on HRQoL parameters [38]. In addition, the patient's perception of the disease, its medication and concerns for long-term complications may also have a negative impact on HRQoL [33, 39].

Most of the surveys of QoL in PAI have been performed with generic questionnaires that are not specific for any particular disease. Recently, an Addison's disease-specific questionnaire was developed called 'AddiQoL-30', which has been validated in a number of European populations [3, 35]. It has been used to assess replacement therapy [36, 40, 41] and to monitor treatment with Plenadren [41], and might be more sensitive to treatment-specific effects in PAI than the generic questionnaires.

Mortality and Long-Term Side Effects

It is well known among physicians who treat patients with PAI that untimely deaths occur in adrenal crisis. Sometimes these patients die undiagnosed, and the diagnosis is made only after death [42]. A national survey in Norway revealed that in two thirds of the cases, the diagnosis was made only after the patient developed an adrenal crisis [5, 43]. Also, after diagnosis, death in adrenal crises is not uncommon [43, 44].

What is more unclear is if mortality is increased due to other factors. A Swedish population study concluded that PAI patients had a 2-fold increased mortality rate due to increased cardiovascular, malignant and infectious diseases; the highest mortality rate was observed in patients who were diagnosed with PAI in childhood [45]. The combination of PAI and type 1 diabetes, found in about 10% of the patients in Scandinavia, increased mortality rates [45]. A follow-up study of the same registry with an expanded observation period reproduced the overall increased mortality rate, but found that cancer deaths were not increased when those diagnosed the first year after PAI were excluded [46]. In contrast, a much smaller case study from Norway did not find an overall increased mortality rate; only for young men was an increment seen, which was most probably due to adrenal crises [43]. Whether overall mortality in PAI is increased or not is still unresolved.

Both the Swedish and Norwegian surveys of PAI revealed daily replacement doses of around 30 mg of HC equivalents per day, which is above the current recommendations (see below). A few small studies have found that Addison's patients have a more unfavourable lipid profile [47, 48], but the changes are subtle. These studies were small, and one used blood donors as controls [49]. There might be genetic or other lifestyle factors involved since Swedish patients using a higher daily dose of HC had a more favourable lipid profile than South African patients [47]. However, the fact that patients on near physiological replacement doses (20 mg/per day) had no changes in lipids as opposed to those on higher doses hints to an impact of the glucocorticoid dose [50]. The altered non-genomic effects of HC caused by non-physiological doses and ways of administration may contribute to an increased cardiovascular risk [51], but this remains speculative at the moment.

Exposure to a higher dose of HC given in the afternoon hours causes a reduction in insulin sensitivity 4–6 h later as demonstrated by a study which gave 50 mg of HC orally in the afternoon [26], which suggests that a dose reduction alone is not enough;

Table 1. Treatment of adrenal insufficiency in major stresses (adapted from [4]).

Procedure	Preoperative needs	Postoperative needs
Major surgery with long recovery time	100 mg of hydrocortisone i.m. just before anaesthesia	Continue 100 mg of hydrocortisone i.m. every 6 h until able to eat and drink; then double oral dose for 48+ h, then taper to normal dose
Major surgery with rapid recovery	100 mg of hydrocortisone i.m. just before anaesthesia	Continue 100 mg of hydrocortisone i.m. every 6 h for 24-48 h; then double oral dose for 24–48 h, then taper to normal dose
Labour and vaginal birth	100 mg of hydrocortisone i.m. just at onset of labour	Double oral dose for 24-48 h after delivery, then taper to normal dose
Minor surgery and major dental surgery	100 mg of hydrocortisone i.m. just before anaesthesia	Double oral dose for 24 h, then return to normal dose
Invasive bowel procedures requiring laxatives	Hospital admission overnight with 100 mg of hydrocortisone i.m. and fluid, repeat dose before start of procedure	Double oral dose for 24 h, then return to normal dose
Other invasive procedures	100 mg of hydrocortisone i.m. just before start of procedure	Double oral dose for 24 h, then return to normal dose
Minor procedure	Usually not required	Extra dose (e.g. 20 mg of hydrocortisone) if symptoms are present
Dental procedure	Extra morning dose 1 h prior to surgery	Double oral dose for 24 h, then return to normal dose
Minor dental procedure	Usually not required	Extra dose (e.g. 20 mg of hydrocortisone) if symptoms are present

when and how the dose is administered could also be decisive. The pattern of HC delivery and the cortisol exposure-time profile may therefore be as crucial for patient outcome as the total daily dose since the hyperglycaemic effect of HC is dependent on interaction with hepatic clock genes and therefore follow a circadian pattern [52]. Using Plenadren reduced 24-hour cortisol exposure by approximately 20% compared to conventional treatment and was associated with a significant reduction in HbA1c compared to thrice-daily treatment [2].

On the other hand, lack of cortisol might increase the risk of hypoglycaemic episodes particularly in patients with type 1 diabetes. Whether glycaemia in the lower level of the reference range may contribute to fatigue remains a question. Some studies have recommended a regular diet regimen and to avoid starvation [53].

Since current glucocorticoid replacement results in large fluctuations in the cortisol levels directly influencing glucose homeostasis, concomitant diabetes mellitus may prove difficult to regulate. This is supported by a German study showing an increased insulin requirement and a tendency towards an increased frequency of severe hypoglycaemia in patients with both Addison's disease and type 1 diabetes as compared to patients with type 1 diabetes alone. Treatment by insulin pump in patients with PAI may be advantageous as insulin administration can then be coordinated with HC dosing. However, more studies are needed to better understand the relationship between cortisol and insulin.

Another feared complication of treatment is osteoporosis. The largest case study to date on Norwegian and British patients showed reduced bone mineral density, but not increased vertebral fractures, in Norwegian patients aged 50 years and older. In contrast, a Swedish population study found a 2-fold increased risk of hip fractures in PAI patients [54]. The fracture risk was highest around the time of diagnosis of PAI (a 4-fold increase) and then decreased; 5 years after diagnosis the hazard ratio was 1.3, indicating that other factors besides replacement therapy were at work. There is not a huge risk of osteoporosis at recommended replacement doses of HC, but bone mineral density should be measured and followed. Use of synthetic and long-acting glucocorticoids such as prednisolone and dexamethasone increases the risk [55].

Taken together, PAI is complicated by an increased risk of mortality in adrenal crises. Whether overall mortality is increased, and what the impact of glucocorticoid treatment is on long-term mortality and morbidity needs further studies.

Replacement Therapy

Basal Replacement Therapy

As a patient with type 1 diabetes needs basal-bolus treatment with insulin, a patient with PAI needs basal and stress treatment with corticosteroids. Conventional treatment consists of multiple daily doses of HC or CA aiming to replace the natural circadian rhythm of cortisol. In addition, the mineralocorticoid fludrocortisone is given to replace the lack of aldosterone. Due to the short half-life of HC and CA, conventional treatment regimens result in several periods of over- and undertreatment over the day [2, 56–58] (fig. 2).

HC is most widely used. It is absorbed rapidly and reaches maximum serum concentrations within 1 h after administration. To comply with circadian variation, the largest dose is given in the morning. On a twice-daily regimen, the next dose is administered in the afternoon around 4:00 p.m., while, on thrice-daily HC, the next doses are given around lunch and in the late afternoon, although not later than 4 h before bed time [56]. Patients particularly affected by morning fatigue could try to administer the first dose while in bed and delay the morning routines by 30–60 min.

An average daily dose of 20 mg of HC or 25 mg of CA is able to produce a cortisol day curve within the normal range [59, 60]. Weight-adjustment of doses improves compliance with the normal range and reduces variability between individuals [61]. However, the thrice-, and in particular the twice, daily regimen gives high peaks and low troughs; the former overwhelms the binding capacity to cortisol-binding globulin, leading to loss of cortisol in urine, and the latter might explain day-time fatigue observed in some patients. Thus, even 4 or 5 doses can be tried if the patient is motivated, which could produce a cortisol serum profile mimicking both circadian and ultradian variations. Actually, patients on 4 daily doses reported better well-being than patients on the common twice-daily replacement regimen in the only double-blind placebo-controlled study to date comparing different dosing regimens using established HRQoL instruments [29]. They found that patients scored better on HRQoL questionnaires after 4-dose treatment compared to 2-dose treatment, and the majority preferred the 4-dose regimen [29]. In support of this, patients on a thrice-daily regimen were more satisfied with their treatment compared to those on twice- or once-daily treatments [62]. However, multiple dosing was seen as problematic, with the major complaint of patients being the necessity to adjust daily activity to the multiple-dose treatment [33, 39].

CA is less frequently used, but in some countries it is the only available glucocorticoid [63]. CA necessitates activation by 11β-hydroxysteroid dehydrogenase type 1 to cortisol [64, 65]. Several factors may affect the conversion and decrease bioavailability of the cortisol, such as growth hormone treatment that reduces the conversion [66]. Unlike HC, however, CA has a longer half-life, reaching the maximum in blood slightly later and with a lower peak than HC, which could be beneficial, especially on a twice-daily regimen. Unfortunately, no head-to-head comparison of CA and HC has been performed so far. Many patients in Norway still use 25 mg of CA in the morning and 12.5 mg in the evening, which according to new assessments is overdosing [4]. Recently, an Australian study described a higher risk of adrenal crises after swapping CA for HC and adjustment according to the current dose recommendation [63]. This retrospective study along with poor management of AC described recently by Hahner et al. [67] underpins a possible pitfall of current dose recommendations.

In an attempt to improve the reduced HRQoL and fatigue felt by many patients and to simplify treatment, Johannsson et al. [2] developed a new extended-release formulation of HC. The Plenadren tablet consists of the outer layer of rapidly releasable HC and a core providing extended release over the next 12–18 h. The only controlled clinical trial comparing once-daily Plenadren with conventional thrice-daily HC revealed 20% lower cortisol exposure on once-daily extended release compared to conventional treatment. Plenadren treatment also lowered body weight, blood pressure and HbA1c values both in non-diabetic and diabetic patients [2]. HRQoL also improved and the participants preferred Plenadren treatment. The latter data should be interpreted with caution since the study was not blinded [2]. These overall promising results have been followed up by an extended prospective observational study documenting excellent safety of Plenadren over a 2-year period [68]. Furthermore, another prospective observational study (median: 202 days) with 26 patients revealed decreased BMI and HbA1c [41]. In conclusion, Plenadren provides a new, safe and simplified treatment concept in adrenal insufficiency, but more studies are needed to document its superiority – and compared to the physiological oscillatory ultradian rhythm, it might not be so physiological after all.

Despite rapidly providing high circulating levels of cortisol, Plenadren (like regular HC) is unable to mimic the late night rise in cortisol. Chronocort was developed to address this problem. By delaying drug release by about 4 h, it can be taken at bedtime and provide increased cortisol levels in the latter part of the night and early morning hours with peak concentrations 8 h after intake [69]. This type of pharmacokinetics could be especially useful for treatment of congenital adrenal hyperplasia where ACTH suppression is important to avoid hyperandrogenism. Thus, by applying a so-called 'tooth brush' regimen with twice-daily Chronocort taken at bedtime and in the early morning, improved ACTH suppression and reduced androgen precursors levels were seen compared to conventional treatment in congenital adrenal hyperplasia [70].

In another alternative to improve 24-hour cortisol coverage and an attempt to avoid administering cortisol by way of the portal circulation, we introduced continuous subcutaneous HC infusion [71]. In a clinical trial comparing continuous subcutaneous HC infusion and conventional HC treatment, the circadian cortisol rhythm was restored and ACTH normalized in many patients [36]. The continuous administration of cortisol even enabled the use of ACTH as a biomarker for dosing. An improvement of HRQoL was also observed, but a similar effect was not seen in another double-blind placebo-controlled study of subcutaneous pump treatment [40]. However, this might be due to high HRQoL scores in the study population being similar to the background population. Pump treatment is cumbersome and costly, and should be reserved for those who function very poorly on conventional or extended-release medication. In the near future, we might learn if pulsatile subcutaneous cortisol infusion mimicking ultradian cortisol variation could be a suitable way of replacing glucocorticoids. Russell et al. [72] showed that it is possible to create cortisol pulses every 3 h in dexamethasone-suppressed healthy volunteers. Development of smarter and smaller pumps would ease the use and hopefully reduce the costs.

Synthetic glucocorticoids such as prednisolone and dexamethasone are long-acting and still in use, especially in the United States [62]. The major problem, especially with dexamethasone, is Cushingoid side effects, and they also lack a mineralocorticoid effect. Prednisolone has a pharmacokinetic profile reminiscent of Plenadren and might provide a cheap alternative.

Mineralocorticoid replacement is quite often underestimated and insufficient [73]. In cases of increased demand for mineralocorticoids, such as hot climate or profound sweating, the mineralocorticoid dosage has to be adjusted. It is important to give sufficient mineralocorticoids to avoid electrolyte disturbances and hypotension. Adequate mineralocorticoid replacement is probably important to normalize HRQoL.

Taken together, promising new and safe alternatives have been added to the treatment tool box that seems to improve HRQoL in patients with PAI, but more and longer studies are needed.

Treatment during Stress

The adrenal gland releases cortisol in response to stress events to meet the enhanced metabolic demands of the organism and to regulate the immune response. The degree of cortisol response to stress depends on the intensity of the stressor (table 1). Current recommendations on stress dosing in adrenal insufficiency are linked to surgical stress [74] (table 1). In severe stress such as abdominal surgery, severe trauma and sepsis, it is recommended to start with 100 mg intravenously, followed by 100–400 mg/24 h [4]. Sustained delivery of doses such as 400 mg/day can create severe hypokalaemia due to the mineralocorticoid effect of HC and should be avoided. In keeping with this, the daily requirement, even during acute stress is probably around 200 mg for most individuals based on calculation of the maximal output of cortisol from the adrenal cortex [75, 76]. Thus, the daily dose should be doubled or tripled as long as the illness lasts, tapering towards regular replacement doses as the condition improves [4, 77, 78]. Similar dosing as in acute stress is recommended when a patient has diarrhoea and vomiting since the oral route is compromised, and without parenteral replacement they can rapidly develop a severe adrenal crisis [79].

While there is general agreement on dosing in severe stress, the best way to tackle mild everyday stress is more controversial. Many patients take frequent extra doses before physical exercise, a stressful meeting or when they feel fatigued, and experience being energized. Others can run a marathon without taking an extra dose. If extra dosing is almost a daily event, it adds to the regular replacement dosing and may lead to overdosing. Currently, no data are available regarding the benefits of stress dosing in this setting, and it is important that the treating physician discuss this with the patients, emphasizing the need to keep stress dosing at a reasonable level.

On the other hand, poor and inadequate treatment of stressful events can lead to adrenal crises [44]. Knowledge about precipitating conditions, early recognition of imminent adrenal crises, availability of glucocorticoids for parenteral use and capability to cope with imminent adrenal crises have been shown to be decisive factors in the outcome [44]. The most important precipitating factors are infections, mainly in the gastrointestinal tract with vomiting and diarrhoea. Unfortunately, many patients still experience that physicians refuse to treat them in an acute situation [67]. Therefore, education not merely of patients and their relatives, but also for care providers is important [80]. Currently, a European emergency card is being implemented in many countries in Europe, and more are following suit [81]. In addition, all patients should be provided with an emergency kit for self-administration of HC [4]. Development of convenient administration of HC in a pen would ease emergency treatment in the future.

Monitoring and Follow-Up

The ideal parameter to monitor glucocorticoid replacement in adrenal insufficiency is lacking. ACTH is only useful when pump treatment is used [36]. Thus, evaluation is based on clinical judgement. The annual regular follow-up relies on clinical evaluation of signs of over- and undertreatment and questions about physical performance and subjective health status.

Whilst recognition of overt overtreatment is quite simple and includes weight gain, the signs of undertreatment are rather unspecific. The current treatment strategy is to find the lowest dose of HC that does not result in symptoms and signs of adrenal insufficiency or put the patient at risk for an adrenal crisis.

History should focus on how the patient tackles professional and private life, energy levels, sleep quality, and daytime sleepiness. Fatigue, weight loss, nausea, joint and muscle pain, hyperpigmentation, salt craving, and orthostatism are symptoms and signs of insufficient medication. Weight gain is a sign of overtreatment. It is important to map how often and in what situations extra doses are taken. Measurement of weight and blood pressure (sitting and standing) is recommended, and evaluation of pigmentation is obligatory. Whether the use of AddiQoL is useful to monitor treatment remains to be seen.

How to tackle an adrenal crisis should be a theme at every annual visit. Re-education of patients and their relatives is essential to decrease the mortality in adrenal crises. Patients' self-help groups can play an important role in education and well-being, providing a forum for discussion and exchange of knowledge. A recent survey on the psychological aspects of adrenal insufficiency revealed that the majority of PAI patients 'hated' and did not trust their treatment, and were worried about side effects of HC [39]. The study emphasizes the importance of a thorough explanation of the basis of the disease, providing a clear rationale for HC treatment and dosage. In some patients, regular psychological support is justified.

A single blood test of either cortisol or ACTH is not helpful since levels are very dependent on when medication is taken. If there is uncertainty as to whether ingested HC or CA is taken up and sufficiently absorbed, or if the patient is non-compliant, a serum or salivary day curve could be useful [82]. It has been suggested that weight-adjusted treatment monitored by a single cortisol measurement 4 h after morning medication might be useful [61].

Urinary cortisol is less suitable. The saturation threshold of cortisol-binding globulin causes marked fluctuation in the free faction of cortisol [83]. Moreover, urinary free cortisol does not reflect changes of HC throughout the day, which is probably important for the patient's well-being.

Since endocrine comorbidities are very common in PAI, annual tests for autoimmune thyroid disease, diabetes, and vitamin B_{12} and iron deficiencies should be performed. Females should be informed of the risk of premature ovarian insufficiency.

Conclusions

Without treatment PAI is a lethal disease. Despite the lack of scientific evidence, current 'unphysiological' treatment is probably a major reason for reduced HRQoL and reduced working capacity. Notwithstanding these limitations, treatment should aim at daily replacement of 15–25 mg of HC for most patients, with occasional stress dosing when needed. The majority should be given fludrocortisone. A thorough annual evaluation focusing on how the disease and its treatment impacts daily life as well as education to tackle crises is important. Hopefully, future research will provide directions for improved treatment.

References

1 Dunlop D: Eighty-six cases of Addison's disease. Br Med J 1963;2:887–891.

2 Johannsson G, Nilsson AG, Bergthorsdottir R, Burman P, Dahlqvist P, Ekman B, Engström BE, Olsson T, Ragnarsson O, Ryberg M, Wahlberg J, Biller BM, Monson JP, Stewart PM, Lennernäs H, Skrtic S: Improved cortisol exposure-time profile and outcome in patients with adrenal insufficiency: a prospective randomized trial of a novel hydrocortisone dual-release formulation. J Clin Endocrinol Metab 2012;97: 473–481.

3 Løvås K, Loge JH, Husebye ES: Subjective health status in Norwegian patients with Addison's disease. Clin Endocrinol (Oxf) 2002;56:581–588.

4 Husebye ES, Allolio B, Arlt W, Badenhoop K, Bensing S, Betterle C, Falorni A, Gan EH, Hulting AL, Kasperlik-Zaluska A, Kämpe O, Løvås K, Meyer G, Pearce SH: Consensus statement on the diagnosis, treatment and follow-up of patients with primary adrenal insufficiency. J Intern Med 2014;275:104–115.

5 Erichsen MM, Løvås K, Skinningsrud B, Wolff AB, Undlien DE, Svartberg J, Fougner KJ, Berg TJ, Bollerslev J, Mella B, Carlson JA, Erlich H, Husebye ES: Clinical, immunological, and genetic features of autoimmune primary adrenal insufficiency: observations from a Norwegian registry. J Clin Endocrinol Metab 2009;94:4882–4890.

6 Hahner S, Loeffler M, Fassnacht M, Weismann D, Koschker AC, Quinkler M, Decker O, Arlt W, Allolio B: Impaired subjective health status in 256 patients with adrenal insufficiency on standard therapy based on cross-sectional analysis. J Clin Endocrinol Metab 2007;92:3912–3922.

7 Ekman B, Blomgren J, Andersson PO, Carlsson M, Arnqvist HJ: Variable sensitivity to the glucocorticoid activity of cortisol in patients with primary adrenal insufficiency: assessment with ACTH profiles. Horm Metab Res 2010;42:961–966.

8 Johannsson G, Falorni A, Skrtic S, Lennernäs H, Quinkler M, Monson JP, Stewart PM: Adrenal insufficiency: review of clinical outcomes with current glucocorticoid replacement therapy. Clin Endocrinol (Oxf) 2015;82:2–11.

9 Øksnes M, Ross R, Løvås K: Optimal glucocorticoid replacement in adrenal insufficiency. Best Pract Res Clin Endocrinol Metab 2015;29:3–15.

10 Stavreva DA, Wiench M, John S, Conway-Campbell BL, McKenna MA, Pooley JR, Johnson TA, Voss TC, Lightman SL, Hager GL: Ultradian hormone stimulation induces glucocorticoid receptor-mediated pulses of gene transcription. Nat Cell Biol 2009;11: 1093–1102.

11 Matthews L, Johnson J, Berry A, Trebble P, Cookson A, Spiller D, Rivers C, Norman M, White M, Ray D: Cell cycle phase regulates glucocorticoid receptor function. PLoS One 2011;6:e22289.

12 Ekstrand K, Boström PA, Arborelius M, Nilsson JA, Lindell SE: Cardiovascular risk factors in commercial flight aircrew officers compared with those in the general population. Angiology 1996;47:1089–1094.

13 Scheer FA, Hilton MF, Mantzoros CS, Shea SA: Adverse metabolic and cardiovascular consequences of circadian misalignment. Proc Natl Acad Sci USA 2009;106:4453–4458.

14 Nader N, Ng SS, Lambrou GI, Pervanidou P, Wang Y, Chrousos GP, Kino T: AMPK regulates metabolic actions of glucocorticoids by phosphorylating the glucocorticoid receptor through p38 MAPK. Mol Endocrinol 2010;24:1748–1764.

15 Linthorst AC, Reul JM: Stress and the brain: solving the puzzle using microdialysis. Pharmacol Biochem Behav 2008;90:163–173.

16 Lightman SL, George CL: Steroid hormones in 2013: glucocorticoids: timing, binding and environment. Nat Rev Endocrinol 2014;10:71–72.

17 Walker JJ, Terry JR, Lightman SL: Origin of ultradian pulsatility in the hypothalamic-pituitary-adrenal axis. Proc Biol Sci 2010;277:1627–1633.

18 Knutsson U, Dahlgren J, Marcus C, Rosberg S, Brönnegård M, Stierna P, Albertsson-Wikland K: Circadian cortisol rhythms in healthy boys and girls: relationship with age, growth, body composition, and pubertal development. J Clin Endocrinol Metab 1997;82:536–540.

19 Raastad T, Bjoro T, Hallen J: Hormonal responses to high- and moderate-intensity strength exercise. Eur J Appl Physiol 2000;82:121–128.

20 Puterman E, O'Donovan A, Adler NE, Tomiyama AJ, Kemeny M, Wolkowitz OM, Epel E: Physical activity moderates effects of stressor-induced rumination on cortisol reactivity. Psychosom Med 2011;73: 604–611.

21 Lightman SL, Conway-Campbell BL: The crucial role of pulsatile activity of the HPA axis for continuous dynamic equilibration. Nat Rev Neurosci 2010; 11:710–718.

22 Esteban NV, Loughlin T, Yergey AL, Zawadzki JK, Booth JD, Winterer JC, Loriaux DL: Daily cortisol production rate in man determined by stable isotope dilution/mass spectrometry. J Clin Endocrinol Metab 1991;72:39–45.

23 Waite EJ, McKenna M, Kershaw Y, Walker JJ, Cho K, Piggins HD, Lightman SL: Ultradian corticosterone secretion is maintained in the absence of circadian cues. Eur J Neurosci 2012;36:3142–3150.

24 Conway-Campbell BL, Sarabdjitsingh RA, McKenna MA, Pooley JR, Kershaw YM, Meijer OC, De Kloet ER, Lightman SL: Glucocorticoid ultradian rhythmicity directs cyclical gene pulsing of the clock gene period 1 in rat hippocampus. J Neuroendocrinol 2010;22:1093–1100.

25 Sarabdjitsingh RA, Spiga F, Oitzl MS, Kershaw Y, Meijer OC, Lightman SL, de Kloet ER: Recovery from disrupted ultradian glucocorticoid rhythmicity reveals a dissociation between hormonal and behavioural stress responsiveness. J Neuroendocrinol 2010;22:862–871.

26 Plat L, Leproult R, L'Hermite-Baleriaux M, Fery F, Mockel J, Polonsky KS, Van Cauter E: Metabolic effects of short-term elevations of plasma cortisol are more pronounced in the evening than in the morning. J Clin Endocrinol Metab 1999;84:3082–3092.

27 Alonso N, Granada ML, Lucas A, Salinas I, Reverter J, Oriol A, Sanmarti A: Evaluation of two replacement regimens in primary adrenal insufficiency patients. Effect on clinical symptoms, health-related quality of life and biochemical parameters. J Endocrinol Invest 2004;25:449–454.

28 Bleicken B, Hahner S, Ventz M, Quinkler M: Delayed diagnosis of adrenal insufficiency is common: a cross-sectional study in 216 patients. Am J Med Sci 2010;339:525–531.

29 Ekman B, Bachrach-Lindström M, Lindström T, Wahlberg J, Blomgren J, Arnqvist HJ: A randomized, double-blind, crossover study comparing two- and four-dose hydrocortisone regimen with regard to quality of life, cortisol and ACTH profiles in patients with primary adrenal insufficiency. Clin Endocrinol (Oxf) 2012;77:18–25.

30 Meyer G, Hackemann A, Penna-Martinez M, Badenhoop K: What affects the quality of life in autoimmune Addison's disease? Horm Metab Res 2013;45: 92–95.

31 Bleicken B, Hahner S, Loeffler M, Ventz M, Allolio B, Quinkler M: Impaired subjective health status in chronic adrenal insufficiency: impact of different glucocorticoid replacement regimens. Eur J Endocrinol 2008;159:811–817.

32 Bleicken B, Hahner S, Loeffler M, Ventz M, Decker O, Allolio B, Quinkler M: Influence of hydrocortisone dosage scheme on health-related quality of life in patients with adrenal insufficiency. Clin Endocrinol (Oxf) 2010;72:297–304.

33 Tiemensma J, Andela CD, Kaptein AA, Romijn JA, van der Mast RC, Biermasz NR, Pereira AM: Psychological morbidity and impaired quality of life in patients with stable treatment for primary adrenal insufficiency: cross-sectional study and review of the literature. Eur J Endocrinol 2014;171:171–182.

34 Kluger N, Matikainen N, Sintonen H, Ranki A, Roine RP, Schalin-Jäntti C: Impaired health-related quality of life in Addison's disease – impact of replacement therapy, comorbidities and socio-economic factors. Clin Endocrinol (Oxf) 2014;81:511–518.

35 Øksnes M, Bensing S, Hulting AL, Kämpe O, Hackemann A, Meyer G, Badenhoop K, Betterle C, Parolo A, Giordano R, Falorni A, Papierska L, Jeske W, Kasperlik-Zaluska AA, Chatterjee VK, Husebye ES, Løvås K: Quality of life in European patients with Addison's disease: validity of the disease-specific questionnaire AddiQoL. J Clin Endocrinol Metab 2012;97:568–576.

36 Oksnes M, Björnsdottir S, Isaksson M, Methlie P, Carlsen S, Nilsen RM, Broman JE, Triebner K, Kämpe O, Hulting AL, Bensing S, Husebye ES, Løvås K: Continuous subcutaneous hydrocortisone infusion versus oral hydrocortisone replacement for treatment of Addison's disease: a randomized clinical trial. J Clin Endocrinol Metab 2014;99:1665–1674.

37 Gurnell EM, Hunt PJ, Curran SE, Conway CL, Pullenayegum EM, Huppert FA, Compston JE, Herbert J, Chatterjee VK: Long-term DHEA replacement in primary adrenal insufficiency: a randomized, controlled trial. J Clin Endocrinol Metab 2008;93:400–409.

38 Alkatib AA, Cosma M, Elamin MB, Erickson D, Swiglo BA, Erwin PJ, Montori VM: A systematic review and meta-analysis of randomized placebo-controlled trials of DHEA treatment effects on quality of life in women with adrenal insufficiency. J Clin Endocrinol Metab 2009;94:3676–3681.

39 Tiemensma J, Andela CD, Pereira AM, Romijn JA, Biermasz NR, Kaptein AA: Patients with adrenal insufficiency hate their medication: concerns and stronger beliefs about the necessity of hydrocortisone intake are associated with more negative illness perceptions. J Clin Endocrinol Metab 2014;99:3668–3676.

40 Gagliardi L, Nenke MA, Thynne TR, von der Borch J, Rankin WA, Henley DE, Sorbello J, Inder WJ, Torpy DJ: Continuous subcutaneous hydrocortisone infusion therapy in Addison's disease: a randomized, placebo-controlled clinical trial. J Clin Endocrinol Metab 2014;99:4149–4157.

41 Quinkler M, Miodini Nilsen R, Zopf K, Ventz M, Øksnes M: Modified-release hydrocortisone decreases BMI and HbA1c in patients with primary and secondary adrenal insufficiency. Eur J Endocrinol 2015;172:619–626.
42 Ringstad J, Rodge S, Løland W, Rode L: Rapidly fatal Addison's disease: three case reports. J Intern Med 1991;230:465–467.
43 Erichsen MM, Løvås K, Fougner KJ, Svartberg J, Hauge ER, Bollerslev J, Berg JP, Mella B, Husebye ES: Normal overall mortality rate in Addison's disease, but young patients are at risk of premature death. Eur J Endocrinol 2009;160:233–237.
44 Hahner S, Spinnler C, Fassnacht M, Burger-Stritt S, Lang K, Milovanovic D, Beuschlein F, Willenberg HS, Quinkler M, Allolio B: High incidence of adrenal crisis in educated patients with chronic adrenal insufficiency: a prospective study. J Clin Endocrinol Metab 2015;100:407–416.
45 Bergthorsdottir R, Leonsson-Zachrisson M, Odén A, Johannsson G: Premature mortality in patients with Addison's disease: a population-based study. J Clin Endocrinol Metab 2006;91:4849–4853.
46 Bensing S, Brandt L, Tabaroj F, Sjöberg O, Nilsson B, Ekbom A, Blomqvist P, Kämpe O: Increased death risk and altered cancer incidence pattern in patients with isolated or combined autoimmune primary adrenocortical insufficiency. Clin Endocrinol (Oxf) 2008;69:697–704.
47 Ross IL, Bergthorsdottir R, Levitt NS, Schatz DA, Johannsson G, Marais AD: Increased cardiovascular risk in South African patients with Addison's disease. Horm Metab Res 2013;45:905–910.
48 Giordano R, Marzotti S, Balbo M, Romagnoli S, Marinazzo E, Berardelli R, Migliaretti G, Benso A, Falorni A, Ghigo E, Arvat E: Metabolic and cardiovascular profile in patients with Addison's disease under conventional glucocorticoid replacement. J Endocrinol Invest 2009;32:917–923.
49 Ross IL, Bergthorsdottir R, Levitt N, Dave JA, Schatz D, Marais D, Johannsson G: Cardiovascular risk factors in patients with Addison's disease: a comparative study of South African and Swedish patients. PLoS One 2014;9:e90768.
50 Filipsson H, Monson JP, Koltowska-Häggström M, Mattsson A, Johannsson G: The impact of glucocorticoid replacement regimens on metabolic outcome and comorbidity in hypopituitary patients. J Clin Endocrinol Metab 2006;91:3954–3961.
51 Henley DE, Lightman SL: Cardio-metabolic consequences of glucocorticoid replacement: relevance of ultradian signalling. Clin Endocrinol (Oxf) 2014;80:621–628.
52 Bass J: Physiology: on time metabolism. Nature 2011;480:466–467.
53 Klement J, Hubold C, Cords H, Oltmanns KM, Hallschmid M, Born J, Lehnert H, Peters A: High-calorie glucose-rich food attenuates neuroglycopenic symptoms in patients with Addison's disease. J Clin Endocrinol Metab 2010;95:522–528.
54 Björnsdottir S, Sääf M, Bensing S, Kämpe O, Michaëlsson K, Ludvigsson JF: Risk of hip fracture in Addison's disease: a population-based cohort study. J Intern Med 2011;270:187–195.
55 Løvås K, Gjesdal CG, Christensen M, Wolff AB, Almås B, Svartberg J, Fougner KJ, Syversen U, Bollerslev J, Falch JA, Hunt PJ, Chatterjee VK, Husebye ES: Glucocorticoid replacement therapy and pharmacogenetics in Addison's disease: effects on bone. Eur J Endocrinol 2009;160:993–1002.
56 Derendorf H, Möllmann H, Barth J, Möllmann C, Tunn S, Krieg M: Pharmacokinetics and oral bioavailability of hydrocortisone. J Clin Pharmacol 1991;31:473–476.
57 Simon N, Castinetti F, Ouliac F, Lesavre N, Brue T, Oliver C: Pharmacokinetic evidence for suboptimal treatment of adrenal insufficiency with currently available hydrocortisone tablets. Clin Pharmacokinet 2010;49:455–463.
58 Blomgren J, Ekman B, Andersson PO, Arnqvist HJ: Non-physiological levels of circulating cortisol in growth hormone-treated hypopituitary adults after conventional cortisone substitution. Scand J Clin Lab Invest 2004;64:132–139.
59 Peacey SR, Guo CY, Robinson AM, Price A, Giles MA, Eastell R, Weetman AP: Glucocorticoid replacement therapy: are patients over treated and does it matter? Clin Endocrinol (Oxf) 1997;46:255–261.
60 Howlett TA: An assessment of optimal hydrocortisone replacement therapy. Clin Endocrinol (Oxf) 1997;46:263–268.
61 Mah PM, Jenkins RC, Rostami-Hodjegan A, Newell-Price J, Doane A, Ibbotson V, Tucker GT, Ross RJ: Weight-related dosing, timing and monitoring hydrocortisone replacement therapy in patients with adrenal insufficiency. Clin Endocrinol (Oxf) 2004;61:367–375.
62 Forss M, Batcheller G, Skrtic S, Johannsson G: Current practice of glucocorticoid replacement therapy and patient-perceived health outcomes in adrenal insufficiency – a worldwide patient survey. BMC Endocr Disord 2012;12:8.
63 Rushworth RL, Torpy DJ: Modern hydrocortisone replacement regimens in adrenal insufficiency patients and the risk of adrenal crisis. Horm Metab Res 2015;47:637–642.
64 Feek CM, Ratcliffe JG, Seth J, Gray CE, Toft AD, Irvine WJ: Patterns of plasma cortisol and ACTH concentrations in patients with Addison's disease treated with conventional corticosteroid replacement. Clin Endocrinol (Oxf) 1981;14:451–458.
65 Nickelsen T, Schulz F, Demisch K: Studies on cortisol substitution therapy in patients with adrenal insufficiency. Exp Clin Endocrinol 1983;82:35–41.

66 Walker BR, Andrew R, MacLeod KM, Padfield PL: Growth hormone replacement inhibits renal and hepatic 11 beta-hydroxysteroid dehydrogenases in ACTH-deficient patients. Clin Endocrinol (Oxf) 1998;49:257–263.
67 Hahner S, Hemmelmann N, Quinkler M, Beuschlein F, Spinnler C, Allolio B: Timelines in the management of adrenal crisis – targets, limits and reality. Clin Endocrinol (Oxf) 2015;82:497–502.
68 Nilsson AG, Marelli C, Fitts D, Bergthorsdottir R, Burman P, Dahlqvist P, Ekman B, Engström BE, Olsson T, Ragnarsson O, Ryberg M, Wahlberg J, Lennernäs H, Skrtic S, Johannsson G: Prospective evaluation of long-term safety of dual-release hydrocortisone replacement administered once daily in patients with adrenal insufficiency. Eur J Endocrinol 2014;171:369–377.
69 Whitaker MJ, Debono M, Huatan H, Merke DP, Arlt W, Ross RJ: An oral multiparticulate, modified-release, hydrocortisone replacement therapy that provides physiological cortisol exposure. Clin Endocrinol (Oxf) 2014:80:554–561.
70 Mallappa A, Sinaii N, Kumar P, Whitaker MJ, Daley LA, Digweed D, Eckland DJ, Van Ryzin C, Nieman LK, Arlt W, Ross RJ, Merke DP: A phase 2 study of Chronocort, a modified-release formulation of hydrocortisone, in the treatment of adults with classic congenital adrenal hyperplasia. J Clin Endocrinol Metab 2015;100:1137–1145.
71 Lovas K, Husebye ES: Continuous subcutaneous hydrocortisone infusion in Addison's disease. Eur J Endocrinol 2007;157:109–112.
72 Russell GM, Durant C, Ataya A, Papastathi C, Bhake R, Woltersdorf W, Lightman S: Subcutaneous pulsatile glucocorticoid replacement therapy. Clin Endocrinol (Oxf) 2014;81:289–293.
73 Quinkler M, Oelkers W, Remde H, Allolio B: Mineralocorticoid substitution and monitoring in primary adrenal insufficiency. Best Pract Res Clin Endocrinol Metab 2015;29:17–24.
74 Chernow B, Alexander HR, Smallridge RC, Thompson WR, Cook D, Beardsley D, Fink MP, Lake CR, Fletcher JR: Hormonal responses to graded surgical stress. Arch Intern Med 1987;147:1273–1278.
75 Salem M, Tainsh RE Jr, Bromberg J, Loriaux DL, Chernow B: Perioperative glucocorticoid coverage. A reassessment 42 years after emergence of a problem. Ann Surg 1994;219:416–425.
76 Nicholson G, Burrin JM, Hall GM: Peri-operative steroid supplementation. Anaesthesia 1998;53:1091–1104.
77 Burke CW: Adrenocortical insufficiency. Clin Endocrinol Metab 1985;14:947–976.
78 Arlt W, Allolio B: Adrenal insufficiency. Lancet 2003;361:1881–1893.
79 Hahner S, Loeffler M, Bleicken B, Drechsler C, Milovanovic D, Fassnacht M, Ventz M, Quinkler M, Allolio B: Epidemiology of adrenal crisis in chronic adrenal insufficiency: the need for new prevention strategies. Eur J Endocrinol 2010;162:597–602.
80 Repping-Wuts HJ, Stikkelbroeck NM, Noordzij A, Kerstens M, Hermus AR: A glucocorticoid education group meeting: an effective strategy for improving self-management to prevent adrenal crisis. Eur J Endocrinol 2013;169:17–22.
81 Quinkler M, Dahlqvist P, Husebye ES, Kämpe O: A European emergency card for adrenal insufficiency can save lives. Eur J Intern Med 2015;21:75–76.
82 Arlt W, Rosenthal C, Hahner S, Allolio B: Quality of glucocorticoid replacement in adrenal insufficiency: clinical assessment vs. timed serum cortisol measurements. Clin Endocrinol (Oxf) 2006;64:384–389.
83 Monson JP: The assessment of glucocorticoid replacement therapy. Clin Endocrinol (Oxf) 1997;46:269–270.

Eystein S. Husebye, MD, PhD
Department of Clinical Science, University of Bergen
NO–5021 Bergen (Norway)
E-Mail eyhu@helse-bergen.no

Author Index

Subject Index